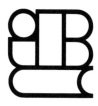

TOTAL
QUALITY
IN HEALTHCARE

Ellen J. Gaucher
Richard J. Coffey

TOTAL
QUALITY
IN HEALTHCARE

From Theory to Practice

Jossey-Bass Publishers · San Francisco

Substantial discounts on bulk quantities of Jossey-Bass books are available to corporations, professional associations, and other organizations. For details and discount information, contact the special sales department at Jossey-Bass Inc., Publishers. (415) 433-1740; Fax (415) 433-0499.

For sales outside the United States, contact Maxwell Macmillan International Publishing Group, 866 Third Avenue, New York, New York 10022.

Manufactured in the United States of America

The ink in this book is either soy- or vegetable-based and during the printing process emits fewer than half the volatile organic compounds (VOCs) emitted by petroleum-based ink.

Library of Congress Cataloging-in-Publication Data

Marszalek-Gaucher, Ellen [date]
    Total quality in healthcare : from theory to practice / Ellen J. Gaucher, Richard J. Coffey.
       p. cm. — (The Jossey-Bass health series)
    Includes bibliographical references and index.
    ISBN 1-55542-534-8
    1. Medical care—Quality control. 2. Total quality management.
3. Health facilities—Administration. I. Coffey, Richard James
[date]. II. Title. III. Series.
RA399.A1M37   1993
362.1'0685—dc20
                                                  92-37677
                                                     CIP

FIRST EDITION
HB Printing   10 9 8 7 6 5 4 3 2 1   *Code 9336*

The Jossey-Bass Health Series

CONTENTS

ix

FIGURES, TABLES, AND EXHIBITS

Figures

Tables

Exhibits

PREFACE

This book is about the University of Michigan Medical Center's Total Quality Management journey and the journeys of our friends at several other organizations. It has been a journey with many successes, false starts, and missteps along the way. It is still in the beginning stages, although much has already been accomplished. There has been great excitement, commitment, skepticism, frustration, and learning as a large academic medical center has struggled to implement a new philosophy of relating to our customers and to each other. As we listened, learned, and experimented, we asked ourselves several questions. First, could the Total Quality Management (TQM) process be applied to healthcare to reduce rework, complexity, and waste in order to achieve cost effectiveness? Second, could this process overcome the organizational inertia that seemed to overwhelm previous attempts at broad-scale organizational change? Third, could TQM be the catalyst for organizational transformation, and through this process could we learn how to work together more effectively and reduce the territorial boundaries that preclude improvement? Fourth, could we become a customer-focused organization? A fifth question we began to ask as we learned more about quality was: Could the process also be utilized to improve patient care? The answer to all these questions is a resounding yes, and throughout the text we will be giving examples of organizational renewal achieved through the TQM process.

Our journey has been anything but smooth. After years of managing with a paralysis-by-analysis approach, we decided to try a Tom Peters "do it, try it, fix it" approach. Consequently we took several steps that were successful, many that needed to be reworked, and some that needed to be totally abandoned. The quality process is complex, and talking about many issues such as organizational culture is much easier than trying to change them. This book will describe both successful and unsuccessful steps.

Our exposure to TQM began in September 1987 when we participated in the National Demonstration Project on Quality Improvement in Health Care, funded by the John A. Hartford Foundation, New York, New York, and the Harvard Community Health Plan, Brookline, Massachusetts. Each of the participating twenty-one healthcare organizations was paired with a quality expert from industry to learn how to apply the tools and techniques of TQM to a healthcare quality problem. The theory of TQM is that it is possible to meet and exceed customer requirements, reduce the cost of poor quality, adopt a new management philosophy, and develop an empowering team-oriented management style that creates a partnership with employees to achieve organizational goals. We began our journey intrigued by the potential and spurred on by new friends in industry and in pioneering healthcare organizations.

At the University of Michigan Medical Center (UMMC), the Total Quality Council established pilot teams, and in early 1988 as these teams began to report their findings, we were energized and excited about the possibilities. Our newly established Total Quality Council celebrated each success and began to dream about a new organization. We envisioned an organization focused on utilizing the philosophy of continuous improvement in all business and clinical functions, the use of teams and team spirit for problem solving, and a continuous striving to meet and exceed customer needs.

We have learned much from our friends in industry who shared freely with those of us in healthcare willing to try their tools and techniques. We have also worked very closely with such hospitals as Alliant Health System, Louisville, Kentucky; Bethesda Hospital, Cincinnati, Ohio; Rush-Presbyterian-St. Luke's Medical Center, Chicago, Illinois; and many others who were early proponents of the Total Quality Processes in healthcare.

TQM represents a major new approach to managing healthcare and other organizations worldwide. Although TQM includes components of many previous management methods, the combination of TQM philosophy, analytical approaches, and people management approaches represents a major paradigm shift. Joel Arthur Barker, a noted futurist and author, defines a paradigm as a "set of rules and regulations (written or unwritten) that does two things: (1) establishes or defines boundaries; and (2) tells you how to behave inside the boundaries in order to be successful" (1992, p. 32). Barker goes further: "The Total Quality Management paradigm has created an epidemic of quality throughout the world. Any organization that doesn't catch this disease may have a difficult time surviving the next twenty years. . . . For these reasons and many more, I predict that the Total Quality Management process will be hailed in the twenty-first century as the most important paradigm shift to come out of the twentieth century" (1992, p. 139). This is a very strong statement given the many fundamental societal and technological changes during the twentieth century, such as the focus on environmental concerns, the development of microcomputers and satellite communications, the women's movement, and cellular phones. Barker is not a TQM expert but rather a futurist looking at all forms of change across all industries and countries.

Healthcare organizations have little choice about beginning the process of organizational renewal. Our customers are demanding that we improve the healthcare system. The pressure for change is growing stronger. The public, the press, and business have taken up the cry for reform. President Bill Clinton has pledged to sponsor healthcare reform. The Joint Commission on Accreditation of Healthcare Organizations (JCAHO) is convinced that continuous quality improvement (CQI) is one of the answers to the cry for change. JCAHO may simply be signaling the increasing expectations of our patients, payers, and other customers.

Barker defines three keys to the success of organizations in the future: excellence, innovation, and anticipation.

> Excellence is at the base of the list because it is the base of the twenty-first century. Many in my audiences justify the importance of excellence (or Total Quality Management, as it is also called) because they believe it will give them a competitive edge in the twenty-first century. I don't believe that. I say it will give them a competitive edge only until the end of the decade. After that, it becomes the necessary price of entry. If you do not have the components of excellence — statistical process control, continuous improvement, benchmarking, the constant pursuit of excellence, the capability of knowing how to do the right thing the first time — then *you don't even get to play the game* [1992, p. 12].

Purpose of the Book

We have written *Total Quality in Healthcare* to share lessons learned during our implementation process. After winning the Healthcare Forum/Witt Award for commitment to quality in April 1990, we received many invitations to talk about our progress. Wherever we traveled people asked: "How did you begin?" "How did you evaluate the teams' efforts?" "How did you design the structure to support the teams?" We have written this book to answer these and many other questions. It is important to stress that we are far from experts; we are still very much learners in the process. Each day we find that our understanding grows and we are able to see things more clearly than the day before. As the term *continuous improvement* indicates, there is no ending point. Writing about our journey may allow others to avoid many of the pitfalls we experienced and perhaps shorten their start-up period. We hope that by helping other healthcare organizations implement quality improvement processes we can add value to the healthcare system.

Audience

The primary audience for this book is administrative and clinical leaders and managers in the healthcare industry. While many books have been written about the theory of Total Quality, few are available that show the application of quality concepts in our industry. This is a "how to" book to guide healthcare organizations as they unfold their quality process. It will be helpful to executives, managers, planners, quality assurance professionals, and staff. We hope that more schools and colleges will begin to teach quality tools and techniques to healthcare professionals as a part of basic education, so that young executives and clinicians are prepared for what we believe will be the organizations of the future.

Overview of the Contents

Chapter One presents a rationale for implementing a TQM process. We also address the question asked most frequently: Why do we have to change? We review healthcare's historic and current environment, the causes of increased cost, and the concerns and complaints of healthcare customers. We address the problems associated with operational definitions of quality and make a case for why quality does not have to cost more. We also discuss JCAHO's current focus on CQI. We attempt to define what Total Quality is and provide some ideas on what your organization can do to overcome the negative perceptions and resistance of physicians and organizations that frequently accompany attempts to implement it. Our belief is that TQM offers a methodology of organizational renewal that can win back the confidence of our customers and achieve a higher level of customer satisfaction.

Chapter Two discusses the basic concepts, terminology, and characteristics of TQM. We view Total Quality as an integration of three elements: a customer-focused continuous-improvement philosophy, analytical knowledge and skills, and interpersonal or "people skills." Characteristics of a TQM process are described along with stages of readiness to implement the required changes and barriers to quality. We describe different quality improvement models, various forms of scientific problem solving, and their relationship to the existing clinical models. Finally, we contrast evolutionary and revolutionary change and describe how quality improvement efforts are most effective in addressing the need for the former.

Chapter Three describes the relationship of TQM to traditional quality assurance (QA) efforts. We begin by describing some common misconceptions about both TQM and QA. Although virtually no healthcare organizations are currently at either extreme, TQM is compared with traditional QA to contrast the characteristics of each. We specifically focus on QA's traditional "eliminate the bad apple" approach, as opposed to aiming to improve the quality of all the apples. We briefly describe how JCAHO's expectations are changing regarding QA functions. Approaches to integrate TQM and QA are presented.

Chapter Four addresses integrating TQM with other previous and current initiatives within your organization. Unless TQM is related to previous efforts, there will be little perceived continuity, and TQM may be viewed as the "program of the year." Similarities and differences of TQM and other common initiatives are presented to help formulate the transition.

Chapter Five presents the critical success factors for TQM implementation. The concepts of leadership and organization are presented with several planning guides and checksheets. The leader's role is discussed as it relates to helping the organization develop its mission, vision, and goals to achieve organizational alignment. A quality audit designed for healthcare and based on the Malcolm Baldrige National Quality Award is included to give you a sense of how your quality process compares to those of Baldrige winners.

Chapter Six offers techniques for creating the organizational culture necessary for quality implementation. We focus on the need for adaptability, innovation, and creativity in today's healthcare environment and discuss the barriers to creating a positive corporate culture. Strategies are presented for cultural assessment, stress management during the transition stage, enhancement of your employee suggestion program, and reduction of barriers that interfere with effective organizational performance. We also discuss the importance of learning to manage and empower today's diverse workforce and the advantages of driving fear out of your organization.

The critical issue for healthcare of gaining physician support is the topic of Chapter Seven. Two guest authors, Eric W. Kratochwill and L. Paul Sonda III, M.D., review the literature and present techniques to gain physician support of TQM. They describe traditional physician resistance to clinical quality improvement efforts, the pressures facing physicians today, and the advantages of CQI for physicians. The chapter concludes with a discussion of UMMC's Clinical Quality Improvement initiative.

Chapter Eight focuses on teams and teamwork. Teams are the building blocks of a quality effort. However, there are many barriers that prevent teams from accomplishing their goals. We suggest strategies and structures for team success and discuss issues that can lead to team failure. The roles and responsibilities of team members are discussed as well as the predictable stages of team development. We conclude by sharing the lessons we have learned.

Chapter Nine presents components of education and training programs to implement TQM in your organization. Characteristics associated with faculty of successful TQM education programs are described. We address key principles of a TQM education program and sample programs from UMMC. Lessons learned about education are described. We conclude with our views on the pros and cons of various methods of educational program development and point out that ongoing education must be in response to learners' needs.

Reward and recognition strategies are discussed in Chapter Ten. Developing an effective reward and recognition system consistent with Total Quality principles is a difficult task. Several frameworks for developing an effective system are reviewed in this chapter.

Chapter Eleven addresses actions to implement TQM as part of your daily work. Actions for managers are presented with examples. Actions for nonmanagerial physicians and staff are suggested. Managers and staff can begin these actions before and concurrent with formal TQM educational programs or quality improvement teams.

Chapter Twelve presents a summary of basic quality improvement methods beginning with a discussion of principles for improvement. Measurement considerations are presented because statistics are meaningless without specified operational definitions and methods. The following quality improvement methods are briefly described, along with guidelines and illustrations: process flowchart, run chart and control chart, brainstorming, multivoting, affinity diagraming, theme selection matrix, checksheet, Pareto chart and histogram, problem selection matrix, cause-effect diagram, countermeasure matrix, barriers and aids analysis, cost-benefit analysis, and teamwork and structures. References are provided for more complete presentations on each subject.

Chapter Thirteen presents a case study of an admission/ discharge process to illustrate application of the methods described in Chapter Twelve. This case study provides a practical, hands-on illustration of the methods, using a process common to all healthcare organizations. For example, an outpatient registration process is very similar to an inpatient admission process.

Chapter Fourteen describes several advanced applications of TQM. The chapter begins with a discussion of cooperation versus competition and potential partnership opportunities. The following advanced applications are described: benchmarking, critical path protocols of care, quality function deployment, hoshin planning, and kansei engineering.

The concepts of TQM are invigorating and uplifting, and people sometimes get blinded by the glitter of the process. In Chapter Fifteen we present strategies for maintaining the momentum. A list of potential barriers is also presented along with aids to overcome them. Barriers include budgetary problems, bureaucracy, and disbelief of TQM philosophy, as well as personal values that conflict with it. As a quality champion in your organization, you must recognize when the process is off the track and requires nurturing.

In Chapter Sixteen, we tie the principles and concepts together and suggest some final advice for those who are undertaking quests for quality.

Acknowledgments

Our Total Quality journey would not have been possible without the assistance of our friends at the National Demonstration Project: Donald M. Berwick, M.D., Paul B. Batalden, M.D., and others on the advisory committee who stimulated our interest and fed our curiosity. Many listened and helped us when our vision became fuzzy and commiserated when the going got tough. Without their encouragement and direction the journey would not have been possible.

The quality team from Alliant Health System in Louisville, Kentucky, kicked off our first training session and provided us much emotional support. Jim Stansbury was never too busy to spare a few minutes explaining why certain steps were necessary and what they had learned in the process.

Caryl Cullen, Bear Baila, and the team from Qualtec, Inc., a Florida Power and Light subsidiary, shared their vast experience in TQM with us. Caryl served as external mentor to us and our facilitators, and continued to push us when we wanted to relax and to praise us when we were doing well.

GOAL/QPC's Bob King and Dona Hotopp expanded our opportunities to learn such new techniques from Japan as quality function deployment, a strategy to build in quality on the front end of product development rather than to inspect it in hindsight. Through their Healthcare Application Research Committee we established a network of friends who wanted to share successes and failures, learn from each other, and develop methods to implement TQM throughout the healthcare industry.

We also wish to thank the members of the Conference Board's U.S. Quality Council who shared their knowledge and expertise freely and helped us learn about Total Quality experiences in other industries.

John D. Forsyth, chief executive officer of the University of Michigan Hospitals; Giles G. Bole, Jr., M.D., dean of the University of Michigan Medical School; and George D. Zuidema, M.D., vice provost for medical affairs, supported our efforts to develop and implement TQM within UMMC.

In addition to the many who offered ideas while we were preparing our manuscript, several have specifically helped us prepare this book. We wish to acknowledge assistance from Hilda Allen, Lana Berry, Lisa L. Cayen, David Chan, Linda Creps, Mindy Eisenberg, Richard E. Finger, John A. "Jack" Germ, Neal E. Gilbert, Karen Good, Connie Hansen, Jennifer L. Hutton, Sharon Jackson, Brent James, Bob King, Eric W. Kratochwill, Patrice Lyons, Monica Mac, Kenneth McClatchey, J. Elizabeth Othman, Larry Poniatowski, Laura Roth, Edward D. Rothman, L. Paul Sonda III, and Kari Tice. We also wish to thank the additional friends and colleagues who reviewed the manuscript and provided valuable ideas to improve the book: Michael O. Bice, Dona Hotopp, Kathryn Johnson, Bob King, Ann Kowlakowski, Glenn Laffel, Rebecca L. McGovern, Lynn O'Neal, Kenneth G. Peltzie, Richard Redman, and Patricia Warner. The UMMC Total Quality facilitators provided valuable input and review comments and have served an extremely valuable role implementing Total Quality. We would like to acknowledge Tamra Bates, Wendy Behnke, Lynne Clevenger, Jim Day, Mindy Eisenberg, Deborah Guglielmo, Tess Kirby, Amy Perry, Larry Price, Steve Raymond, Jacqueline Robinson, Jean Robinson, Carol Wesolowski, and our part-time facilitators.

Additionally, there are all the people at UMMC: staff, physicians, managers, supervisors, top leadership, our customers, and our suppliers — the team leaders, the facilitators, and all the team members who embraced the theory and made it work. We extend our thanks to the housekeepers, dietary workers, security staff, finance staff, door attendants, clerical staff, nursing and medical staff, our students, our customers, and everyone else who contributed to our learning. We thank the organization's facilitators and team leaders who stepped up, took a risk, and have energized the process. We are grateful that staff trusted the vision from the beginning and are making it a reality in our organization. We hope you enjoy hearing about their progress and find helpful the practical quality stories they have to tell.

Finally, we thank our families, who were understanding of our passion to write this book. We appreciate their support. They demonstrated great patience, particularly given the time we had devoted to our first book and commitments to tell others about TQM. We hope that in some small way this book will serve as an inspiration to our children as they pursue their creative interests. We would like to dedicate this book to our families: Oneta, Todd, and Tonya Coffey, and Steve Gaucher and the Marszalek/Gaucher children.

Ann Arbor, Michigan   Ellen J. Gaucher
March 1993   Richard J. Coffey

THE AUTHORS

Ellen J. Gaucher is senior associate hospital director and chief operating officer of the University of Michigan Hospitals in Ann Arbor, Michigan, an 886-bed academic health center with several satellite facilities and over $550 million in annual revenues. She holds faculty appointments in the University of Michigan's School of Nursing and School of Public Health. Gaucher is a registered nurse who received her B.S. degree (1975) from Worcester State College in nursing and her M.S.P.H. degree (1977) from Clark University. She has completed additional postgraduate education at Boston University and at the University of Michigan.

She has been leading the Total Quality Management (TQM) process at the University of Michigan Medical Center since 1987. Gaucher served on the advisory board of the National Demonstration Project on Quality Improvement in Health Care funded by the John A. Hartford Foundation and the Harvard Community Health Plan. She serves on the United States Quality Council II of the Conference Board. Gaucher also serves on the Federal Quality Advisory Board and is a judge for the Malcolm Baldrige National Quality Award. She serves on the editorial boards of *Health Care Competition Week* and *QI/TQM*, and is associate editor of *Quality Management in Health Care*, a new journal published by Aspen Systems.

Gaucher has sixteen years of experience in senior management positions in healthcare organizations. Her previous positions were director of nursing and associate hospital director of ambulatory care at the University of Michigan, and assistant director of nursing and director of ambulatory care at the University of Massachusetts Medical Center. She has published numerous articles and book chapters. Her book *Transforming Healthcare Organizations: How to Achieve and Sustain Organizational Excellence* (1990, with R. J. Coffey) received the 1992 James A. Hamilton book-of-the-year award from the American College of Healthcare Executives. She serves as a consultant on TQM and lectures internationally on continuous quality improvement, hospital management, and systems development.

Richard J. Coffey is director of management systems at the University of Michigan Hospitals, Ann Arbor, and an adjunct assistant professor in industrial and operations engineering at the University of Michigan. He received his B.S.E. degree (1967) from the University of Michigan in industrial engineering and his M.S. degree (1971) from the University of Arizona in systems engineering. He holds an M.S.E. degree (1972) and a Ph.D. degree (1975), both from the University of Michigan, in industrial and operations engineering.

Coffey's current activities include development, training, and project support for UMMC Total Quality Process and decision support services for senior managers within the University of Michigan Medical Center. He has performed operations analysis and planning and market research projects in many university, consulting, government, insurance, and private organizations within the healthcare industry since 1963, both in the United States and abroad. He received an industrial engineering Alpha Pi Mu honor membership in 1966, a special research fellowship from the National Center for Health Services Research and Development from 1971 to 1974, and a first-place literature award from the Hospital Management Systems Society in 1979 (with K. G. Bartscht) for "Management Engineering—A Method to Improve Productivity," in *Topics in Health Care Financing.* Coffey has authored over thirty published articles and a chapter in the book *Health Care Delivery Planning* (1973). His book *Transforming Healthcare Organizations: How to Achieve and Sustain Organizational Excellence* (1990, with E. J. Gaucher) received the 1992 James A. Hamilton book-of-the-year award from the American College of Healthcare Executives. He has given many presentations at regional and national conferences in addition to his extensive project presentations.

TOTAL
QUALITY
IN HEALTHCARE

PART ONE

Setting the Stage

Chapter One

Why Implement
Total Quality Management?

Why implement a Total Quality Management (TQM) program in your institution? Primarily because it works! The University of Michigan Medical Center (UMMC) and a variety of other healthcare organizations have found that the tools and techniques of TQM can be the foundation for organizational transformation and renewal. A TQM approach can help you define quality, establish measures of customer satisfaction, improve upon those measures, and simultaneously reduce your cost per unit of service.

Why do you have to change? It is clear that the American public is not satisfied with the healthcare industry and their discontent grows each day. The popular press is full of stories about the crisis in healthcare and what should be done about it. The intensity of concern indicates that if the people inside healthcare cannot fix the system, the people outside *will*. Improving quality while reducing cost is not an easy task, but your organization's survival may depend on your ability to do so. Rosabeth Moss Kanter said it well: "The years ahead will be the best of all for those who learn to balance dreams and discipline. The future will belong to those who embrace the potential of wider opportunities but recognize the realities of more constrained resources—and find new solutions that permit doing more with less" (Kanter, 1989b, p. 18).

The customers of healthcare—patients and their families,

business and industry, insurance companies, and the federal government—believe their needs are not being met, on an access, cost, or quality basis. Our customers are telling us that they want value for their healthcare dollar. What is value? According to Stephen Shortell: "Value embodies the concept of cost, productivity, and quality. Adding value requires hospitals to change the nature of both their internal and external relationships. It requires a rethinking of what it means to be a hospital in the healthcare environment of the future" (1990, p. 19). We believe that the hospitals and healthcare organizations that can provide high-quality services and meet customer requirements at a reasonable price will compete very effectively. The problem is that learning how to elicit customer requirements is not an easy task for an industry that has always assumed it knows what its customers need.

While it is clear to all healthcare managers that the financial incentives have changed and the "golden days" of medicine are over, answers about how to respond to the crisis are few and far between. Some believe that this fiscal crisis is a blessing that will help unfreeze the attitudes of those who feel that the crisis in healthcare is temporary. Perhaps the unfreezing of attitudes will lead to the development of creative models of delivery and successful approaches to cost containment.

The Voice of the Customer

The Depressing Statistics

There is an urgent need to improve the value of healthcare services by improving quality and cost effectiveness. Healthcare costs are escalating rapidly and consuming a growing proportion of the nation's resources. Figure 1.1 shows that healthcare spending as a percentage of the gross national product (GNP) has risen from 5.3 percent in 1960 to 13 percent in 1991 and will continue to rise to a projected 17.3 percent in the year 2000. If the current rate of escalation continues, by the year 2030 healthcare costs may be equal to 35 percent of the GNP. Figure 1.2 shows that per capita healthcare expenditures have risen to

Figure 1.1. Real per Capita National Health Expenditures (in 1992 Dollars).

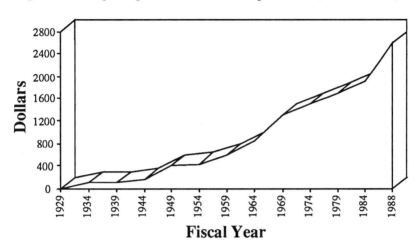

Fiscal Year

Source: The Advisory Board Company, 1991b, p. 3; Health Care Financing Administration, Office of the Actuary.

well over $2,500 per person. Some may argue that such costs are justified because healthcare contributes to the maintenance of a healthy society and workforce. However, our healthcare outcome statistics are no better than those of countries who spend far less per capita. "Life expectancy in the United States is shorter than 15 other nations and infant mortality is worse than 22 other countries" (Hilts, 1991, p. 4–1). The issue, then, is not whether we are spending enough on healthcare, but rather *how* are we spending valuable healthcare dollars.

Evidence of Discontent in the Press

The public outcry concerning these issues is growing. In the March 11, 1991, issue of *USA Today*, the headline story was entitled "Health Care Costs More, Serves Fewer!" The story was the first in a continuing series by Kevin Anderson that looked at why healthcare costs are so high and seem to defy free market economics. The emphasis of the series was that while the crisis in healthcare costs seems recent, costs have actually exceeded the

Figure 1.2. Health Spending Projections from 1960 to 2000.

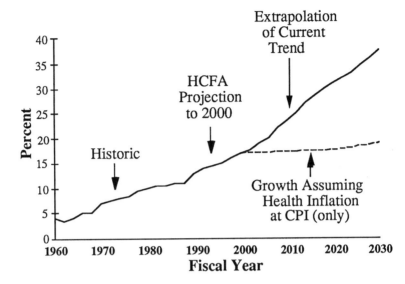

Source: The Advisory Board Company, 1991a, p. 8; Health Care Financing Administration, Office of the Actuary.

consumer price index for twenty-five years. The author states: "For those it serves best, it offers the most sophisticated, innovative and effective medical care in the world. But, it is an expensive welter of inefficiency that excludes more and more people even as it consumes an ever growing chunk of our national resources" (Anderson, 1991, p. B1).

The May 19, 1991, issue of the *Wall Street Journal* featured a story entitled, "Say Ouch: Demands to Fix U.S. Health Care Reach a Crescendo." The story, by Philip J. Hilts, compared our system to other healthcare systems in the world. He found that since 1986 healthcare expenditures as a portion of GNP rose faster in the United States than in other countries such as Canada, Germany, Japan, France, and Great Britain. A large gap also exists between dollars spent and services provided. Figure 1.3 compares the healthcare expenditures of the United States and other countries. Hilts also believes that "healthcare has become a political problem that will be difficult to solve without leadership from the White House, which so far has little to say on the issue" (Hilts, 1991, sec. 4, p. 1). Will the politicians continue to stand on the sidelines, or will some type of governmental restructuring be the next attempt to reduce healthcare costs?

In the May 1991 issue of *Money* magazine, readers were asked what suggestions they could offer as solutions for the healthcare crisis. Hundreds of readers sent in letters, which were printed in the July 1991 issue. The letters called for a federal takeover and reorganization of the healthcare system, reduction in malpractice coverage, and increased taxation to pay for the uninsured. The article emphasized that if we do not take the initiative to redesign the system, the federal government will! The article also carried advice from five healthcare authorities invited to a roundtable discussion. They described how medical costs can be reduced and how to be a smarter, more aggressive consumer The experts' advice paralleled the advice from readers.

Figure 1.3. Comparison of 1989 per Capita Healthcare Expenditures by Country.

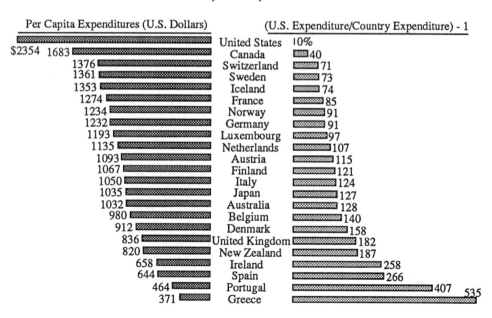

Source: Schieber and Poullier, 1991, p. 113.

The July 1991 issue of *Fortune* carried a special report called "A Cure for What Ails Medical Care." The author referred to the problem in healthcare as a disease. The symptoms: unchecked healthcare spending and too many uninsured. His answer was to introduce more marketplace logic into the system (Smith, 1991, p. 44).

Many healthcare professionals are also speaking out. Heinz Galli, the president and chief operating officer of the Harvard Community Health Plan, said: "Despite the greatness of its achievements American medicine is paying a huge price for poor quality. I sometimes have felt the system was designed to produce waste, rework, and inefficiency, the hallmarks of poor quality." He blames the problem on the cloak of mystery that surrounds medical care. This mystery creates not "bad" medicine but very expensive black box medicine (Galli, 1991, p. 1).

Major employers are beginning to demand that healthcare organizations adopt Total Quality programs. Bruce A. Mueller, vice president and corporate director of personnel administrative management, Motorola Corporation, told a group of healthcare administrators at a Chi Systems Conference on TQM in Healthcare: "If you don't implement Quality Improvement Programs, I'll be talking to your successors" (June 24, 1991). We believe that many payers, such as Motorola, Ford, IBM, Xerox, and others, will demand that healthcare organizations meet the same quality standards as their other suppliers.

One Final Note on Customer Requirements

The call for reform of the healthcare system is coming from many constituents. W. Edwards Deming, a leader of the quality improvement movement, has listed the high cost of healthcare as one of the seven deadly diseases that stand in the way of the American industry's quality transformation (Deming, 1986, pp. 97–98; as cited in M. Walton, 1986, p. 19).

1. *Lack of constancy of purpose.* A company that is without constancy of purpose has no long range plan for staying in business. Management is insecure and so are employees.

2. *Emphasis on short-term profits.* Looking to increase quarterly dividends undermines quality and productivity.
3. *Personal review system.* The effects of these are devastating— teamwork is destroyed, rivalry is nurtured. Performance ratings build fear and leave people bitter, despondent and beaten. They also encourage defection in the ranks of management.
4. *Mobility of management.* Job-hopping managers never understand the companies they work for and are never there long enough to follow through on long-term changes that are necessary for quality and productivity.
5. *Running a company on visible figures alone.* The most important figures are unknown and unknowable—the "multiplier" effect of a happy customer, for example.
6. *Excessive medical costs for employee healthcare, which increase the final cost of goods and services.* High medical costs contribute to the high prices of American goods and services, which decrease our international competitiveness.
7. *Excessive cost of warranty, fueled by lawyers who work on contingency fees.* High legal fees, like high healthcare costs, decrease our competitiveness.

The factors in this list affect the ability of all American industry to compete effectively in global markets.

Why Healthcare Costs Are Rising

There are many reasons why healthcare costs have been rapidly escalating. Some selected examples include new technology, our aging population, medical malpractice, overspecialization, cost of poor quality, and a lack of public policy establishing rationing mechanisms. These will be briefly described to illustrate differing reasons for the need to change. A more complete explanation was provided by Marszalek-Gaucher and Coffey (1990, pp. 19–40).

New Technology

Technology is defined here to include all forms of advancement of medical science, due to the application of new equipment, drugs, or other forms of science. Many new healthcare technologies are less invasive, reduce length of hospital stay, reduce complications, and return the patient to work more quickly. Laproscopic surgery, lithotripsy, laser surgery, balloon angioplasty, and the new drugs TPA and streptokinase are examples of changes that reduced the length of stay and hastened the recovery process. However, much new technology supplements rather than replaces old methods and makes it difficult to determine the effectiveness and cost benefits of the new procedures. One need look no further than the radiology department to see a proliferation of the old and the new: magnetic resonance imaging (MRI), computerized axial tomography (CAT), positive emission tomography (PET), and the standard radiological tests. Few hospitals have protocols to serve as guidelines or gatekeepers to approve the use of tests. Therefore, as hospitals attempt to use the latest technology, tests overlap, are unnecessary, and drive up the cost of healthcare.

Another issue that adds to the demand for new technology is coverage in the popular press. The American press writes about new drugs and technologies, often before the technology is available. Patients and families then demand these latest therapies. Many physicians feel compelled to respond to these requests whether the technology or the drug is required or not (Eisenberg, 1986).

We are approaching a situation in which the rate of development of new technologies is exceeding society's willingness or ability to apply them to all people who may want or could potentially benefit from them. Politicians are beginning to debate the national and international issues of resource allocation priorities and the rationing of healthcare services.

Aging Population

The most rapidly growing age groups are those over sixty-five, and this will be accentuated as the large population group of post–World War II baby boomers begins reaching sixty-five by 2010. One out of every nine Americans is over sixty-five; by the year 2010, the proportion will be one in five (Coile, 1986; Schick, 1986). While life expectancy has been extended, more than 80 percent of those over sixty-five have at least one chronic illness (Coile, 1986). We have no ability to predict accurately how the aging of the population will affect healthcare costs. However, most experts predict that it will mean increased services and costs.

Medical Malpractice

There is built-in bias to order more procedures for the protection of both the patient and the physician. Currently in the United States, many people bring suits against healthcare organizations, physicians, and other healthcare providers whenever there is a question about the clinical decision, procedure, or outcome. Insurance companies increasingly are denying payment for services and products considered "unnecessary," without regard to any legal implications. A healthcare organization or provider's reputation can be severely damaged by the mere public notice of a suit, whether founded or not. There is strong pressure to order diagnostic and treatment procedures for legal protection alone. This is an example of Deming's seventh deadly disease, "Excessive cost of warranty, fueled by lawyers who work on contingency fees" (M. Walton, 1986, p. 19). Traditionally, such practice has been referred to as defensive medicine.

Overspecialization

Given the expanded level of expertise and new professions accompanying the expansion of technology, there has been a tendency for overspecialization among physicians and other providers. There are too few family practitioners and primary care providers, and too many specialists and subspecialists. Another example of overspecialization is in allied health professions. There are many new specialties, each with a narrowly defined scope of responsibility, adding to the complexity of care.

In an era of shrinking resources, we must examine what services and providers are necessary to satisfy and effectively care for our customers. Healthcare organizations must undertake work re-design efforts to reduce the amount of overspecialization.

The Cost of Poor Quality

The cost of poor quality (COPQ) is the cost incurred when things are not done correctly the first time. It can also be caused by not doing the right things or doing the wrong things, errors of omission or commission. There are many examples of COPQ in our daily work: the x-ray that must be retaken because the patient was not positioned correctly, the pharmacist who must call the physician because the prescription could not be read, the procedure that must be canceled because the patient is not adequately prepared, and the patient and physician who must wait in the clinic and delay treatment because the record is lost. At times, the examples seem endless.

Experts estimate the COPQ in well-managed organizations runs about 25 percent of the revenues. Philip Crosby says, "you can spend 15–20% of your sales dollar on the cost of poor quality without even trying hard" (Crosby, 1979, p. 18). Many managers are unaware of the magnitude of poor quality on the bottom line. The cost of poor quality is never addressed on the balance sheet mainly because in most organizations it remains hidden and unknown. For our organization, with current revenues of over $550 million annually, the impact of poor quality is impressive. Utilizing the 15–25 percent of sales dollar as a target, we could save $82–$137 million a year if we are successful in reducing the COPQ. Teaching all employees how to eliminate the COPQ in their daily work is an essential part of TQM education. Rework, complexity, and waste must be eliminated by applying the tools and techniques in every area and in every job in the organization. The concept of continual improvement means a commitment to identifying critical processes and improving them across the organization. It is a long-term strategic commitment.

While the COPQ is a very important concept, we do not

recommend spending large amounts of resources to calculate it. It is better to spend the same effort to make improvements.

Rework and Waste

The American healthcare system is of very high quality, and yet we allow a very large amount of rework (see Figure 1.4). The desired outcome is to produce a service, product, or information acceptable to both the supplier and the customer and producing a satisfied or delighted customer.

If the service or product is unacceptable to the supplier or provider, the question is whether rework is cost-effective. This question is asked explicitly in most industrial organizations. If there is a warp in a television picture tube, for example, it is not cost-effective to rework the picture tube, so it is discarded. This process leads to formally acknowledged waste. In healthcare, however, we seldom even ask the question, and just do the rework. An example is an x-ray that is unacceptable to the radiology technologist or radiologist. The x-ray must be re-

Figure 1.4. Illustration of Rework and Waste.

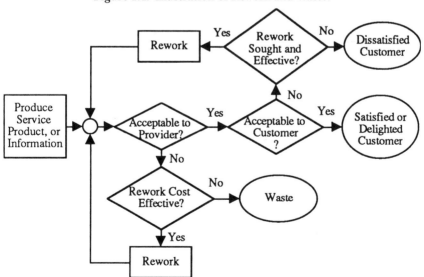

peated, which costs more in technologist time, radiologist time, equipment time, additional film, administrative time, and delays for other patients, increasing dissatisfaction.

If acceptable to the provider, the next question is whether the service or product is acceptable to the customer. Continuing the x-ray example, the patient may be charged for both of the x-rays, the rework may delay a visit to the physician or another diagnostic service, and the patient may have to pay more for parking. If the customer is not satisfied, the question is whether any correction is sought by the customer. There is substantial market research to suggest that most people will not complain to the physician, nurse, or other healthcare provider about unacceptable service, a situation that leads to an unhappy customer. This is the worst alternative, because the customer will not return, and research suggests the customer will tell approximately nine other people about the unacceptable service. If correction is sought by the customer, this once again leads to rework, but at least there is a good possibility that you can satisfy the customer. For the x-ray example, the patient may complain to administration about additional delay and parking cost or complain to patient accounts about the bill. There will be additional clerical and administrative time to make corrections. In contrast to industrial organizations, few hospitals formally measure or even acknowledge the amount of waste and rework that occurs within their organizations. Consequently, they miss the opportunity to make improvements. Rework and waste are so common that many employers just accept them as "the way things are done."

Errors

Errors are also a problem for hospitals and other healthcare organizations. For example, the number of medication errors in a typical hospital is far too large. At UMMC we have heard many excuses such as, "Most of the errors are only the wrong time and those errors do not hurt anyone." This is faulty thinking. Errors cost money and take extra staff time. Every time an error is made, it must be reported. The reporting alone is rework that takes a nurse away from the patient. Medication systems need to be revamped in ways that make distributing medications easier and as error-free as possible. We should keep in mind that Motorola has a goal of tenfold improvement (six sigma, or 3.4 defective parts per million). How would your hospital's error rate measure up against this goal?

Variation in Practice

There is tremendous variation in healthcare practice due to a lack of standards. Granted each patient is an individual and response to treatment may differ, but there are as many different treatment plans as there are physicians. John E. Wennberg points out, "most people view the medical care they receive as a necessity provided by doctors who adhere to scientific norms based on previously tested and proven treatments" (Wennberg, 1984, p. 7). His research has shown that variations in practice style have had profound implications for both the patient and the payer of care. There is major variation in practice from physician to physician, hospital to hospital, and state to state. Resource utilization for a specific diagnosis may vary up to two to three times. Wennberg proposed in the same article that "physicians when given effective data will accept responsibility for the outcome of the practice variation phenomenon" (p. 23). Malpractice fright is also utilized as an excuse for overutilization. The tools and techniques of TQM are effective and proven methods for communicating standards, variation, countermeasures, and results. It is our hope that physicians, managers, staff, and professional organizations can work together to reduce unnecessary variation through the appropriate application of clinical standards and Total Quality principles. We will not achieve quality improvement goals for healthcare until medical practice variation is dramatically reduced.

No Incentive to Control Cost

The American healthcare system evolved in such a way that there is little incentive to contain cost. Bills for care were paid by third parties, not those receiving services, so patients were not price sensitive. During the 1940s and 1950s, the Hill Burton Act encouraged hospital construction through federal matching funds. Hospitals were frequently built based on a local politician's need for reelection rather than on community need. During World War II, wage freezes led to enhancements in healthcare benefits. Once benefits were gained by employees in bargaining, healthcare emerged as a standard part of compensation. The growth in healthcare services was accentuated by the cost-based reimbursement system initiated by Blue Cross and other payers during the 1950s and drastically expanded by Medicare and Medicaid in 1965. The more a healthcare organization spent, the more it was paid for covered services. The most costly inpatient services were covered, while outpatient and preventive services normally were not covered. This policy did not result in a widespread, intentional misuse of resources. But both providers and patients pursued any and all healthcare services for the benefit and convenience of the patient, with little regard for value. In the past, physicians were not questioned about utilization. Hospitals were, as some have said, a "doctors' workshop." This is complicated by the overutilization resulting from malpractice protection discussed earlier. As a result, due to overcapacity, technology, increased access, and overutilization, the healthcare system has consumed a steadily increasing percentage of GNP each year. Major employers and payers are now establishing strong incentives to control costs, but to be effective these must be integrated with protections for healthcare providers related to malpractice claims.

Definitions of Healthcare Quality

Customers Are Unable to Judge Quality

One of the problems for our industry is that the definitions of quality change based on who is defining the term. Our customers include healthcare providers, patients and their families, the payers, and society at large. Many times nonprovider customers are not competent to judge what constitutes quality in healthcare relative to the technical and scientific aspects of care. The professionals within the industry, however, have not helped to define technical measures of quality care and demonstrate how our multiple customers should evaluate healthcare services. Most quality measures are indicative of quality failure. For example, we measure mortality, morbidity, hospital-acquired infection rates, and unplanned readmissions, all indicators of process failure. These measures are not customer-focused or focused on excellence. There are very few patients who come to a hospital expecting any of these complications to occur.

Traditionally Quality Means Doing More

From the providers' perspective, the traditional way of viewing quality within healthcare is "quality means doing more"—using greater technology, doing more tests, giving more intensive care, making that last-ditch effort to save a life. When the first national efforts to hold down the cost of healthcare were proposed, providers and administrators alike were concerned and worried about the impact on quality of care. Whether it was prospective payment and the advent of Diagnosis Related Groups (DRGs) or the arrival of Health Maintenance Organizations (HMOs), healthcare professionals expressed fear that there would be a reduction in quality of care. Those fears were never realized. Several research studies have investigated the relationship of cost and quality indicators such as medical surgical death rates and post-operative surgical complication rates. The findings suggest there is no tradeoff between efficiency and high-quality care. In fact, performing unnecessary tests and procedures exposes patients to avoidable medical risks along with unnecessary costs.

Americans Are Willing to Pay for Quality

There is much evidence to confirm that the American consumer is willing to pay more for quality products. The knowledgeable professionals in healthcare should define the characteristics of quality care and prepare the customers to better evaluate services. Intermountain Health Care, for example, in 1990 was able to obtain an HMO contract with large employers at costs 6 percent higher than a competing HMO by demonstrating both a current high quality of care and actions to increase quality further in the future.

Quality Does Not Have to Cost More

It is a myth that quality always costs more! Many American corporations have proven that focusing on quality can save money. As J. M. Juran and F. M. Gryna point out: "Confusion arises when the word 'quality' is used without making it clear whether the speaker is referring to quality of design or quality of conformance. Generally speaking, quality of design can be attained only at an increase in costs, whereas higher quality of conformance can often be attained with an accompanying reduction in costs" (Juran and Gryna, 1980, p. 2). Achieving quality through reducing defects reduces the cost of the product or service. Achieving quality through added features often increases costs.

There is also a need to understand the components of quality, such as quality in fact and in perception. Quality in fact occurs when an organization meets professionally established specifications. Quality in perception, on the other hand, is quality defined by the patients or other customers based upon their perception of whether a product or service is as good or better than it was expected to be. A successful quality organization will consider quality from all aspects.

Approaches to Improve Quality

There are three distinctly different approaches to improve quality, as illustrated in Table 1.1. Our only method of measurement in the past has been quality by inspection. We try to identify and remove unacceptable services, products, or information or find the persons who made the mistake and punish them. This type of quality approach is retrospective and involves rework. For example, most hospitals review surgical infection rates. A better

Table 1.1. Approaches to Improve Quality.

Approach	*Impact*
• Inspection	• Identifies and removes unacceptable services, products, or information
	• Almost always creates rework, delays, and additional cost.
• Prevention	• Improves processes causing poor quality
	• Reduces rework, waste, delays, and costs
• Planning and design	• Plans processes and designs to meet and exceed customers' requirements
	• Reduces unnecessary activities, reduces costs, and increases revenues

approach would be to determine what measures can be applied to prevent surgical infections. In healthcare we also set up systems because we expect existing ones to fail. Two examples of this type of practice were uncovered by our Admission/ Discharge Team. Because we had long waits in our admission lounge, we provided meals to patients and family members to make their stay more acceptable. We also assigned staff to bring delayed patients a flower and an apology from the hospital administration after they were admitted. These were systems set up to cover a system failure. The right answer was not to feed or apologize to patients but to reduce their wait times. Through Total Quality we realized that we needed to cure the root causes of problems, not just attack the symptoms.

Healthcare organizations must improve quality by prevention, improving the systems that are causing poor quality. This will eliminate rework and reduce costs while simultaneously enhancing quality. By utilizing the voice of the customer in the planning and design of systems and services we have the best chance to affect both quality and price.

Joint Commission on Accreditation of Healthcare Organizations

Beginning in 1992, JCAHO began focusing on continuous improvement. The plan is to make a shift from the current standards to new standards over a two-year period. A recent article by the editor of the *QI/TQM Newsletter* said: "Hospitals not working in a Total Quality environment by 1992 will find themselves seriously out of step with the Joint Commission for Accreditation of Healthcare Organizations. And those that aren't well into continuous quality by 1993 may be unable to retain accreditation" (*QI/TQM Newsletter*, 1991, p. 1). The article quoted William F. Jesse, M.D., vice president for quality management at Humana, Inc., Louisville, Kentucky: "Clearly the Joint Commission is pushing organizations in the direction of QI and TQM."

What Is Total Quality Management?

"Total Quality is a new approach to quality improvement. It encompasses all systems and processes, clinical and non-clinical, with actions directed towards processes to improve the quality of all services and products for patients and all other customers" (Coffey, Eisenberg, Gaucher, and Kratochwill, 1991, p. 23). TQM is a process for meeting and exceeding customer requirements. It extends the concept of customers to include employees within the organization as a critical customer group. It is both a philosophy and a new way of doing business. TQM is a participative team-oriented process. On a step-by-step basis, through the application of a scientific problem-solving methodology, the organization learns to manage with fact rather than intuition. A TQM approach allows you to enhance all critical systems and processes in the organization. It helps managers focus on long-term strategies rather than a quick-fix approach. Each employee is taught how to listen to the voice of the customer, continually improve those essential services, reduce cost, and ultimately help the organization to compete more effectively. Experience shows that high quality and return on investment usually go together. "In the long run, the most important single factor affecting a business unit's performance is the quality of its products and services, relative to those of the competitors. Quality leads to both market expansion and gains in market share. Excellent service translates to satisfied customers who will use the organization again and recommend it to their friends" (Buzzell and Bradley, 1987, p. 7).

The New Quality Philosophy: Does It Work?

When we were first exposed to the concepts of Total Quality and studied the work of Deming, Juran, and others, we were not sure that the philosophy would apply in healthcare. Could we simultaneously improve quality and reduce cost? Would improved quality translate into improved productivity? Could we reduce rework, complexity, and waste and ultimately the cost per unit of service? Could we reduce the barriers to quality improvement? Could we adopt the new philosophy? As we listened to W. Edwards Deming at our first four-day seminar, we heard him say: This is what I told the Japanese in 1950. If you improve your quality, you improve your productivity automatically—it is a chain reaction. You do this by lowering waste, lowering restarts, lowering rework. When this happens you can then capture markets with higher quality and lower cost of goods and services. This will allow you to stay in business and provide jobs. It's that simple. The relationship of quality, productivity, and cost can be represented as a chain reaction, illustrated in Figure 1.5.

We have not found it quite so simple. An analytical approach alone will not yield the necessary change. The culture must support the concepts of teamwork and employee involve-

Figure 1.5. Deming Chain Reaction.

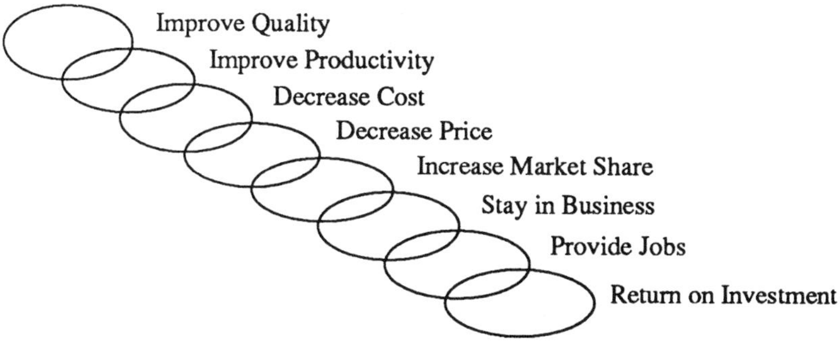

Improve Quality
Improve Productivity
Decrease Cost
Decrease Price
Increase Market Share
Stay in Business
Provide Jobs
Return on Investment

ment. All critical business functions, clinical as well as administrative, must be involved. Our initial approach was to begin looking at those functions that were closest to the production function in industry, such as the operating rooms or the admitting or billing functions. There were some quasi-clinical issues, such as drug utilization studies or the Surgical ICU project where they developed and implemented a new nurse extender program, but these were the exception rather than the rule.

Still Not Convinced?

The U.S. General Accounting Office (GAO) produced a report detailing the effect of quality improvement activities on corporate performance. The report, *Management Practices, U.S. Companies Improve Performance Through Quality Efforts,* is based on the responses of twenty of the twenty-two companies that were finalists for the Malcolm Baldrige National Quality Award in 1988–89. The report concentrated on five categories of success: improved market share, improved profitability, greater customer satisfaction, quality and lower cost, and better employee relations. The results were consistently positive: market share was boosted an annual average of 13.7 percent, customer complaints dropped by 11.6 percent, employee turnover was reduced by 6 percent, and defects declined by 10.3 percent.

The report states:

- Companies that adopted TQM practices experienced an overall improvement in corporate performance. In nearly all cases, companies that used total quality practices achieved better employee relations, higher productivity, greater customer satisfaction, increased market share, and improved profitability.
- Each of the companies studied developed its practices in a unique environment with its own opportunities and problems. However, there were common features in their quality management systems that were major contributing factors to improved performance.
- Many different kinds of companies benefited from putting

specific TQM practices in place. However, none of these companies reaped those benefits immediately. Allowing sufficient time for results to be achieved was as important as initiating a quality management program (U.S. General Accounting Office, 1991, pp. 2–3).

Quality Results at UMMC

When UMMC initiated the TQM process in 1987, our major focus was improving quality through meeting customer requirements and improving the quality of work life. We did not implement TQM as a means to reduce cost. We did understand that Deming's chain reaction promised that when quality issues were addressed, cost could simultaneously be decreased. We also believed that the COPQ in our institution was high because of our size and complexity and felt that it could be reduced. We made no formal effort to calculate costs and benefits until 1991. There were many skeptics who questioned the time and energy the organization was dedicating to TQM. The leadership decided to undertake an analysis of the cost benefit and return on investment from the nineteen Quality Improvement Teams completed between July 1987 and June 1991. The analysis covered only the team reports; none of the other improvements made by managers or staff as they applied the TQM approach in daily work were considered. Our approach was to identify only incremental costs and benefits because it is our expectation that all managers and staff will use TQM methods for all work and it will be impossible to separate how much time each person spends on quality.

The methodology included information on net marginal or incremental costs and benefits after accounting for payer mix, insurance allowances, and bad debt. Costs were counted for only two years, even though many projects will produce revenue or savings for many years. Costs and benefits were calculated in the year the recommendations were implemented.

In addition to numerous quality improvements, most teams achieved significant savings. Seventeen of the nineteen quality improvement teams showed a financial benefit equal to

Table 1.2. Present Value of Incremental Financial Costs and Benefits.

Description	Amount ($ in millions)	Percentage of $550 M Budget
Total benefits (savings and additional revenues)	$17.7	3.2%
Incremental costs	(2.5)	0.4%
Incremental benefits	15.3	2.8%
Costs of training time	(1.5)	0.3%
Incremental benefits minus training costs	13.8	2.5%
Benefits/costs return ratio, excluding training time costs	7.2	
Benefits/costs return ratio, including training time costs	4.5	

Note: Annualized value of one-time savings and capital costs were calculated at an interest rate of 8.5 percent per year. The present value of costs and benefits in fiscal year 1990–91 dollars was also calculated using an 8.5 percent discount rate.

Source: University of Michigan Medical Center, 1992a.

or exceeding the costs. For seven of the nineteen teams, benefits exceeded costs by more than $100,000. The net financial benefit over the four-year period equals 2.8 percent of the hospitals' $550 million budget. The present value of the benefits was 7.2 times, or 720 percent, the present value of costs (University of Michigan Medical Center, 1992a, p. 2). The present value of incremental financial costs and benefits are illustrated in Table 1.2. The incremental centralized and project costs and benefits from July 1987 through June 1991 are summarized in Table 1.3.

Fourteen of the nineteen required negligible resources to implement their recommendations. Two teams required $1,800 and $7,600 respectively. Most team recommendations were within existing resources. Although incremental dollars were not used for training, these costs at an estimated cost per hour per attendee were calculated as a cost. The training dollars for 1987 to 1991 were $1,461,321 of direct labor time. Even with these costs allocated, the return on investment is substantial.

Table 1.3. Incremental Costs and Benefits of TQM Implementation, 1987–1991.

Description	Costs	Savings and Revenue Increases
Centralized Costs		
Incremental salaries/consultants	$1,000,000	
Training	113,000	
Leadership audits	94,000	
Incremental equipment	61,000	
Miscellaneous	44,000	
Centralized Benefits		
Honoraria/site visit fees	$0	$41,000
Individual QI Projects		
Operating rooms	$785,000	$13.1 million
Nursing resource pool	227,000	1.5 million
Continuing care – placement days	0	1.1 million
Admission/discharge	0	580,000
Commercial insurance holds	0	394,000
Medicaid pending	0	337,000
Surgical intensive care unit	0	313,000
Stockroom	0	140,000
Security – quality of work life	7,600	71,000
Cefazolin usage evaluation	0	69,000
End-stage renal disease billing	0	68,000
Nursing work redesign	0	8,200
Patient accounts – telephones	125,000	0
Clinician communication	1,800	0
Blue Cross authorizations	0	0
Blue Cross verifications of coverage	0	0
Diagnostic coding/attestations	0	0
Charge processing errors	0	0
Operating rooms – gynecological surgery	0	0
Total	$2.5 million	$17.7 million

Source: University of Michigan Medical Center, 1992a.

Chapter Two

Understanding TQM

Since readers will have a wide range of knowledge and experience with TQM, this chapter describes the basic concepts and sets the stage for TQM implementation within healthcare organizations. However, even those with a sound basic knowledge of TQM may want to skim over these concepts to familiarize themselves with the terms and operational definitions we will be using.

Many people have difficulty understanding what TQM is. Because TQM is a very comprehensive process with many component parts, a complete understanding of it may be difficult to grasp. This difficulty relates to the perspective from which one views TQM. If one looks at its components, one finds that many of its concepts, tools, and techniques are familiar; they have been around for years. In fact, virtually every organization has successfully implemented some portion of TQM. However, if one looks at TQM as a whole, its combination of philosophy, knowledge, and skills is uniquely effective in accomplishing major organizational change through improvement in quality, cost effectiveness, and human relations. In the case of TQM, the whole is more powerful than the sum of the parts in transforming an organization. Throughout the book, we hope to provide you with the strategies to integrate the different components of TQM.

Total Quality Requires Integrating Several Skills

Total Quality Management is an integrated effort focused on customers. The purpose and success of an organization is based on its internal and external customers. TQM is the integration of a customer-focused, continuous-improvement philosophy, analytical skills, people skills, and a structure and organization, within an internal and external culture affected by leadership, as illustrated in Figure 2.1. This integrated model, developed at UMMC, is helpful in visualizing the larger picture. The power of TQM comes from the integration and balance of these components. An overemphasis on any one portion of the model will fail to achieve the potential benefits of TQM.

1. *Customer-focused, continuous-improvement philosophy.* TQM is grounded in a philosophy of meeting and exceeding customer-defined requirements and working for continuous improvement. The fourteen points of W. Edwards Deming (1986), summarized in Exhibit 2.1, are examples of elements of this

Figure 2.1. UMMC Integrated TQM Model.

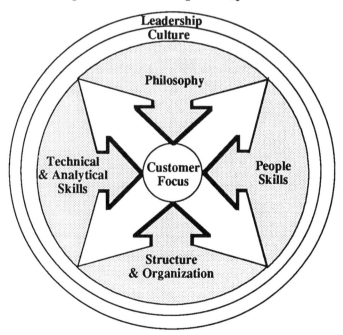

Source: Copyright © 1992, University of Michigan Medical Center, Ann Arbor, Mich.

philosophy. Its basic tenets are that employees want to do their best, that they know the most about their own jobs, and that they should be involved in planned improvements. For many managers, who have accomplished their responsibility by making most decisions and controlling everything, this represents a major shift in thinking. Clearly there is a minority of employees, suppliers, and others who do not want to do their best, but it is counterproductive to develop a whole management philosophy and system to address the nonperformers. This is an example of focusing on the "bad apple" theory, described by Donald M. Berwick (1989, pp. 53–56). Often staff who have wanted to do their best have been beaten down by barriers in the system, and have lost initiative. In adopting the new philosophy, management concentrates on removing barriers that prevent employees from doing their best.

2. *Analytical knowledge and skills.* The concept of making business decisions based on the use of data and analytical tools and techniques is very important to a TQM process. Engineers, business managers, quality control staff, and others have used measurement, graphs of data, control charts, statistics, and other quantitative techniques for years. However, these skills have not been widely used by healthcare managers and staff to improve organizational performance. Another issue is that certain people who advanced due to strong analytical skills may lack effective interpersonal skills. They tend to be very task oriented.

3. *Interpersonal or "people" skills.* Work is accomplished by people, and involvement of everyone in the organization is critical to success in a highly competitive environment. Better ideas are generated and changes implemented faster if staff closest to the process are involved in the analysis and decision-making process. Human resources staff and others have encouraged the participative management style, continuing education and training for all staff, and other people-oriented skills for years. However, they often failed to demonstrate quantitatively to results-oriented top leadership the effectiveness of these ap-

Exhibit 2.1. Deming's Fourteen Points.

The following is a summary of the fourteen points for management pre-scribed by W. Edwards Deming (1986, pp. 23–86). Selected healthcare exam-ples related to the fourteen points were also discussed by Marszalek-Gaucher and Coffey (1990, pp. 125–131).

1. "Create constancy of purpose for improvement of product and service" (p. 23).
2. "Adopt the new philosophy" (p. 23).
3. "Cease dependence on inspection to achieve quality" (p. 23).
4. "End the practice of awarding business on the basis of price tag alone. Instead, minimize total cost. Move toward a long-term relationship of loyalty and trust" (p. 23).
5. "Improve constantly and forever the system of production and service to improve quality and productivity, and thus constantly decrease costs" (p. 23).
6. "Institute training on the job" (p. 23).
7. "Institute leadership. The aim of supervision should be to help people and machines do a better job" (p. 23).
8. "Drive out fear, so that everyone may work effectively for the company" (pp. 23, 59).
9. "Break down barriers between departments" (p. 24).
10. "Eliminate slogans, exhortations, and targets for the work force asking for zero defects and new levels of productivity" (p. 24).
11. "Eliminate work standards (quotas). . . eliminate management by objec-tive" (pp. 70, 75).
12. "Remove barriers that rob the hourly worker of his right to pride of workmanship" (p. 24).
13. "Institute a vigorous program of education and self-improvement. . . . Encourage education and self-improvement for everyone" (pp. 24, 86).
14. "Put everybody in the company to work to accomplish the transforma-tion" (pp. 24, 86).

proaches in day-to-day management. Creating an organiza-tional culture for TQM is further addressed in Chapter Six.

4. *Structure and organization.* A supportive structure and organization should be established to ensure the success of a wide range of quality improvement efforts ranging from formal Quality Improvement Teams through daily quality improvement efforts of every employee. If quality improvement is to become an organizational focus, it must be actively led by the organiza-tion's leaders. Organization and leadership are further dis-

cussed in Chapter Five, and teamwork is further discussed in Chapter Eight.

5. *Culture and environment.* It is important to understand that, although the principles remain the same, TQM must be tailored to the unique internal and external culture and environment of every organization. TQM should be integrated into your organization's quality assurance and other initiatives, as described in Chapters Three and Four.

6. *Leadership.* This is shown as the outer circle, because over time leadership drives the process and creates the pressure for cultural change within the organization, which can significantly influence the external culture.

The uniqueness and power of TQM is in the integration and balance of these components, not in the use of individual parts. The key to organizational goal achievement is people, especially in a labor-intensive industry like healthcare. Inattention to people and cultural change are the most common reasons for the failure of change strategies and excessively long periods for implementing changes. It is important to recognize that very few healthcare professionals have a combination of analytical and people skills today. Training programs with skill-building opportunities are essential to help people develop and combine these skills.

Terminology and Characteristics

There is a wide range of terminology associated with Total Quality Management. Many healthcare providers are turned off by the jargon of the TQM movement. We will introduce terms as they are used. Operational definitions vary substantially from person to person and organization to organization. In this book, we have not differentiated Total Quality Management (TQM), continuous quality improvement (CQI), or other common terms because the components and methods of implementation are virtually the same for all of them. The Joint Commission on Accreditation of Healthcare Organizations (JCAHO) and other organizations have used the term continuous quality improvement (CQI). Total Quality Control (TQC) is a more common terminology in Japan, but the Japanese interpretation of control is broader than the common U.S. one. To the extent practical, you should try to use terms similarly to their general use, but it is very important that you establish and widely communicate the terms and operational definitions used *within* your organization.

The terminology selected is an important decision because it can affect how your TQM effort is perceived by patients, physicians, staff, and others. Try to avoid terms that have a negative connotation within your organization. Some sample terms used to describe an issue are:

- Process improvement. A basic tenet of TQM is that improving processes will achieve far greater results than finding the "people" who are causing the problems. Hence, the term is used frequently.
- Problem. Everyone understands the word *problem*, but it often also carries the connotation of finding the guilty person, the one responsible for it. There may also be a tendency to stop looking for improvements when people stop complaining about problems. The way the word is used and the way managers act may create different meanings in different organizations.
- Opportunity. The use of the word *opportunity* has a more positive connotation than the word *problem* and is more oriented toward continuous improvement philosophy.

At UMMC we use all three words but try to focus on opportunities for improvement, and then look for process improvements as the first step toward improvement.

Many action steps are highlighted throughout this book to suggest possible specific actions you and others can take to continue implementing TQM within your organization.

Action Step: Clearly state and demonstrate your commitment to change the organizational culture and processes to implement TQM as an approach to serve better your patients and other customers, including staff.

Action Step: Develop and communicate operational definitions for terms used in your TQM process, so that everyone in your organization can communicate effectively.

Customer and Customer Requirements

As you introduce Total Quality within your organization, the term *customer* may be controversial. When we initiated Total Quality at UMMC in 1987, some physicians, nurses, and other staff had major difficulty accepting and understanding the term *customer*. And, of those who accepted the term, many associated it with patients, referring physicians, and external customers solely, and did not initially recognize internal customer relationships. We found that as we repeatedly explained the term customer as a relationship there was greater acceptance. Today the words *customer* and *customer requirements* are regularly used throughout the Medical Center.

"*Customer* is an all-inclusive term that is much broader than *patient*; it includes patients' families, physicians, nurses, other healthcare professionals, co-workers, professional associations, third party payers, and students. A simple way of visualizing the supplier-customer relationship is illustrated in Figure 2.2. For any transaction involving a product, service, or information, the person or organization at the tail of the arrow is the supplier, and the person or organization at the head of the arrow is the customer. For any transaction in which you are providing something to someone else, that person is the customer" (Marszalek-Gaucher and Coffey, 1990, pp. 84–85). The customer at one step in a process normally becomes the supplier to another customer at the next step in the process. Everyone is a supplier and a customer at different times. The supplier and customer relationship is different for each transaction and has nothing to do with money. This model has been used effectively to communicate the terms and their relationship and has

Figure 2.2. Supplier-Customer Relationship.

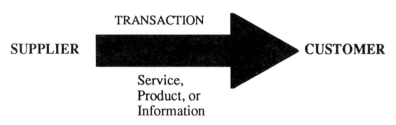

decreased resistance to the terms. Some choose to place particular emphasis on external customers who are purchasers.

Customer Requirements. Once your external and internal customers have been identified, the next step is to define valid customer requirements for each customer by talking directly with them. There may be some confusion among terms like needs, wants, expectations, and requirements. As defined here, valid customer requirements include any needs, wants, and expectations of customers for which an agreement has been reached between the supplier and customer. Some suggestions related to establishing customer requirements are illustrated in Table 2.1. Directly ask customers about their requirements.

The following refinements to customer requirements are offered.

Table 2.1. Suggestions Related to Establishing Customer Requirements.

Do:	*Do Not:*
• Encourage staff to identify all customers for each service	• Assume you know customer requirements
• Talk directly with customers	• Treat initial requests as fixed
• Understand customer needs and desires	• Try to establish all requirements at once
• Start with most important requirements	
• Negotiate, if appropriate	
• Offer better alternatives	
• Establish measures for requirements	

1. *Link internal and external customer requirements.* Requirements of internal customers should be linked to those of external customers. If an internal requirement does not in some way help meet external customer requirements, then its value should be questioned. For example, if an internal management report does not include information relevant to meeting the requirements of patients, payers, referring physicians, or other external customers, it may not add value.

2. *Link to needs and health status of community.* The ultimate objective of the healthcare system is to improve health. Yet most "healthcare" organizations focus almost exclusively on treating sick patients that come to them for care. Using data from state or local health departments, the healthcare needs and health status of your community or service area should be estimated. These serve as indicators of the extent to which your organization and others are collectively improving health status. If a healthcare organization looks only at those people currently served, it may experience two major omissions. First, it may exclude people in its community or service area who are not served appropriately by any healthcare provider. We may be providing high-quality, high-technology services to our patients, while others do not have basic services like prenatal care. Second, there may be opportunities to improve healthcare and health status that are outside of our current scope of services. For example, senior citizens may need home care services not currently available in order to avoid hospitalization for more serious conditions later. Another example might relate to strokes. Early diagnosis and treatment with a blood thinner may avoid a stroke, years of disability, and costly hospital and nursing home care. A comprehensive analysis of health status and needs may lead to the ability to serve customers better and to improve health within your service area.

3. *Customers may not verbalize all requirements.* When asked, customers will verbalize their perceived requirements. Noriaki Kano, Nobuhiro Seraku, Fumio Takahashi, and Shinichi Tsuji (1984, pp. 39–48) and Noriaki Kano (1984, p. 6) described three

Figure 2.3. Kano Model of Quality Measures.

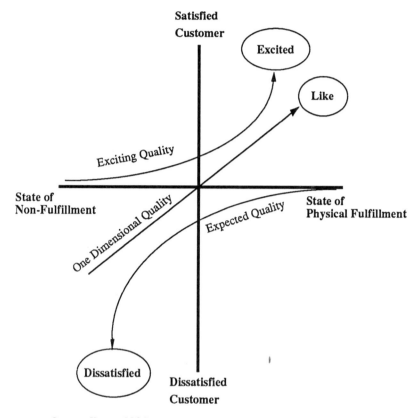

Source: Kano, 1984.

different measures of quality, as illustrated in Figure 2.3: one-dimensional quality, attractive or unexpected quality, and must-be or expected quality. One-dimensional quality measures, such as waiting time, are readily perceived, and customers are often sensitive to such measures. As the measure is better fulfilled, customer satisfaction steadily increases. These measures are normally mentioned when customers are asked about their requirements. On the other hand, the other two types of quality measures will seldom be mentioned when customers are surveyed. Attractive or unexpected quality, such as a staff person stopping work to assist a lost visitor, is seldom mentioned during surveys or interviews because the customer may not have experienced this type of service before. Yet this type of quality produces delighted customers. Must-be or expected quality is also seldom mentioned during surveys or interviews because the customers expect this level of service. For example, patients will seldom mention the avoidance of a hospital-acquired infection as a measure of quality because patients expect they will not acquire an infection while in the hospital.

You must consider not only requirements expressed by patients and other customers but also expected and unexpected quality items not expressed by customers. For example, healthcare professionals normally establish professional standards related to expected quality, such as clinical and housekeeping procedures, which patients are unaware of.

Quality

We define *quality* as meeting or exceeding valid customer requirements. Because each organization is unique, developing your own operational definitions is essential. One of the first tasks of your leadership group should be the definition of quality for your organization, as described in Chapter Five.

Characteristics of TQM

To help clarify the concept of TQM, some of its important characteristics are described here.

Focus on Continuous Improvement

The focus is on continuous improvement rather than achieving fixed goals. There must be improvement every year. This is contrary to traditional quality assurance efforts, in which the same thresholds may have been used for years. Thresholds are difficult to establish, may be inaccurate, and once reached may receive little additional attention. For example, if 1.8 percent of your surgical patients acquire post-operative deep wound infections this year, the organization should seek to reduce the percentage next year, even though the rate is already below the national average. Since TQM focuses on continuous quality improvement, you are beginning on a never-ending journey. Total Quality will not be completed next month, next year, or next decade. We seek to improve continually, with quantitative measurements to demonstrate that improvement. Probably more important is that what our patients, physicians, and other customers perceive as excellent care, service, and value today will be perceived as ordinary in the near future and may be perceived as unacceptable later, as other providers improve. In an analogy to high jumping, the customers and other providers keep raising the bar. Changes in knowledge, technology, and expectations will cause ever-increasing expectations.

TQM Is a Means, Not an End

TQM is not an end in itself. The objective is to improve performance continually, as judged by internal and external customers. TQM provides an approach and methods to help us accomplish our goals. However, some managers and consultants today are selling TQM as a panacea or almost as an end in itself. The aim is to accomplish the vision, values, mission, and goals of your organization through meeting and exceeding the requirements of your customers. Leadership should reinforce the aim regularly.

TQM Requires a Paradigm Shift

Everyone recognizes that the healthcare industry is experiencing major changes. The concept of a paradigm shift may be helpful in understanding both the changes and how to address them. There are many definitions of paradigms, but the one offered by Joel Barker is particularly helpful: "A paradigm is a set of rules and regulations that: 1) defines boundaries; and 2) tells you what to do to be successful within those boundaries. (Success is measured by the problems you solve using these rules and regulations)" (Barker, 1989, p. 14). The way you saw events and acted in the past may have been a successful paradigm at that time, but will it be the right model for the future? We suggest not. Given the current and future workforce, a major paradigm shift is required. Managers must become leaders and focus on developing new skills, as illustrated in Figure 2.4. To create a work environment in which everyone in a more diverse workforce contributes to his or her potential, your approach should shift from controlling to coaching, from quantity to quality, from opinion to data-based decisions, etc. The words *manager* and *leader* here refer to behavior or leadership styles, not to job titles.

This paradigm shift is very difficult to accomplish for two important reasons. First, people who have been successful with one management paradigm may not see the need for change. They have been successful by virtue of their current behaviors. The way they view the environment, their staff, and their customers is filtered by their paradigm of management. For example, if managers view staff as lacking knowledge, they are not likely to acknowledge good suggestions from staff members. Second, "New paradigms put everyone practicing the old paradigm at great risk. And, the higher one's position, the greater the risk. The better you are at your paradigm, the more you have invested in it. To change your paradigm is to lose that investment" (Barker, 1989, p. 32). Yet it is these very healthcare leaders that must recognize the need for change, and lead the change by

Figure 2.4. Paradigm Shift from Managing to Leading.

Managing	⟹	Leading
Control	⟹	Coaching
Quantity	⟹	Quality
Opinion	⟹	Data
Resistance to Change	⟹	Open to Change
People as Commodities	⟹	People as Resources
Suspicion	⟹	Trust
Compliance	⟹	Commitment
Internal Focus	⟹	Customer Focus
Individual	⟹	Team
Detection	⟹	Prevention

changing their behaviors first. *This is very difficult.* In this book we propose a number of practical methods to implement change.

Healthcare providers are being attacked on many fronts because the patients and payers perceive a lack of value for the money being spent on healthcare. Minor changes are not likely to change that perception. We must seek whole new paradigms of care, management, and financing. Joel Barker offers a challenge particularly applicable to healthcare organizations now: "What do I believe is impossible to do in my field, but, if it could be done, would fundamentally change my business?" (Barker, 1989, p. 74).

Requirements for Positive Vision

People are not motivated by a negative vision of the future. Motivation is an inherent incentive to do something. You are motivated to do something if it makes you feel better or if the situation becomes better because you do something. When something motivates you, you want to do it more. Yet many of the changes that we implement today in our organizations represent negative visions for most people: cutting costs, increasing productivity, and searching for the unacceptable few who "caused the problem" or "fail to meet the quality standards." We do these things because we must, but we certainly are not inherently motivated to do them. For most people these are considered necessary evils; they represent negative visions of the future.

You can, however, motivate people to positive visions. People want to improve quality for their patients and other customers and of course for themselves. Similarly, we are motivated to reduce rework and waste and to improve our working environment. These are common goals of TQM. Another aspect of the future vision is a different role for managers, as reflected by the paradigm shift from managing to leading. The challenge is to communicate this vision so that it is viewed positively rather than negatively.

Although not initially evident, if you pursue these positive visions of quality improvement, you gain improved cost effec-

tiveness as a byproduct. You may initially question this statement because many of us have been taught that quality always
costs more. However, the results from UMMC discussed in Chapter One demonstrate that improving quality often costs less, not
more.

It is also important that the vision be communicated. If a
positive vision of the future exists, it is often held only by a few
people at the board, administration, and medical staff leadership level. That vision is seldom communicated to all staff.
There are two problems with this approach. First, the people
within and participating with your organization will not know
the vision. Hence, they will not understand how their position,
role, and activities should support the organization's vision. As a
consequence, most people define their own vision of the future,
independent of the remainder of the organization, and it is pure
luck if these visions are the same. Second, without knowledge of
the positive vision of and benefits for the future, people see only
the pain of changes and are therefore likely to resist them.

Barriers to Quality

There are many barriers to quality and quality improvement.
Some sample barriers are summarized here.

1. *Lack of common direction.* Few organizations have a well-
communicated common direction that is understood by all
employees. This common direction is described by statements
of values, vision, mission, guiding principles, goals, and expectations and must be demonstrated through the actions of organizational leaders.

2. *Loss of key leaders.* If your organization loses one or
more key leaders of your TQM implementation, particularly
within the first few years, it can cause the implementation to
slow down or stop. Since the average tenure of chief executive
officers within U.S. hospitals now averages about three years, this
raises the question of who must "carry the flame." We would
propose that the organization's board must carry the flame by

recruiting new leaders who share the commitment to TQM and the organization's common direction. Another behavior that produces similar stalls in TQM implementation is leadership that vacillates in its active support and promotion of TQM.

3. *Poor communication.* Probably the single biggest barrier to continuous improvement is poor communication. It may begin with the supplier's not fully understanding customer requirements. Most processes in healthcare organizations have many steps. A relay race provides a good analogy. Each person is trying his or her hardest, but if the baton is dropped, the race is lost. In the case of healthcare processes, the analogy of the dropped baton is some form of miscommunication: the patient's scheduled admission time is wrong, the bed is ready for the admission but no one is told, or the operating room is cleaned but the patient has not been called from the inpatient unit.

4. *Too many steps in a process.* When a process becomes very complex, it typically has a high failure rate. As an example, consider a process with twenty-five steps in sequence. If each step in the process has a 99 percent probability of meeting requirements the first time, the system as a whole has only a 78 percent probability (.99 to the 25th power) of meeting all requirements the first time. It will fail to work correctly the first time 22 percent of the time. Examples of the impact of reducing steps in a process will be illustrated in Chapter Eleven. Therefore, a serious effort should be made to eliminate process steps that do not add significant value.

5. *Dysfunctional culture.* One of the key barriers to change is the conscious or unconscious retention of old beliefs and actions that discourage innovations, creativity, empowerment, diversity, or other components of TQM. The first step is to identify and raise these to the attention of the people involved. One approach used at UMMC was a leadership for Total Quality education program, which included assessment of managers' management styles by their subordinates and colleagues. These evaluations provided unexpected, and in some cases shocking,

insights into each manager's actions. As part of the program, managers then developed action plans to change part of their dysfunctional actions.

6. *Lack of integration and balance.* There are many components of implementing TQM in a healthcare organization which must be integrated and balanced to be successful. For example, an overemphasis on the analytical tools and techniques of TQM without a balanced emphasis on the cultural changes and people skills needed will be less effective than an integrated, balanced approach including all of the components. Examples of components of a TQM process that must be integrated and balanced during implementation are:

- Customer-oriented, continuous-improvement philosophy, analytical skills, people skills, and structure, as illustrated in Figure 2.1.
- Quality assurance and quality improvement
- Suppliers, your healthcare organization, and your customers
- Your healthcare organization, your medical staff, and other key groups
- Factors that may initially be viewed as paradoxes:
  - Passion for quality improvement and objectivity
  - Standardizing processes and innovation
  - Patience with process and impatience to improve results
  - Individual excellence and group commitment and synergy
  - Delegation/empowerment and control

Quality Improvement Implementation Models

There are many different models for implementing quality improvement (QI), although most of them include similar characteristics. Some sample quality improvement models are described here to illustrate this point and some alternatives that are available.

Hospital Corporation of America, FOCUS–PDCA. The

QI process developed at Hospital Corporation of America (HCA), Nashville, Tennessee, includes nine steps: FOCUS–PDCA (Hospital Corporation of America, 1989a).

Find a process to improve
Organize a team that knows the process
Clarify current knowledge of the process
Understand causes of process variation
Select the process improvement
Plan: improvement, data collection
Do: improvement, data collection, data analysis
Check: data for process improvement and customer outcome, lessons learned
Act: to hold gain, to reconsider owner, to continue improvement

The FOCUS–PDCA process has been used very effectively by several HCA hospitals, the Henry Ford Health System, Detroit, Michigan, and other healthcare organizations. Many other healthcare organizations have adopted this model because HCA has encouraged others to use it.

Joiner Associates, Madison, Wisconsin, uses a five-stage plan for process improvement (Scholtes and others, 1988).

1. Understand the process. Describe the process, identify the customer needs and concerns, and develop a standard process.
2. Eliminate errors. Work to eliminate errors in the process.
3. Remove slack. Streamline the process and eliminate steps that do not add value.
4. Reduce variation. Reduce variation in measurement systems and the process and bring both the measurement systems and process into statistical control.
5. Plan for continuous improvement. Conduct the Plan-Do-Check-Act process on the changes made.

Juran Institute, Wilton, Connecticut, uses a process called Juran's "Journey," which is composed of the following steps

(Juran, 1989, pp. 60–61; Joint Commission on Accreditation of Healthcare Organizations, 1991a, p. 56).

The Diagnostic Journey. This portion of the problem-solving process moves from the evidence of the problem toward identifying its cause. At least these three activities are involved:

1. Understanding the symptom. This step requires not only noting the words and findings that indicate a problem exists, but investigating to learn, as specifically as possible, the symptoms.
2. Theorizing as to causes. Juran suggests that those affected by the problem brainstorm and organize the various theories that result.
3. Testing the theories. This testing may require small-scale or large-scale data collection and analysis and should result in identifying the symptoms' cause or causes.

The Remedial Journey. This journey moves from the causes to their remedy. The activities involved include these three:

1. Stimulating the establishment of a remedy. Although the project team itself may not establish the remedy, Juran suggests that the team "follow up and stimulate until the remedy has been established."
2. Testing the remedy under operating conditions. This activity involves implementing and observing the remedy under day-to-day conditions. Juran encourages project teams to make sure "the cure is not worse than the disease."
3. Establishing controls to hold the gains. Juran reminds us that "[some] changes are reversible." Whatever procedures are necessary to make sure improvement is maintained should be implemented.

Organizational Dynamics, Inc. (ODI), Boston, Massachusetts, uses a quality improvement model known as FADE (Organizational Dynamics, Inc., 1990, pp. 12–13; Joint Commission on Accreditation of Healthcare Organizations, 1991a, pp. 56–59).

Focus. Generate a list of problems, select one problem, and verify/define the problems, which lead to a written statement of the problem.

Analyze. Decide what you need to know, collect data on baselines and patterns, and determine influential factors, which lead to baseline data and a list of most influential factors.

Develop. Generate promising solutions, select solution, and develop implementation plan, which lead to a solution for the problem and a plan for implementation.

Execute. Gain commitment, execute the plan, and monitor the impact, which lead to organizational commitment, an executed plan, and a record of impact.

Analog Devices Seven-Step Problem-Solving Model.
Analog Devices has successfully used a seven-step process to implement quality improvements (Center for Quality Management, 1991, p. 25).

1. Select theme. Select theme or specific problem to address, based on weighing what is most urgent, will give quickest payback for effort, or is most important.
2. Data collection and analysis. Data can take numerical and non-numerical forms.
3. Causal analysis. Identify and verify the root cause of the problem.
4. Solution planning and implementation. Identify solutions that reverse root causes.
5. Evaluation of effects. Collect and analyze data and compare with prior results.
6. Standardization. Standardize improvements and use in Standardize-Do-Check-Act cycle.
7. Reflection on process. Ask whether the process or problem was chosen for improvement and how the improvement process itself can be improved.

To our knowledge, this specific process has not been used by healthcare organizations, but it is very similar to other QI processes.

Qualtec Seven-Step QI Process. The process developed at Florida Power and Light, and marketed by Qualtec, Inc., includes seven steps (Qualtec, Inc., 1989a, 1989b):

1. Reason for improvement. Identifies a theme or problem area and the reason for working on it.
2. Current situation. Selects a problem and sets a target for improvement.
3. Analysis. Identifies and verifies the root causes of the problem.
4. Countermeasures. Plans and implements countermeasures that will correct the root causes of the problem.
5. Results. Confirms that the problem and its root causes have been decreased.
6. Standardization. Standardizes to prevent the problem and its root causes from recurring.
7. Future plans. Plans what to do about any remaining problems and evaluates the team's effectiveness and how to replicate the countermeasures elsewhere.

This process has been used very effectively by many team and individual QI efforts at UMMC and has been used by all formal Quality Improvement Teams (QITs). This model has also been used effectively at Methodist Medical Center of Illinois, Peoria, Illinois; Franciscan Sisters Health Care Corporation, Mokena, Illinois; St. Joseph's Health Care Corporation, Stockton, California; Middle Tennessee Medical Center, Murfreesboro, Tennessee; and Alliant Health System, Louisville, Kentucky.

UMMC Seven-Step QI Process. As the UMMC Total Quality Process has progressed, we have developed a new seven-step QI process to meet the unique requirements of healthcare organizations and to address issues that our teams have experienced (University of Michigan Hospitals, 1992). The seven steps are:

Recognize the process. To identify customers and major work processes and to analyze those work processes.
Organize the data. To collect and stratify data to identify

specific problems resulting in a detailed statement reflecting the quality gap.

Analyze root causes. To identify and analyze contributing factors (causes) to the process flow (effect).

Determine options. Select options (proposed solutions) that will decrease or eliminate the identified significant root causes of the quality gap.

Measure the change. Measure results and success of the proposed option(s).

Apply to workplace. Standardize and maintain successful options from quality improvement process to prevent recurrence of root causes.

Plan for the future. Generalize improvements to other areas, investigate additional improvements, and celebrate achievements.

Based on the experiences at UMMC and other organizations, the following are sample improvements included within the implementation of this model. More emphasis is placed on the selection of topics for Quality Improvement Teams. Many of our teams were given very broad issues to deal with and had substantial difficulty selecting appropriate opportunities for improvement. After pilot studies were completed, a number of our teams had difficulty maintaining the gain and standardizing to other areas of the organization. The new model also more explicitly addresses the relationship between TQM and quality assurance.

Similarities and Differences of TQM Models. Different organizations develop different models and methodologies to tailor the approach to their needs. Each healthcare organization should also tailor TQM for its environment and requirements. All of the TQM models have these similarities:

- Focus on internal and external customers.
- Use scientific problem-solving approach.
- Identify the root causes of problems or opportunities for improvement.
- Pilot test new approaches to improve quality.

- Include staff who do the work in the QI effort, although this step is not explicitly stated in the steps of the models.

The differences among the TQM models are more in the statement of the models than in actual differences of implementation. These include:

- Scope of the model. Some models focus exclusively on problem solving, while other models include a broader range of TQM activities.
- Treatment of variation. Some models explicitly list steps to reduce variation of the process; other models do not. However, underlying the improvements of all models will be reduced variation.
- Removing slack or steps that do not add value. This is not listed in several of the models but is normally addressed during the process of identifying improvements.

Similarities to Traditional Clinical Models. Although some of the terminology is different, there are strong similarities between the QI problem-solving process and traditional clinical models because they are all based on the scientific process. UMMC developed the following analogies to sample clinical models in order to illustrate their similarities.

1. Medical practice model. The similarities of the seven-step quality improvement model to the medical practice model are discussed in Chapter Seven.
2. Nursing care process. The assessment and nursing diagnosis are similar to step 2, current situation, in the quality improvement process, as illustrated in Figure 2.5. The care plan is similar to step 3, analysis, and the intervention is similar to step 4, countermeasures. The evaluation is similar to step 5, results, and any revision is similar to step 7, future plans.
3. SOAP-IER charting process. Dr. Lawrence Weed developed a charting process known by its acronym SOAP. A later revision had the acronym SOAP-IER. The *Subjective* customer perception is similar to step 1, reason for improve-

Figure 2.5. Nursing Care Process Compared to UMMC QI Process.

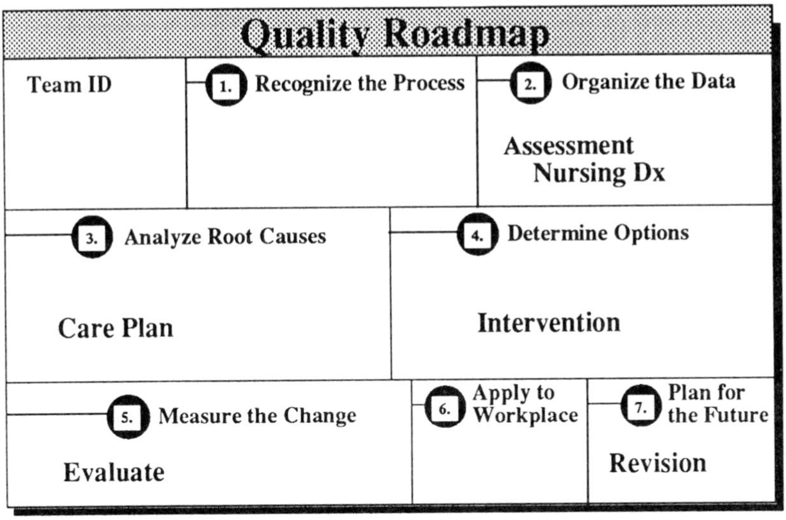

Quality Roadmap		
Team ID	1. Recognize the Process	2. Organize the Data **Assessment** **Nursing Dx**
3. Analyze Root Causes **Care Plan**	4. Determine Options **Intervention**	
5. Measure the Change Evaluate	6. Apply to Workplace	7. Plan for the Future **Revision**

ment, in the quality improvement process, as illustrated in Figure 2.6. The *O*bjective data and *A*ssessment are similar to step 2, current situation. The *P*lan of care is similar to step 3, analysis, and the *I*ntervention is similar to step 4, countermeasures. The *E*valuation is similar to step 5, results, and the *R*evision is similar to step 7, future plans.

Implementation Processes. There are also a number of implementation processes.

GOAL/QPC Ten-Element Model. GOAL/QPC, Methuen, Massachusetts, has developed ten elements of a TQM implementation model, including (GOAL/QPC, 1992, p. 29):

1. TQM decision
2. Customer focus
3. Critical processes
4. Initial teams
5. Five-year plan
6. Managing momentum
7. Hoshin planning

Figure 2.6. SOAP-IER Charting Process Compared to UMMC QI Process.

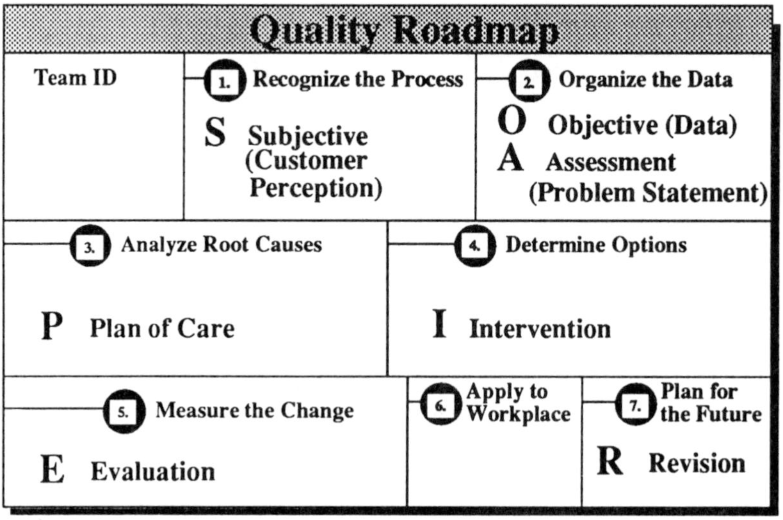

Quality Roadmap		
Team ID	1. Recognize the Process S Subjective (Customer Perception)	2. Organize the Data O Objective (Data) A Assessment (Problem Statement)
	3. Analyze Root Causes P Plan of Care	4. Determine Options I Intervention
	5. Measure the Change E Evaluation	6. Apply to Workplace 7. Plan for the Future R Revision

8. New teams
9. Daily management
10. Evaluating progress

This process addresses an overall TQM implementation, not just the quality improvement process. This model has been used effectively by Bethesda Hospital, Cincinnati, Ohio; Bryn Mawr Hospital, Bryn Mawr, Pennsylvania; Our Lady of Lourdes Medical Center, Camden, New Jersey; and other organizations.

The Juran Quality Improvement Journey. Juran Institute, Inc., Wilton, Connecticut, has identified the following five phases and key steps of the quality journey (Juran, 1991, pp. 9-3 to 9-11). See also the Juran quality improvement process steps in Figure 9.1 in Chapter Nine.

1. Decide to pursue total quality.
    —Determine why you need to change.
    —Understand your options.
    —Select total quality.
2. Prepare for the journey.

—Educate upper management.
—Form a quality council of upper managers.
—Prepare plans and objectives.
—Communicate actions.
3. Start the journey.
   —Conduct pilot quality projects.
   —Build basic infrastructure of support.
   —Communicate results.
4. Expand effort.
   —Include all organizational units.
   —Add more quality teams.
   —Include teams for quality improvement, planning, control, cross-functional business processes, and benchmarking.
   —Provide adequate training.
   —Develop measurement of quality indicators throughout organization.
5. Integrate the entire organization.
   —Set systematic quality goals from the strategic to the individual.
   —Involve everyone.
   —Manage key business processes cross-functionally.
   —Review and audit results.

Crosby Fourteen Steps. Philip Crosby Associates, Winter Park, Florida, developed a fourteen-step process (Crosby, 1979, pp. 112–119).

1. Management commitment.
2. Quality improvement team.
3. Quality measurement.
4. Cost of quality evaluation.
5. Quality awareness.
6. Corrective action.
7. Establish an ad hoc committee for the zero defects program.
8. Supervisor training.
9. Zero defects day.

10. Goal setting.
11. Error cause removal.
12. Recognition.
13. Quality councils.
14. Do it all over again.

The QI models and implementation processes described above, with the exception of the GOAL/QPC ten-element model, focus on evolutionary, incremental improvements. Staff and managers of the many different supplier-customer relationships work to identify process improvements. However, there is also a need to plan for more revolutionary changes.

Evolutionary Change Versus Revolutionary Change

Although the QI models work very well to make evolutionary, incremental improvements, the models have weaknesses related to revolutionary changes, which may not be perceived or implemented by the people involved in the current process. There is a strong need to integrate continuing research and strategic planning with QI efforts. For example, a QI team working on how to improve surgery for kidney stones is unlikely to conceive of a lithotripter, which dissolves the kidney stones within the body without surgery. Laser surgery radically changed the practice of ophthalmology. Those working to rehabilitate stroke patients, for example, may not address new approaches to prevent strokes through better health management. These revolutionary changes represent major shifts in technology, clinical practice, or management. Also, customers seldom mention unexpected quality characteristics when surveyed (see Kano model, Figure 2.3). Revolutionary changes are normally discovered by scientists or professionals; some represent complete paradigm shifts. Joel Barker points out that people who identify whole new paradigms are normally outsiders or people on the fringes; they are not part of the mainstream of the professions, organizations, technologies, or practices traditionally involved (Barker, 1989, pp. 25–27). The developers of new paradigms tend to be young graduates, older scientists shifting fields, or tinkerers. They do not view things in traditional ways and are not threatened by any resulting changes. Hence, QI efforts should be supplemented with a continuing search for revolutionary ideas that could change your whole business.

One way of thinking about the difficulty of implementing a Total Quality Process is that, although the analytical process improvements are evolutionary in nature, the required cultural changes are perceived as revolutionary by the people involved.

As we define TQM, it includes quality planning to address revolutionary changes, in addition to quality improvement and quality operations. TQM includes techniques such as quality function deployment (QFD) and hoshin planning, which can address the more revolutionary changes. These are addressed in Chapter Fourteen.

It should be clear to everyone that provision of care and management on a daily basis will continue to require some immediate decisions in which there is no time for a team problem-solving approach. This is most evident in emergency medical situations. Although a formal process is not followed, often similar problem-solving steps are done mentally while reaching a quick decision.

Tailored Implementation

Each organization should tailor implementation of TQM to its own environment, organization, and history. The principles, tools, and techniques are generally applicable anywhere, but the specific approach and speed of implementation must be tailored to your organization. TQM implementation will take place in the context of existing knowledge, skills, and relationships of the physicians, staff, management, and community. The types and perceptions of previous programs will also affect the success of TQM. The relationships of TQM to previous programs should be described, as discussed in Chapter Four. A "cookie-cutter" approach, using the same exact implementation plan in different organizations, is generally ineffective. You should be cautious of those who suggest an approach not substantially tailored to your organization.

Chapter Three

Integrating TQM and Quality Assurance

One of the commonly asked questions about TQM is how it relates to the existing quality assurance or assessment (QA) process. There are several misconceptions and fears among people working on both TQM and QA. We hope to clarify some of the differences between the two and demonstrate how QA is an integral part of an overall TQM process.

This chapter discusses the relationship of QA and TQM and the rationale for and alternative approaches to their integration. As TQM is introduced to a healthcare organization, there is typically substantial confusion about how it relates to the organization's existing QA program. Every healthcare organization has a QA program for internal quality control and because it is mandated by external organizations such as JCAHO. In many organizations, one of the common initial responses to beginning TQM is that "we already do quality improvement; we have a quality assurance program."

Common Misconceptions

It may be helpful to review some common *misconceptions* about the relationship between QA and TQM.

Either QA or TQM. Some people perceive QA and TQM as an "either-or" situation. Thus the QA staff may view TQM as threatening their existence, and TQM staff may view QA staff as related to an old paradigm. This should not be the case but occurs because TQM is often initiated by non-QA managers who do not recognize the role of or involve QA staff. Many TQM processes begin by looking at nonclinical issues, which are of little interest to traditional quality assurance functions. Also, some traditional QA staff are oriented to detailed audits with a "bad apple" focus and lack a broader process or organizational focus.

TQM does not include any QA activities. W. Edwards Deming's third point, "cease dependence on inspection to achieve quality" (Deming, 1986, p. 23), is taken by some to imply that there will be no inspection or quality assurance activities. This is not true. Deming is urging that organizations cease dependence on inspection as the *primary* method to achieve quality, such as following up on every drug error as though it had an assignable cause. Inspection is a very costly approach because it leads to large amounts of rework and waste. However, some amount of inspection, quality control, or quality assurance is always part of a TQM process.

TQM should be led by QA staff. Quality is most effectively achieved the first time something is done by the person who provides the service, product, or information. Quality cannot *effectively* be the responsibility of any centralized QA or TQM staff. For a quality approach to be effective, quality must become everyone's priority job, from executive leadership to every employee throughout the organization. Changes of this magnitude must be led by the organization's executives. Of course, the QA staff can serve as key resource staff to implement TQM as well as QA, but cannot effectively lead the TQM effort.

TQM does not include QA staff. On the other hand, some organizations don't recognize the role QA staff can play in the TQM effort. This perception ignores the knowledge, experience, and important relationships of the current QA staff, as well as the fact that some level of quality control or quality assurance is part of every complete TQM process. To be an effective part of the TQM team, however, QA staff must develop a broader understanding of customers, customer requirements, and quality improvement tools and techniques. In particular,

QA staff cannot have a "fill-out-the-form" attitude and approach, or TQM leaders may not include them as key support staff for the TQM effort. Similarly, those leading the TQM effort should draw on the knowledge and skills of experienced QA staff. QA staff bring firsthand knowledge of opportunities for improvement, especially in clinical areas, and knowledge about issues related to data collection, reliability, and validity useful for an integrated TQM/QA effort.

Comparison of Traditional QA and TQM

Since every healthcare organization's quality assurance program is different, it is impossible for us to compare TQM with your individual QA program. Virtually no healthcare organizations have completely traditional QA programs or have fully implemented TQM processes; most are somewhere in the middle. However, it is beneficial to understand the similarities and differences between traditional QA and TQM before looking at how to integrate the approaches. Therefore, we will contrast the characteristics of a traditional QA program and those of a fully implemented TQM process.

Similarly, the requirements of QA as defined by the JCAHO have also evolved. From its formation in 1953 until 1974, there were general references to assessing and improving care, but no specific methodologies or standards. In 1975 the Quality of Professional Services standard was published, requiring hospitals to "demonstrate that the quality of patient care was consistently optimal by continually evaluating care through reliable and valid measures," mostly through time-limited audits of care (Joint Commission on Accreditation of Hospitals, 1975; Joint Commission on Accreditation of Healthcare Organizations, 1991b, p. 7). In 1985 JCAHO replaced the problem-focused approach with a requirement for systematic monitoring and evaluation of important aspects of patient care (1991b, p. 8). Then JCAHO began developing its now well known ten-step monitoring and evaluation process outlined in Table 3.1 (1991b, pp. 39–54). This ten-step process, like other quality improve-

Table 3.1. JCAHO Ten-Step Monitoring and Evaluation Process.

Step	Description
Step 1	Assign responsibility
Step 2	Delineate scope of care and service
Step 3	Identify important aspects of care and service
Step 4	Identify indicators
Step 5	Establish means to trigger evaluation
Step 6	Collect and organize data
Step 7	Initiate evaluation
Step 8	Take actions to improve care and service
Step 9	Assess the effectiveness of actions and assure improvement is maintained
Step 10	Communicate results to relevant individuals and groups

Source: Joint Commission on Accreditation of Healthcare Organizations, 1991b, p. 41.

ment processes described in Chapter Two, can be used as a common approach for quality improvement.

The key characteristics of a traditional QA approach compared to TQM are illustrated in Table 3.2. There are several differences, but three key factors are:

- The focus on everyone as customers and suppliers in a process
- The emphasis on improving the processes for everyone rather than identifying only the problems and unacceptable few
- Continuous improvement rather than static thresholds for quality indicators

For any given quality measurement, QA focuses on those individuals who exceed the appropriate upper or lower threshold, as illustrated in Figure 3.1. One of the key deficiencies in traditional QA programs is that no action is taken regarding the 90 + percent of the people or outcomes that fall within the thresholds. Eliminating the people in the lower, upper, or both tails of the distribution improves the average very little if at all. There may be some improvement when people know they are

Table 3.2. Comparison of Traditional QA and TQM.

Characteristic	Traditional Quality Assurance	Total Quality Management
Purpose	Improve quality of patient care for patients	Improve quality of all services and products for patients and other customers
Scope	Clinical processes and outcomes	All systems and processes—clinical and nonclinical
	Actions directed toward people studied	Actions directed toward process improvement
	Mandated by JCAHO and others	Optional, but in order to meet JCAHO performance measurement, some aspects of TQM needed
Leadership	Physician and clinical leaders: chief of clinical staff, QA committee	All clinical and nonclinical leaders
Aims	Problem solving	Continuous improvement, even if no "problem" identified
	Identify individuals whose outcomes are outside specified thresholds—implies special causes	Addresses both special and common causes—most attention toward common causes
Focus	Peer review vertically focused by department or clinical process—each department does its own QA	Horizontally focused to improve all processes and people that affect outcomes
	Unacceptable few—education or elimination of those who do not meet standards	Improve performance of everyone, not just the unacceptable few
	Inspection	Prevention and design to improve the processes—then inspection to monitor process
	Outcome-oriented	Process- and outcome-oriented
Customers and Requirements	Customers are professionals and review organizations—patient is focus	Customers are patients, professionals, review organizations, and others—everyone
	Measures and standards established by healthcare professionals only	No long-term fixed standards—continuously improving standards established by customers and professionals

Table 3.2. Comparison of Traditional QA and TQM, Cont'd.

Characteristic	Traditional Quality Assurance	Total Quality Management
Methods	Chart audits Nominal group technique Hypothesis testing Indicator monitoring	Indicator monitoring and data use Brainstorming Nominal group technique Force field analysis Coaching/mentoring Flowcharting Checklist Histogram/Pareto chart Cause-effect, fishbone diagram Run/control chart Stratification Quality function deployment Hoshin planning
People Involved	QA program and appointed committees Actions decided by committees appointed for specific periods Limited involvement	Everyone involved with process Actions decided by team of people familiar with process—no time period specified Total institutional involvement
Outcomes	Includes measurement and monitoring May improve performance of the few individuals addressed Creates defensive posturing	Includes measurement and monitoring Improves performance of everyone involved in process Focus on process improvement—reduces threat to individuals, promotes team spirit, and can break down turf lines Includes QA efforts
Continuing Activities	Monitor for deviations from thresholds/standards Follow up when there are special cause deviations	Monitor processes for deviations (QA) and continually improve standards (QI) Follow up when there are special or common cause deviations

Source: Coffey, 1991.

Figure 3.1. QA Addresses Unacceptable Few.

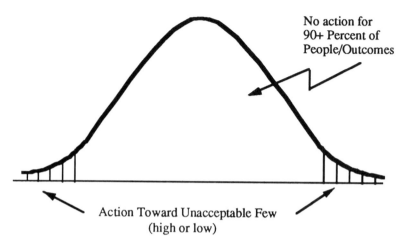

Source: Coffey, 1991, p. 10.

being studied, due to their desire not to fall outside the thresholds (this is known as the Hawthorne effect). However, these changes do not represent process improvements and tend to be temporary. Alternatively, TQM focuses on improving the process, which improves the performance of everyone, not just those in the tails of the distribution, as illustrated in Figure 3.2. Thus process improvements achieve performance increases for everyone. By focusing on process improvements first, you identify and eliminate the legitimate process failures first, so when you do reach a conclusion that an individual provider is a problem, there is a high probability that you are correct. This is much better than the traditional approach when QA committees inappropriately challenge an individual physician or other provider, only to have that provider demonstrate that there are problems with the data collection or supportive process. This approach wastes a lot of time and causes angry, defensive providers.

QA Areas That Can Be Improved with TQM

We see the current quality assurance processes as a valuable function, and QA staff as having important knowledge, skills,

Figure 3.2. TQM Improves Process to Shift Distribution.

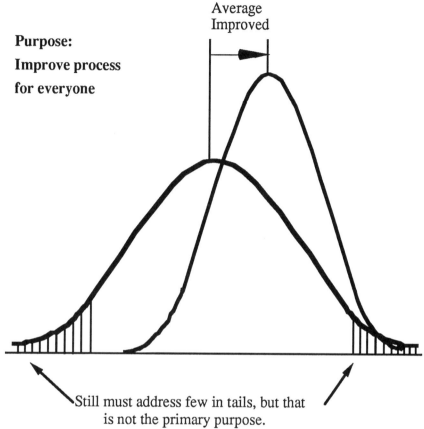

Purpose:

Improve process

for everyone

Average
Improved

Still must address few in tails, but that
is not the primary purpose.

Source: Coffey, 1991, p. 10.

and relationships. However, a number of QA functions can be improved by using a TQM approach. Some examples follow.

Broader Definition of Quality. For most QA programs, quality is defined in terms of clinical outcomes or services that directly affect clinical outcomes. This definition ignores many other characteristics of care which are important to our patients, their families, the referring physicians, staff, payers, and other customers. TQM has a much broader definition; quality is meeting valid customer requirements, for *all* customers. Thus, for TQM, quality encompasses all clinical and nonclinical services, products, and information. Indicators are based on the require-

ments of patients, families, physicians, payers, and other customers, in addition to traditional professionally defined quality
indicators. As an example, patient satisfaction information
could be included in QA, TQM, and operational management
reports.

Extension Beyond Clinical Performance. The performance
of a physician, nurse, or other clinician is heavily influenced by
supportive and administrative processes as well as the clinician's
personal decisions. For example, a physician orders a laboratory test and the results are delayed or incomplete. This may
lead to delayed clinical decisions and treatment. It may also
require rework. The physician may be forced to order the same
laboratory test on a stat basis. Delays can lead to an undesirable
clinical outcome and excess use of services, for which the physician is criticized during the QA process. Yet can the physician be
judged separately from the performance of the rest of the
healthcare organization's processes? TQM extends consideration to the whole process, not just clinical performance.

Application of TQM Methods to Improve QA. TQM has
several useful methods and techniques that have been developed and refined in many product and service industries. These
methods can facilitate the QA process, which exists to identify
problems with individual or system performance but does not
include any particular methods to improve performance. TQM
includes several group-process and analytical methods that can
be used to direct attention to the most important quality improvement issues, to focus on data rather than opinions, to ask
the correct questions, and to reduce defensive posturing. Several of these methods will be described in Chapter Twelve.

Evolution of Positive Approach. The history of QA implementations in most healthcare organizations has been both a
negative and a punitive approach. Thresholds for unacceptable
outcomes or behavior are established using standards from
other organizations or a group decision process. These thresholds are seldom statistically based on the measured outcomes of
the current process, are infrequently updated, and may not be
consistent with local practice. The thresholds are then used to
identify the unacceptable few. Berwick refers to this as the "bad

apple" approach (1989, p. 53). Those people are then challenged regarding their behavior. Given this challenge and the drive to defend themselves, the accused bring forward all possible reasons why the outcome is not due to their personal actions. These issues must then be addressed. Neither the people being challenged nor those on the QA committee find this to be a positive experience. Seldom can one individual change the process in order to improve results. Eighty-five percent or more of opportunities for improvement are through process improvements, leaving 15 percent or less due to people, as illustrated later in Figure 10.1. Yet traditional QA programs attack people first. The TQM approach is much more positive; it attacks the process first in order to improve quality. There is no personal attack but rather a team approach to improving processes for everyone. Certainly there will be some occasions when personal actions are unacceptable, but they will arise in the context of evaluating a wide range of possible improvements, and will arise only after process problems have been identified.

   Standards Based on Process Capabilities Rather Than Opinion. Most QA standards or thresholds are based on data from other organizations or on opinions relating to acceptable performance held by members of the respective QA committees. QA standards are seldom based on the capabilities of the current process. This leads to two situations. The first is that the thresholds are set too narrowly, and virtually everyone easily meets the thresholds. Alternatively, the thresholds may be set too widely, and the QA committee spends a lot of time investigating individual performances that simply reflect that the overall system is incapable of meeting the thresholds.

   By using a TQM method called a control chart, the control limits are based on the measured outcomes, or capabilities, of the current process. This allows managers, teams, or the QA committee to ask the appropriate questions about whether the process measurements are due to a special/assignable cause, in which case the reason for that outcome is investigated individually. If, on the other hand, the measurements are within the control limits, attention is focused on how to improve the processes so everyone's performance can be improved. There is no investigation of individuals or possible special causes in this situation. Certainly, it is helpful to identify the best possible performance, or "stretch goals," by using the processes from other organizations as benchmarks or establishing goals for improvement within your own organization. However, the focus of this investigation is finding better processes and developing plans to improve your processes, not identifying individuals who do not meet those goals.

Dynamic Quality Improvement. Most healthcare organizations establish QA standards or thresholds, then use the same standards for multiple years. TQM, on the other hand, stresses continual improvement. Quality levels are expected to improve each year.

Prevention and Design Rather Than Inspection. Quality assurance is based on inspection as the primary approach to identify problems for resolution. TQM, on the other hand, is primarily based on prevention and design of new or improved systems to prevent quality problems. This type of approach can help your QA process move away from inspection as a primary means to achieve quality. Your QA process will cost less and achieve better results. You will, however, still need a mechanism to identify and take action on the few people who are below the desired performance level and need personal attention.

Changes in External Expectations

External customers, including patients, referring and staff physicians, payers, and business and industrial organizations, are changing their expectations relating to quality service, quality assurance, and Total Quality Management.

Changes in JCAHO Expectations

JCAHO has undertaken a multiyear effort to direct much more attention toward quality improvement through performance improvement. These expectations are very important to most healthcare organizations, since reimbursement for care by Medicare, Medicaid, Blue Cross, and other payers is based on

JCAHO accreditation. The new emphasis on QI by JCAHO represents a substantial change in expectations but is consistent with the worldwide paradigm shift toward TQM principles. Your organization should contact JCAHO for specific expectations, but examples of new expectations for 1992 through 1994 include:

- **1992:** The leaders of the board, administration, medical staff, and nursing "set expectations, develop plans, and implement procedures to assess and improve the quality of the organization's governance, management, clinical, and support processes" (QA.1). For 1992, only the first of the six expectations, "The leaders undertake education concerning the approach and methods of continuous quality improvement" (QA.1.1), will be judged (Joint Commission on Accreditation of Healthcare Organizations, 1991b, p. 66; 1991c, p. 139; 1992c, pp. 140–141). For 1992, this will be scored based on participation in educational activities and knowledge of CQI (1991d, p. 3).

- **1993:** The leaders will be expected to meet more of the QA.1 criteria, in addition to other organizational CQI requirements:

  QA.1.1 "The leaders undertake education concerning the approach and methods of continuous quality improvement."

  QA.1.2 "The leaders set priorities for organization-wide quality improvement activities that are designed to improve patient outcomes."

  QA.1.3 "The leaders allocate adequate resources for assessment and improvement of the organization's governance, managerial, clinical, and support processes," including personnel, time, and information systems.

  QA.1.4 "The leaders assure that organization staff are trained in assessing and improving the processes that contribute to improved patient outcomes."

QA.1.5 "The leaders individually and jointly develop and participate in mechanisms to foster communication among individuals and among components of the organization, and to coordinate internal activities."

QA.1.6 "The leaders analyze and evaluate the effectiveness of their contributions to improving quality" (1991c, p. 139; 1991b, p. 66).

- **1994:** The planned 1994 standards will continue increased focus on QI, with a transition to focus on key processes rather than departments (1992a). The accreditation manual will be organized around the following planned key functions:

  a. Part A: Care of the patient functions
     - Patient rights
     - Admission to the setting or service
     - Patient evaluation
     - Nutritional care
     - Nonoperative treatment selection and administration (such as medication)
     - Operative and other invasive procedures
     - Patient and family education
     - Continuity of care

  b. Part B: Organizational functions:
     - Leadership
     - Human resources management
     - Health information management
     - Environmental management
     - Quality assessment and improvement

  c. Part C: Essential structural components:
     - Governing body
     - Management and administration
     - Medical staff
     - Nursing

Changes in Business/Insurance Payer Expectations

More important in the long run than changes in accreditation standards will be increasing expectations by major businesses, industries, and insurance payers who direct their employees and subscribers to healthcare organizations based on their perceived value. Ford Motor Company, General Motors, Motorola, Xerox, and many other organizations are now stating that they will expect healthcare organizations to meet the same quality monitoring and quality improvement processes and standards that they expect of their other suppliers. In our opinion, healthcare organizations have only about two to five years to implement such Total Quality Processes within their organizations or face loss of patients from those business, industry, and insurance organizations. These organizations know that TQM works to improve quality, cost effectiveness, and value for their organizations, and that they must demand similar improvements from all their suppliers to remain competitive in the world market. The U.S. automobile manufacturers, for example, regularly point to their healthcare costs as a significant factor in their total cost. They spend more money on Blue Cross than on any other single vendor, including steel, plastics, or tires.

The federal government, state governments, industrial and business organizations, and insurance payers have increasingly refined measures of cost. They are developing crude measures of quality, from which they can judge value. If healthcare organizations, especially the medical centers and others with higher costs, do not want to be subjected to the measures and judgments of these other organizations, we are challenged to:

- Increase our quality and cost effectiveness continuously and substantially.
- Develop and demonstrate measures of clinical and service quality, upon which value judgments can be based along with cost data.
- Demonstrate that our organizations meet the quality assessment and quality improvement requirements established by industrial and business organizations. Examples include Ford Motor Company's Q-101 standards (1990) and General Motors' Targets of Excellence (1990).
- Participate in joint efforts with the payers, community orga-

nizations, and insured people to improve health and reduce medical costs.

Action Step: Meet with major businesses and insurance payers in your area to share information on TQM methods and projects, and discuss their expectations of your organization.

Approaches to Integrate QA and TQM

Transition from quality assurance or assessment to a fully implemented TQM process will take time, and can be accomplished by many different approaches. Most organizations will go through multiple stages of relationships between QA and TQM as the two are gradually integrated.

Experiences in Integrating QA and TQM

Virtually everyone agrees that the goal is to integrate the QA functions with the TQM functions. Yet most healthcare organizations have found integration very difficult. *Why has integration been so difficult?* The answers may be helpful in understanding and planning TQM implementation and the integration of QA and TQM within your organization.

Limited resources. All organizations undertaking TQM have been faced with limited resources, including time of the leaders, manager and staff time, availability of technical and training staff to support the effort, and of course money. This has discouraged broad-scale implementation of TQM, including clinical and nonclinical staff, and integrating it with current QA activities.

Lack of data and information. Both QA and TQM efforts are hindered by a lack of useful data and information. Especially for clinical care, much of the information is located in manually documented medical records. Substantial improvement in data collection and information systems will be required for QA and TQM to be individually or collectively successful and cost-effective.

Skepticism of efforts led by others. Many quality improvement efforts led by administrative staff have met with skepticism, caution, and even distrust by the physicians and other clinical staff. They often take a "wait-and-see" attitude. Similarly, quality improvement efforts led by physicians have been met by a "wait-and-see" attitude by management. Union leaders and members may be cautious of efforts led by either group. The key to overcome this caution is to involve people in projects that directly affect them.

QA leadership is threatened. The current leaders of the QA process may be threatened by the TQM process. The perceived threat may be substantial if they are not included in the development and education associated with TQM, and if it is not clarified that TQM will always include a QA component.

Industrial analogies. Some of the initial TQM efforts in the healthcare industry, such as the National Demonstration Project on Quality Improvement in Health Care, which started in 1987, used industrial quality experts as consultants. Their experience and industrial examples were most relevant to similar processes within healthcare organizations. Berwick, Godfrey, and Roessner pointed out: "The first projects chosen by NDP teams tended to be on nonclinical processes, such as business systems, information systems, registration and access systems, and systems for deploying staff. This trend was disappointing to some who hoped that quality improvement might tackle clinical issues directly" (1990, p. 154). Part of the reason for this was the existence of industrial analogies.

Physicians and clinical staff time requirements. Physicians and other clinical staff have very little available time, and in many organizations have not been available to work on Quality Improvement Teams in addition to their QA commitments. Most clinical demands on physicians and other clinical staff cannot be delayed to allow them to attend training or a quality improvement project team meeting. Often staff working in an office setting can schedule time for training or a team meeting, and the work can be completed at a later time.

Stages of Integrating QA and TQM

There are four stages of relationships that may occur between QA and TQM during the integration of the two approaches.

The *first stage* is a quality assurance process by itself, with no use of TQM tools and techniques, as illustrated in Figure 3.3. This was the starting point for all healthcare organizations through 1986 and for many organizations through 1991. As of 1992, however, JCAHO set an expectation for hospitals to at least undertake training with respect to continuous quality improvement or TQM, as described above.

The *second stage* is the independent coexistence of the QA process and the newly emerging TQM process, as illustrated in Figure 3.4. Depending upon the alternative used, an organization may not enter this stage. If TQM is initiated by a person in your organization who is not a key figure in your current quality assurance program, you are likely to experience independent QA and TQM activities for some period, as we did initially at UMMC. The QA process will continue to function, as it must, while the TQM process is developing separately. Another common approach is that the TQM effort is developed with major involvement of your QA leadership and staff. The two processes could still function independently, but there is a greater tendency with this approach to begin early education of QA staff and use of TQM tools and techniques within the QA process. The approach used will depend upon the emerging TQM leaders within your organization and their relationship to the traditional QA process and its leaders.

Figure 3.3. Stage 1: Quality Assurance Program Only.

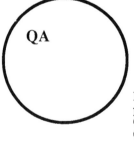

Focus is high-volume, high-risk,
problem-prone areas;
Clinicians lead program;
Outcome-oriented monitoring and
evaluation activities.

Figure 3.4. Stage 2: Independent Quality Assurance and TQM Processes.

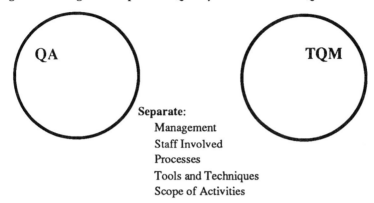

Separate:
Management
Staff Involved
Processes
Tools and Techniques
Scope of Activities

The *third stage* involves an increasing overlap and integrated development of the QA and TQM processes, as illustrated in Figure 3.5. These overlaps include:

- The same people are involved in QA and TQM processes.
- TQM tools and techniques are used by QA committees.
- Clinical Quality Improvement Teams are formed to improve processes and outcomes identified by QA committees as requiring improvement.

Figure 3.5. Stage 3: Related QA and TQM Processes.

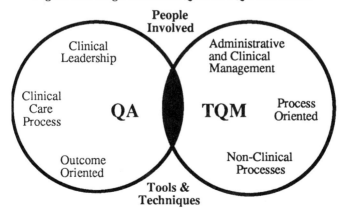

- Quality Improvement Teams develop quality measures for use in the QA process.

The GOAL/QPC Healthcare Application Research Committee investigated both independent and integrated development of QA and TQM and concluded that an integrated approach is more effective.

> Integration of clinical and operational TQM efforts means that all professionals in both clinical services and operations share a common philosophy and process for implementing organization-wide continuous improvement. Clinical leaders are involved in the TQM planning process from its inception, process improvement teams include clinicians and operations personnel, and efforts to meet and exceed customer needs are aligned and unified. Some health care organizations have achieved outstanding successes using methods of implementation that are solely clinical or operational in nature. The committee contends, however, that an integrated approach to TQM is the most effective. An integrated approach more likely ensures the long-term success of a TQM program, and will more likely result in a complete metamorphosis to a new health care paradigm [GOAL/QPC, 1992, pp. 7-8].

The *fourth stage* is full integration of QA and TQM, as illustrated in Figure 3.6. TQM is broader than QA for two reasons. First, TQM includes internal and external customers of all services, products, and information. Second, TQM includes planning, design, and prevention activities in addition to inspection. Hence, TQM is shown as the larger circle, with QA integrated within it. Depending upon the operational definition adopted by your organization, QA may expand beyond its current scope to include monitoring of nonclinical processes. It is our prediction that the emphasis on monitoring of quality will

Figure 3.6. Stage 4: Integrated QA and TQM Processes.

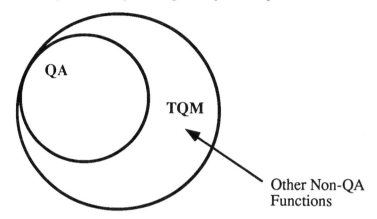

increase as businesses and insurance payers continue efforts to reduce costs. They will, therefore, need quality measurements to estimate value. In addition, JCAHO and others will increase emphasis on plans for continuous improvement, with measurement to determine whether improvement was achieved.

Over time, many organizations may drop the distinction between QA and TQM and simply call the whole process something like "quality excellence," with staff groups helping develop and monitor the processes, while staff providing services, products, and information personally determine their customers' requirements and monitor performance against mutually agreed upon requirements.

Actions to Integrate QA and TQM

Each organization must develop an approach consistent with its current situation, plans, and resources. The following are suggested actions to facilitate the integration of QA and TQM.

Communicate relationship of QA and TQM. Probably the most important action is for the organization's leaders and the Total Quality steering group to describe and communicate the planned relationship and integration of QA and TQM. This will communicate the intent that they will be integrated, although they may continue to function independently for some period of time because of resource or other constraints. Fortunately, at UMMC the leaders of our QA process were also leaders in the TQM process. We communicated the intent that the two would become integrated, but we could have done a better job communicating to the staff working on QA and TQM how and when this would be accomplished.

Action Step: Communicate the similarities and differences of TQM and your traditional QA program. Develop and communicate plans for integration.

One useful approach to communicate the relationship of QA and TQM is to use the P-D-C-A and S-D-C-A cycles illustrated in Figure 3.7. The outer cycle is the Plan-Do-Check-Act, or P-D-C-A, quality improvement process. This approach is used when a process is being studied for improvement. The inner cycle is the Standardize-Do-Check-Act, or S-D-C-A, cycle. Once a process is improved, it should be standardized to minimize the variation among different people performing the process. The quality assurance process then continues to monitor for compliance with the established standards. If special causes are identified, the QA committee may investigate and resolve the issues. If, on the other hand, a systematic quality gap is identified, a Quality Improvement Team may be established. One or more of the QA committee members or staff may be part of the quality improvement team. The situation jumps back and forth between the P-D-C-A cycle for improvement and the S-D-C-A cycle for quality assurance or control.

Consolidate leadership of QA, TQM, and operations. One of the most important changes is to make sure the leadership of QA, TQM, and daily operations have a common direction and are coordinated. All three should report to the same leadership body. If the three report to different leaders, it will be very difficult to maintain an integrated plan, direction, and priorities. At UMMC this required changes in the leadership team for all three. Now QA, TQM, and daily operations all report through the same leadership group.

Figure 3.7. QA Relationship to P-D-C-A and S-D-C-A Cycles.

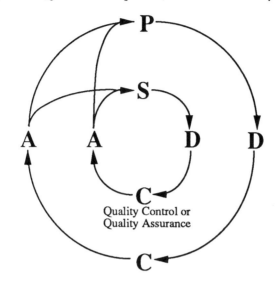

Source: Adapted from King, 1989b, pp. 1–18.

Include QA management and staff in the development, education, and implementation of TQM. You will meet much less resistance if your QA staff are informed and involved. The QA leaders and staff should be included in all TQM education programs. Even if TQM is not formally introduced into the QA process, the tools and techniques will begin to be used. We have found that this is an effective, nonthreatening approach.

Cross-educate QA and TQM leaders and staff. Educate QA staff in the use of quality improvement methods. It is particularly important to train QA leaders and staff as TQM team leaders and facilitators. Similarly, it is important to educate TQM leaders and staff about the QA processes, data sources, and staff capabilities.

Provide diversified opportunities for TQM training. Given the restricted time availability of clinical staff, involving them in TQM training may require providing diversified training opportunities. Sample approaches used at UMMC included providing TQM orientation training sessions on all days of the week and all shifts, providing videotapes of training programs, presenting TQM at regularly scheduled clinical departmental and staff meetings, and distributing a wide variety of reading materials on TQM in general and quality improvement projects in the Medical Center.

Select TQM pilot project from QA process. An effective approach to begin integrating QA and TQM is to use the QA process to select one of the pilot TQM projects. One of the early quality improvement projects will then yield an improvement visible to QA leaders and staff.

Use QA organization and resources rather than duplicate them. Physicians and other clinical staff have very limited time available. The QA organization and resources can be used to identify important quality improvement projects. Some of the clinical and QA staff may also serve on some of the quality improvement projects.

Integrate the indicators used for QA and TQM. By integrating the indicators, the relationship of QA and TQM will be more evident to all.

Based on the work at UMMC and other healthcare organizations, you must be very sensitive about time requirements of physicians, clinical staff, and others. Physician time commitment has always been an issue, but the need for physician participation and to conserve physician time on quality improvement teams has become even more important since the Resource Based Relative Value System (RBRVS) was introduced by the federal government in January 1992. We have found that staff support is required to expedite the progress of physician-led and -dominated teams. Unless there is significant perceived progress, physicians will not continue to participate.

Caution

When moving ahead to implement TQM and develop a new integrated quality process for your organization, you must continue to meet the requirements of external accrediting and review agencies. In *Striving Toward Improvement: Six Hospitals in Search of Quality*, JCAHO highlighted implementation of TQM processes in six sample organizations (1992b). One of those hospitals received a conditional accreditation by JCAHO while the book was being prepared. In the hospital's effort to establish a new process focused on TQM, it had neglected to continue to meet current JCAHO requirements for monitoring and evaluation of key quality characteristics.

Chapter Four

Integrating TQM
with Other Initiatives

A common difficulty when introducing any new change process or program to a healthcare organization is that customers, managers, staff, and suppliers may not understand the relationship to previous processes, programs, or initiatives and why the change is necessary. Therefore, the new process or program may be viewed as an unrelated new "program of the year" and of questionable long-term viability. The same response can be expected when TQM is introduced, if it is not related to and integrated with previous undertakings of your organization. Leadership must clarify these relationships and demonstrate over time the commitment to TQM.

Action Step: When introducing TQM or any other new process or program within your organization, communicate its relationships to previous processes and programs.

Action Step: Include all levels of managers, staff, and physicians in the planning of any new process or program. Ask them what questions they have about the new program and its relationship to past or existing programs.

Most organizations have some elements of a Total Quality approach in place. For example, guest relations is a building block for a customer-oriented approach. Explaining similarities can illustrate the progression, moving from a past program to a more encompassing and integrated one. In addition, the similarities will allow a translation of useful knowledge and skills that already exist within your organization.

On the other hand, there may be many differences, and in some cases conflicts, between components of previous and current programs and a TQM process. These differences should be carefully explained, along with the reasons for changing to TQM. Remember, you must answer at least two questions for *every person* in your organization: *Why change at all?* and *Why change to a TQM approach?* If you do not address the differences between previous and new approaches and the reasons for change, customers, staff, and suppliers are likely to view the leaders and managers as inconsistent and contradictory. One month managers tell you an action is appropriate; the next month they tell you the same action is inappropriate. Such inconsistencies, without an explanation, break down trust and commitment. Merely stating changes will not be sufficient. Consistency in management actions, follow-through on commitments to employees, and admitting mistakes are critical to successful change.

Comparison of TQM with Other Programs

This section contrasts the characteristics of a TQM process with those of other programs and processes commonly implemented by healthcare organizations.

Clearly there are many operational definitions and characteristics of programs that vary from organization to organization. Operational definitions may also vary among people within an organization, and program characteristics may change over time. For example, the University of Michigan Hospitals has changed the organizational structure and operational definitions of its Total Quality Process multiple times since the process began in 1987. Similarly, we have changed suggester eligibility, types of suggestions accepted, and reward structures of our employee suggestion program over the years. Programs with the same names may differ in each organization and over time within each organization.

Quality Circles and TQM

In the early 1980s, many healthcare organizations implemented a quality circles program. Most organizations experienced a fair to modest initial success; later the program failed. The University of Michigan Hospitals, for example, implemented quality circles within the Ambulatory Care Services Division. Substantial resources were expended on training, yet over several years interest in the program decreased and the program failed. Three things occurred that caused a decrease in employee participation:

1. The mid-level managers and first-line supervisors were not part of the process. Top management was trained along with employees, but the first-line and mid-level supervisors were bypassed. A consultant at the time had recommended that the focus be on the employees, with little attention to managers and supervisors.
2. When quality circle teams made recommendations to top management, mid- and front-line supervisors failed to make the required changes. There may have been good reasons, but since management was not involved with the team, the team was unaware of the reasons and perceived the inaction as a lack of support for the staff. Without management *and* employee input, unrealistic expectations may come forward. On the other hand, one team with management and employee involvement continued to meet and be productive after the pilot was concluded.
3. Other topics, which management did spent time on, were perceived to be of greater importance than the quality circle activities.
4. During the process, we moved to a new facility and the process lost steam.

These are important lessons to be mindful of while implementing TQM. If your management treats TQM in this manner, the outcome is likely to be the same. Employees will remember how management acted during the quality circles program and ask, how is TQM different?

Some typical similarities and differences of quality circles and a TQM process are:

Quality Circles' Similarities with TQM	*Quality Circles' Differences with TQM*
• Focus on customers. • Tools and techniques. • Teamwork to solve problems. • Training for team members. • Focus on quality improvement. • Involve those closest to the process.	• Mid- and first-line managers were not personally involved. • Quality circles teams involve only staff, presenting recommendations to top management. TQM teams include staff and managers. • Without management involvement with quality circles, it is difficult for teams to work on processes involving multiple areas.

If your organization previously implemented a quality circles program or currently has one, you should do at least the following three things:

1. Communicate the similarities and differences between your previous quality circles program and your TQM process. A single communication will be inadequate and will not reach everyone. Repeated communications in different formats are necessary, including meetings, organization's newspaper, and other written communications.
2. Demonstrate management commitment to TQM by including TQM on all meeting agendas, including time on your calendar for TQM, and including managers as active participants on Quality Improvement Teams. Your staff will be

watching to see whether management really commits personal time to TQM.
3. Use and build on the knowledge and skills gained by em-
    ployees during quality circles training. Many of the ana-
    lytical tools and techniques are the same, such as flowcharts,
    run charts, and control charts. Make an effort to build on
    the previous learning.

Employee Involvement and TQM

Employee involvement efforts have been much more varied than
the quality circles efforts, and therefore it is more difficult to give
a good comparison model. Each organization that has implemented an employee involvement (EI) program will have to
develop a unique comparison.

Some typical similarities and differences of EI programs
and a TQM process are:

EI's Similarities with TQM	*EI's Differences with TQM*
• Broad employee involvement.	• Managers' involvement varies.
• Seek employee ideas.	• Prescribed methodology for improvement may not exist for EI.
• Encourage employee involvement.	• Depending upon design, EI may encourage individual "ownership" and competitiveness rather than cooperation.

Guest Relations and TQM

Many healthcare organizations, including UMMC, have implemented guest relations programs. As an example, the guest
relations house rules for UMMC are illustrated in Exhibit 4.1.
Most of the guest relations rules are equally applicable in a TQM

Exhibit 4.1. UMMC Guest Relations House Rules.

1. Greet the guest.
2. Introduce yourself (and function, such as nurse or transporter).
3. Call the guest by name (Mr., Mrs., Ms., Miss).
4. Knock or announce yourself before you enter.
5. Smile.
6. Help those who need assistance.
7. Exceed expectations.
8. Listen carefully.
9. Maintain eye contact.
10. Communicate in a language the guest will understand.
11. Communicate to let the guest know what to expect.
12. Respond quickly.
13. Patient information is confidential—keep it that way.
14. Maintain a professional look (neat, clean, and unwrinkled).
15. Keep our facilities beautiful.

process. A guest relations model is a good building block for a customer focus.

Some typical similarities and differences of guest relations programs and a TQM process are:

Guest Relations' Similarities with TQM	*Guest Relations' Differences with TQM*
• Focus on patients and visitors.	• Guest relations focuses on external customers; TQM focuses on external and internal customers.
• Focus on customer-oriented philosophy.	
• Guest relations rules are similar to TQM actions.	• No improvement process as part of guest relations.
• Focus on good interpersonal skills and courtesy.	• Guest relations is usually a top-down set of expectations.

The guest relations house rules at UMMC, for example, are still taught during new employee orientation, along with an orientation to our Total Quality Process. Supporting TQM did not mean we were dropping guest relations. The principles and practices of good guest relations are important to good customer and staff relations as part of the TQM process. However, this must be communicated to staff, or they may view the two as completely different.

Employee Suggestion Programs (ESPs) and TQM

Employee suggestion programs have been around for many years, with highly varied participation, processes, and results. According to the National Association of Suggestion Systems (1990), employee participation in suggestion programs in healthcare organizations ranges from 1 to 35 suggestions per year per 100 eligible employees. At UMMC we have had an employee suggestion program since 1983. It is seen as part of our reward and recognition system as described in Chapter Eleven. There has been a steady increase in the number of eligible employees and the scope of suggestions accepted. The key characteristics of the UMMC employee suggestion program during fiscal year (FY) 1991–92 are listed in Exhibit 4.2. The number of suggestions, awards, and benefits to the organization has steadily increased, with the number of suggestions ranging from 137 in FY 1981–82 to over 400 in FY 1991–92. The net first-year savings during FY 91–92 were almost $400,000. Although this level of participation yields important employee contributions and financial benefits, it is far from that experienced by some Japanese industrial organizations. ESP is one of several ways in which employees can contribute their ideas. Suggestions are often completely out of the normal scope of an employee's job. As a result, it is unlikely that the employee would develop these changes through a normal team process.

Some typical similarities and differences of an ESP and a TQM process are:

ESP's Similarities with TQM	*ESP's Differences with TQM*
• Seeks employee ideas for improvement.	• ESP focuses on individuals rather than teams, although teams may submit ideas.
• Provides recognition for employee contribution.	

Exhibit 4.2. Key Characteristics of UMMC Employee Suggestion
Program, FY 1991–92.

- "All University of Michigan Medical Center (UMMC) regular, temporary, and student employees, including Medical and House Staff, can participate in the Employee Suggestion Program (ESP)" (University of Michigan Medical Center, 1991a).
- Suggestions are accepted that reduce costs, increase revenues, or make significant improvements in quality of operations or patient care.
- Awards are:
  - 10 percent of the first year's net savings/revenue generated through adoption of the suggestion, with a minimum award of $25 and a maximum of $10,000.
  - $100 for suggestions that result in a significant quality improvement but no financial benefit. A substantial percentage of suggestions accomplishes both.
  - $1,000 annual awards for the most significant suggestion in each of the three categories: cost savings, revenue increase, and quality improvement.
  - A recognition process for managers who provide timely evaluations of suggestions.
- "Suggestions submitted are individually considered for award eligibility based on the suggestion's merit and its relationship to the defined job responsibilities and specific assignments of the suggester. For those staff members who are above the level of first line supervisor, the specific suggestion must be outside of the scope of the suggester's job (as defined by the suggester's position description and interpreted by the suggester's supervisor) to be eligible for a tangible award. For those employees who are first line supervisors and below, the suggestion, to be eligible for a tangible award, must not be a result of a direct and specific assignment by his/her supervisor" (University of Michigan Medical Center, 1991a).
- Suggestions go through two levels of review and evaluation. Initially the suggestions are evaluated by the coordinator of the ESP for completeness, overlap with previous suggestions, and basic logic. The more detailed evaluations are done by managers in those areas affected by the suggestion.
- The cost of awards and a 5 percent surcharge to pay for annual awards and promotion are charged proportionately to the departments benefiting from the suggestions.
- The suggestions, suggesters, and awards are regularly recognized in several forms, including announcements at meetings; regular publication in the organization's daily publication, *Bulletin*, and newspaper, *Hospital Star*; and announcements on check stubs.

Source: Compiled from University of Michigan Medical Center, 1991a.

- Breaks down barriers by encouraging cross-organizational cooperation.
- Emphasizes improvement, not fault or blame finding.
- Drives out fear by providing a secure route for promoting change.
- Positive assumption of individual's ability to contribute.
- Acts on basis of factual analysis and feedback.

- ESP offers individual financial rewards; TQM normally provides no individual or team awards.
- Can cause conflict of individual incentives and cooperative team efforts.

There are a number of characteristics of employee suggestion programs related to a TQM process that may conflict with a TQM process.

- *Participation.* Virtually all ESPs depend upon voluntary participation. Most TQM processes include a combination of assignment and volunteer participation in quality improvement efforts. Consequently most suggestion programs have had relatively small percentages of total employees participate. The UMMC employee suggestion program will allow groups of employees to submit suggestions, but not if they have been assigned to a Quality Improvement Team working on that topic.
- *Individual versus group reward and recognition.* Individual recognition and reward through the ESP can conflict with group recognition and reward through Quality Improvement Teams, natural work teams, and individual efforts.
- *Personal financial benefits.* There are direct personal financial benefits to individuals through ESP, as opposed to none or limited ones to employees through the TQM process. UMMC has initiated a gainsharing program to provide collective benefit to employees when the organization exceeds its budgeted financial performance. However, this is paid

after the end of each fiscal year and does not have as much immediate benefit for an individual's contribution.

There are different approaches to implementing a TQM process, with different relationships to employee suggestion programs. At UMMC, we have used a number of process-focused Quality Improvement Teams and natural work teams, and more recently quality improvements on each person's daily job. We have retained the employee suggestion program, with the rules defined in Exhibit 4.2. Pat Townsend, on the other hand, proposes that every employee be assigned to a Quality Team of approximately ten people each. Given this TQM approach, he proposes:

> The suggestion system would have to be eliminated. If the two systems—the suggestion system and the Quality Teams—were allowed to coexist, some rather confusing scenarios could be the result. If, for instance, a Quality Team discussed a particular problem without reaching a conclusion and adjourned until the next meeting with the agreement that all the team members would think about the problem, what would prevent a team member from hustling to the nearest suggestion box with the problem and his or her individual solution? Trying to decide if a particular idea belonged to an individual or to a team would require the second coming of Solomon [Townsend, 1990, p. 30].

We do not fully agree with Townsend's position; different avenues for employees to contribute can be simultaneously effective.

Innovation Programs and TQM

A small percentage of healthcare organizations have implemented innovation programs. Although the characteristics of such programs vary widely, they tend to focus on the longer-term development of whole new services and products. The Innovation Program at UMMC functions by providing guidance, support, and financial resources for intrapreneurs (Pinchot, 1985). A request for proposals was announced, and then the proposals with the greatest promise were selected for support. UMMC provided a range of support based on the requirements for the individual project, including: staff support, release time for the employee, videotape production, prototype design and production, and clinical trials.

Some typical similarities and differences of innovation programs and a TQM process are:

Innovation Program's Similarities with TQM	*Innovation Program's Differences with TQM*
• Seeks employee ideas for improvement. • Empowers employees to maximize potential in a manner that benefits organization.	• Innovation programs focus on individuals rather than teams. • Innovation projects tend to deal with new venture ideas.

One aspect of the Innovation Program that was tried early on did not work well — assigning corporate leaders to help mentor innovators. The intention of having a corporate mentor was good, but the relationships did not prosper. A true mentoring relationship must build over time between people through their mutual interests and respect.

Management by Objectives and TQM

Many healthcare organizations have implemented some form of management by objectives (MBO) programs. The intent of some individual program objectives may be inconsistent with TQM principles. The most important potential conflict is the TQM requirement that there must be plans for process improvement developed to meet continually increasing customer requirements. Many MBO objectives are established with no plan or process improvement to achieve them, which is inconsistent with the principles of TQM. The transition from an MBO program to a TQM process can be facilitated with a major change of focus toward the development and implementation of process improvements to accomplish the planned objectives.

There are many different forms of MBO programs, and the similarities and differences depend upon the implementation. In particular, some MBO programs may address specific plans to accomplish the objectives, although many do not. Some typical similarities and differences of MBO programs and a TQM process are:

MBO's Similarities with TQM	*MBO's Differences with TQM*
• Focuses on improvement. • Both use indicators to measure progress toward goals.	• MBO focuses on specific objectives; TQM focuses on process improvement. • MBO objectives are typically set without plans to accomplish them. TQM goals must include specific plans for accomplishment. • There are specific tools and techniques for TQM, but not for MBO. • MBO emphasizes individuals more than teamwork; TQM emphasizes teamwork.

Cost Reduction and TQM

Probably the most difficult relationship exists between cost-reduction programs and the TQM process. The conflict arises from the approach and timing of changes. Medicare, Medicaid, and other payers are restricting reimbursements to less than the market increases in commodity and labor costs. Many HMOs require a competitive bidding process to provide services. In addition, the reduced number of admissions and decreases in length of stay are resulting in falling inpatient occupancy rates for many healthcare organizations. The combination of these and other factors is requiring most healthcare organizations to implement programs that will substantially reduce budgets and costs, increase cost effectiveness, and increase value to customers. Although quality improvement projects can be demonstrated to improve cost effectiveness, the rate of change may not be sufficient to meet the externally imposed requirements to improve cost effectiveness. A common comment is, "How can you talk about quality when you are cutting costs?"

Some common barriers to relating a TQM process to a past or current program to substantially increase cost effectiveness are described in Table 4.1, along with some approaches to reduce the barriers. People typically go through the same stages related to cost reduction as they do for other major changes, as described in Table 6.1: denial, anger, resistance, exploration, and commitment. Therefore, the first issue that must be dealt with is the *why*. Why is improved cost effectiveness required? A major question from employees is, how can you be talking about quality improvement and cost reduction at the same time? Spend time illustrating how the tools of quality improvement can assist in a cost-cutting process. It is the cost of poor quality that should be attacked. As one learns more about the approach, tools, and techniques used in TQM, it becomes clear that the same approach and methods are effective at increasing cost effectiveness.

Whenever there is a reduction or restructuring of an organization, fear is rampant. Fear is detrimental to implementing a TQM process. Steps must be taken to reduce fear, as discussed in Chapter Six on organizational culture.

Two issues that have faced us at UMMC concern the relationship between our cost effectiveness program and our Total Quality Process. First, most managers become so consumed with the short-term requirements to plan and implement the cost effectiveness changes that they reduce priority on the TQM approach and methods. Second, some managers still do not see the two undertakings as related or compatible. One approach used to address these issues is to develop a multiyear cost effectiveness plan directed toward the expectations of our external payers. Another is to measure and communicate the financial benefits that have accrued as a byproduct of quality improvement projects.

Some typical similarities and differences of cost-reduction programs and a TQM process are:

Cost Reduction's Similarities with TQM	*Cost Reduction's Differences with TQM*
• Improves cost effectiveness and value. • Uses same tools and techniques. • Work redesign and re-engineering are effective approaches.	• Cost reduction focuses on costs; TQM focuses on customer requirements and quality. • Reduces staff as an objective. • Cost-reduction approach tends to overlook customer requirements and possible reduced workload by eliminating things not desired by customers.

Alternative Strategies for Implementation. There are different strategies to implement a cost effectiveness program and a TQM process, depending upon the financial situation of your organization and where you are in your TQM implementation.

One strategy used by some organizations is to make cost reductions swiftly, with little employee input, then to begin implementing a TQM process to help the healing process after the reductions. This works best if you have not yet begun your TQM process. The advantage of this approach is that there is a relatively short period of very high stress and tension. The disadvantages are that good employees are laid off, and you communicate little commitment to your employees. Increasing cost effectiveness by doing more work with the same staff nor-

**Table 4.1. Common Barriers to Relating TQM Process
to Cost-Reduction Program.**

Barrier to TQM Cost Effectiveness Program	Approaches to Reduce Barrier
• Why is cost reduction necessary? This is a particular problem if the organization is still profitable.	• Communicate widely the projected costs, revenue restrictions, and other factors, so staff can understand the risks of not cutting costs. Focus on decreasing cost per unit of service.
• Fear of losing job, income, or stature.	• Commitment of employment if possible, but may be unrealistic. • Develop and implement attrition management plan to reduce positions of people who voluntarily leave. • Create fund for retraining staff for different jobs. • Distinguish the person and the job he or she currently performs. • Provide supportive services for employees, to demonstrate commitment to them as individuals, such as outplacement services.
• Short-term focus of cost effectiveness program.	• Maintain and communicate long-term commitment to vision, mission, and quality. • Develop multiyear cost effectiveness plan, linked to strategic and quality plans. • Develop human resources plan to coordinate job requirements with available people and skills.
• Focus on costs and revenues only.	• Evaluate cost effectiveness proposals in terms of all organizational goals, not just financial goals.
• Approach of reducing staff and commodities rather than making process improvements to meet customer requirements.	• Incorporate TQM process improvement tools and techniques to improve cost effectiveness. • Do not allow cost-reduction goals without a plan for accomplishment. • Formally identify customers and their requirements, to identify services and products that are not required.

Table 4.1. Common Barriers to Relating TQM Process
to Cost-Reduction Program, Cont'd.

Barrier to TQM Cost Effectiveness Program	Approaches to Reduce Barrier
• Cost effectiveness and TQM are perceived as totally different, and possibly even opposites. Cost reductions will damage quality.	• Communicate cost effectiveness improvements of TQM efforts, in addition to quality improvements. • Demonstrate that TQM methods improve cost effectiveness. • Communicate that quality service and satisfied customers are absolutely necessary for future survival and prosperity. • Acknowledge that some top-down cost reductions may be necessary in response to key external customers and need for quick action.
• Proportion of leader and manager time spent on cost effectiveness program, compared to time spent on TQM, employee development, etc.	• Plan time for the TQM process, no matter how pressing the cost effectiveness effort is. • Include quality on all agendas, even cost effectiveness agendas.
• Performance evaluation not linked to TQM principles.	• Integrate TQM expectations into performance review and evaluation.

mally takes longer because of the time needed for workloads to grow.

Another strategy is to use the TQM approaches and methods to the maximum extent possible. This will require a major effort to manage attrition and retrain staff for other jobs. The advantage is that you minimize the number of people laid off and maximize your commitment to employees. The disadvantage is that there will be a prolonged period of very high stress. In the case of UMMC, we developed a four-year cost effectiveness program. Because managers and staff realized their jobs may be in jeopardy for multiple years, we created a job retraining fund and pledged that no member of a team that recommended changing his or her job would be displaced. Our goal is systems and work redesign. The approximate number of staff to be reduced may be known years in advance. However, no one knows which staff will be affected because that depends upon who leaves and who transfers and upon the amount of workload increases, if any. If your TQM has been successful, the improved quality, service, and customer satisfaction may result in increased customers and workload handled by the same staff and costs, rather than having to decrease staff and costs to increase cost effectiveness.

The best approach, if your payers are not demanding more radical cost reductions, is to achieve your cost effectiveness improvements as a byproduct of a continuing series of quality improvement efforts. This may be possible for some organizations, and if so, we recommend getting started as soon as possible. The other two alternatives can exacerbate fear and create a major barrier to TQM implementation.

Integrating TQM with Other Initiatives

The key to integrating TQM effectively with previous and current programs is understanding the relationship and communicating progress. Each organization begins with a different history, culture, environment, and set of past and current management initiatives. You must first understand those initiatives and their relationship to your TQM process; then, using many different media, communicate this information regularly to the board, managers, physicians, employees, customers, and suppliers.

The following actions are recommended to document, understand, and communicate the relationships of the TQM process to previous and current programs.

1. List all major programs and processes undertaken by your organization within the last five years.

2. Prepare a table listing and comparing the characteristics of TQM and the programs and processes listed above. A sample table is illustrated in Exhibit 4.3.

**Exhibit 4.3. Comparison of TQM with Previous and Current
Programs and Processes.**

TQM Characteristic	Similarities and Differences Compared to TQM				Action Plan
	Program 1	Program 2	· · ·	Program N	

3. List the similarities and differences between TQM and the other programs and processes, and highlight the key ones.

4. List the reasons for change. Remember, you must answer the question "Why change?" for everyone, so they can relate the changes to their customers and their job. In some cases, there may be major changes from previous or current programs to the principles and actions of TQM. It is generally better to identify the changes and to focus on the similarities and improvements rather than to discredit previous efforts.

5. Develop an implementation plan to address the transition from past and current programs and practices to the TQM process. This may slow implementation of TQM initially but will greatly reduce confusion in the long run. Special attention should be directed toward the key managers and staff who implemented the previous and current programs. They are

likely to be the most vested in those programs and may have difficulty making the paradigm shift. These are committed people who can help make TQM successful also.

6. Prepare several different communications to address the highlights of the similarities, differences, reasons for change, and the implementation plan. Sample communications include the organization's newspaper, special publications, posters, special presentations, and regular staff meetings.

7. Prepare handout materials for managers to share with every employee showing the similarities, differences, reasons for change, and implementation plan.

The important thing to remember is that your organization, every person working in your organization, your customers, and your suppliers have been affected by previous and current management practices. All need to understand the reasons for change and how the changes will affect them.

PART TWO

Creating a TQM Culture

Chapter Five

Organization and Leadership

The implementation of TQM requires extraordinary leadership, energy, patience, and skill. It is so easy to say, "we're going to turn the pyramid upside down and allow customer requirements to drive our organization." However, just determining where to start to make this dream of a customer-driven organization a reality is a complex assignment.

This chapter focuses on the type of leadership required to challenge the business-as-usual environment and lead a quality process. It addresses the major challenges that have caused many quality processes to derail and presents strategies to deal with issues of organization. It is our hope that, by sharing what worked for us, your implementation time will be shortened.

Creating the Tension for Organizational Change

As illustrated in Chapter One, there are many pressures that will continue to make change the only constant in healthcare. In the midst of this change, we are challenged to develop an organization that is flexible, friendly, and delivers customer-oriented services. How do we inspire the changes necessary to allow us to compete on a quality and cost basis? How do we invite everyone within the organization to do better than we have ever done before? The first step is to create the rationale for why the institution should change at all. We found it helpful at UMMC to discuss the phases of organizational development in order to make the case for TQ implementation. In *Enlightened Leadership*, Ed Oakley and Doug Krug express a theory that every organization is at some phase of a development cycle. They believe that each organization, like each product, has a life cycle. While not all companies pass through the life cycle phases in the same fashion, there are many similarities. Some companies remain in one cycle longer than others, some jump from one cycle to another, and some organizations will not survive. According to their model: "There are four potential phases, entrepreneurial, growth, and decline or renewal" (Oakley and Krug, 1991, p. 13). Any crisis, internal or external, may lead to decline. Without a planned intervention that leads an organization to the renewal phase, decline may be inevitable. Figure 5.1 illustrates the phases of business development.

The first phase of the model is the entrepreneurial period, the time of formation of the business. This is the infancy stage in which the organization is searching to find its market niche. The characteristic behavior of the organization in this phase is one of energy and excitement. Once the market niche is found and the company is firmly established, the organization moves to the next phase, growth. The growth phase is divided into two parts, early and late. In the early growth phase, there is still tremen-

Figure 5.1. Phases of Organizational Development.

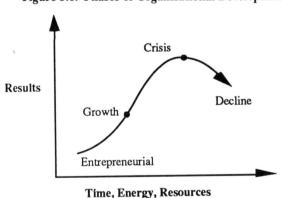

Time, Energy, Resources

Source: Oakley and Krug, 1992, p. 13.

dous energy and excitement, but there is a definitive shift from an entrepreneurial culture to a culture of management control. There is a tendency to insert rules and regulations in order to control growth. This focus intensifies in the late growth phase, which is categorized by many levels of managers between the employee and the chief executive officer, low energy, bureaucratic style, and the breakdown of communication. Oakley and Krug point out that "every growth cycle has a peak. If we stay locked onto this curve past the peak, we move into decline" (1991, pp. 17–21).

Given the chaos in the current healthcare environment, many organizations have already reached the decline phase. Revenues have fallen below expenses, customer satisfaction is at an all-time low, medical staff seem to be at odds with the administration, administration is unhappy with productivity and profit margins, and staff express an anxiety about the future. Decisions seem to be made by political pressure rather than rational thinking. These changes are not unusual; they are predictable. Peter Drucker warned: "Unless challenged, every organization tends to become slack, easy going, diffuse. It tends to allocate resources by inertia and tradition rather than results" (1980, p. 41). In other words, if we in healthcare keep on doing what we have always done, we will become mired in the decline phase. Even the most successful companies that keep on doing the same thing may find themselves in a state Robert Kriegel and Louis Patler call "plateauing." This happens when an organization stops growing and moving upward. They name several companies such as "IBM, DEC, Cusinart, and Heineken who tried resting on their laurels and found plateauing can quickly be followed by plunging" (Kriegel and Patler, 1991, p. 71).

Organizational renewal is a potential antidote for decline. Oakley and Krug describe their renewal phase as a:

- Reawakening, revitalization
- Closeness to customers and markets
- Willingness to take risks
- Change-friendly mindsets
- Quality orientation

- Rekindling of the entrepreneurial spirit
- Openness and flexibility (1991, p. 20)

We believe that this is the essence of the transformation Deming encourages management to make. UMMC and others have demonstrated that an organization can reposition itself and enter the renewal phase by utilizing quality principles and techniques. The cost of poor quality can be reduced, productivity and relationships enhanced, and organizational renewal can begin to take hold. Renewal of an organization requires the renewal of its people. There must be a means to energize and excite people to create a stronger, more effective organization, something that makes them want to establish new standards of excellence. In our organization TQM has been a people-energizing process. Our employees have found the process challenging and enjoyable. Communication has improved, employee suggestions are at an all-time high, and many more employees are participating in improving critical processes and solving common work problems. With a quality improvement process in place, employees can challenge the status quo and introduce changes that continue to motivate and create the potential for continuous renewal, as illustrated in Figure 5.2.

Figure 5.2. Continuous Organizational Renewal.

Time, Energy, Resources

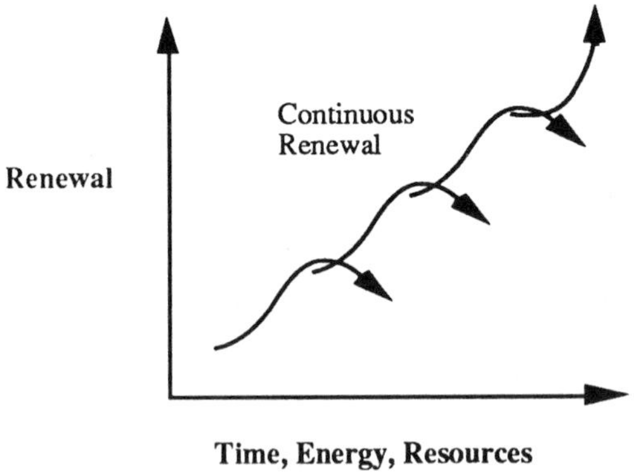

Source: Oakley and Krug, 1992, p. 23.

Critical Success Factors for Organizational Renewal

While many can see the need to create a renewed organization, the steps to get from where you are to where you would like to be are not very clear. There are many tasks required as implementation begins, and their number may become overwhelming. Many hospital executives have asked us which tasks are the most critical. We believe there are four critical success factors that the Total Quality Council must take into consideration as an organization begins its quality journey. If these tasks are not accomplished, there is a great probability of a stalled or failed process. Critical success factors are illustrated in Figure 5.3.

Clear Customer-Focused Vision

Once the organizational leadership is committed to implementing a quality improvement process, a customer-focused vision statement and a strategic plan to align the organization behind the vision are required. The vision must be positive, motivating, and inspiring. People cannot become motivated by a basically negative vision such as cost reduction. The vision should say to the organization: we can and must change! A quality environment does not seem to be anything new to many managers or employees. Many of the tools and techniques of quality improvement have been used for years, and on the surface it seems like commonsense management. However, Brian Joiner, a noted quality consultant and former Malcolm Baldrige judge, has been credited with saying that TQM is actually counterintuitive. If it were commonsense management, every corporation in America would be competing effectively in the global marketplace.

Figure 5.3. Critical Success Factors.

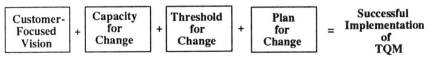

The best way to accomplish the visioning process is by scheduling a top management retreat, away from the operations, where full attention can be paid to the task. Visioning should be a creative process where brainstorming is an essential tool. Previous meetings with customers, suppliers, and employees should provide the executives with a variety of suggestions about consensus for a desired future. The main question the executives must answer is what type of organization do we wish to become? Richard Whiteley suggests that "the leaders of the organization should ask the following questions to develop the vision:

- What kind of company (or group within the company) do we want to be?
- What will the company be like for our customers and us when we achieve this vision?
- What do we want people to say about us as a result of our work?
- What values are most important to us?
- How does this vision represent the interest of our customers and values that are important to us?
- What place does each person have in this vision of the future?" (Whiteley, 1991, p. 27).

The vision statement should emphasize how the organization will differ from past performance and focus on what the organization will become in the future. The visioning process starts with divergent thinking, capturing as many ideas as possible; then convergent thinking is used to narrow down the list. The vision statement is then crafted from the remaining key statements. When the executives are pleased with the draft of the vision, they should share it with the next level of management, and changes should occur based on feedback. The final vision statement should be shared broadly with the organization, after all levels have had a chance to comment and provide insight.

A clear vision by itself, however, will not accomplish the goal of organizational transformation. The vision requires appropriate strategies for goal achievement and followers who commit to the vision and wish to make it a reality. Once the final vision statement has been created, it must be communicated at all levels throughout the organization. Each department must review the organizational vision and plan how they will contribute to making the vision a reality. When you communicate the vision and align the organization behind it, you have created a powerful force. When every person is marching to a different drum, there is no synergy, no common purpose. When a revitalized mission, vision, and values statement is developed and shared broadly, there is a feeling of unity and common purpose. Then the energy of employees is focused on achieving common goals.

The organization's progress toward achieving the vision should also be communicated frequently to all staff. At UMMC we developed the concept of a Vision Report Card to communicate what measures we were going to utilize to evaluate our organizational progress toward achieving our vision. These measures are evaluated on a semi-annual basis. A more detailed report including the actual measurement of each element is being developed by our CEO. He plans to share this data with all employees through the organizational newsletter, the *Hospital Star*. Exhibit 5.1 is a summary of the report elements.

Action Step: Establish a motivating vision and a plan for organizational alignment. Frequently update all levels of the organization on progress toward the vision.

Capacity and Capability for Change

The type of broad organizational change required for TQM implementation will not happen without a support system that provides people with the capacity and capability for change. For example, the vision must be seen as attainable by the people in the organization or there will be no energy for change. Leadership must be visibly committed to TQM or the process will languish. We have seen many hospitals where the executives say quality is important, but their personal agendas show no commitment. They delegate responsibility to a quality department

Exhibit 5.1. Vision Progress Report for UMMC, 1991.

Vision Statement	Measurements
• Provider of choice	• Customer satisfaction surveys • Quality assurance studies • Quality indicators (institutional and departmental) • Patient comment cards • Referring physician surveys • Payer surveys
• Preeminent in teaching and advancing medical science	• Increasing number of funded research grants • Attraction of highly qualified students • Achievement of goals for house staff match • Student surveys • Financial support of graduate medical education
• Employer of choice	• Employee/medical staff surveys • Cultural survey • Retention rate • Employee feedback • Wage/benefit studies • Safety/security reports • Educational offerings • Communication strategies

and then wonder why there is no organizational momentum. A task team should assess the organization's capacity for sustaining the process. What tools and aids will be required?

Organizational capacity and capability are enhanced by a strong educational curriculum. The curriculum must include time for appropriate skill building and a chance to practice these skills in a safe environment. Leadership must learn to lead by example and reinforce the desired new behaviors. The creation of an appropriate structure for quality, with the top leadership driving the process, will provide not only resources but the type of emotional support required to sustain the capacity. As the process expands, the structure must expand as well. As the institutional knowledge base grows, new tools, techniques, and methods will be required to ascend to the next learning plateau. Each organizational success requires flexibility and sustained growth to stay in the continuous renewal loop.

A complete educational program must be tailored to the organization's needs, as described in Chapter Nine. Learning needs assessments should be completed at least every six months in order to adjust the educational process. We have found it helpful to survey by category, such as mid-level or senior-level management, and by role in the quality process, such as team leader or team member. The key to success is to accelerate organizational learning, to reach a new series of plateaus, and to compete more effectively.

Tools and aids also help build organizational capability and capacity for change. A partial list of tools created at UMMC is included in Exhibit 5.2. These tools are discussed in depth throughout the book. Please see the Index for further information about each tool.

Action Step: Assess the organizational structure for quality, educational process, tools, and aids to determine the capacity and capability for change.

Information systems also can provide capability and capacity. As quality indicators are developed, the data systems must support the rapid collection and analysis needed to adapt to customer requirements.

A Threshold for Change

Most organizations do not change until they have to. They wait until they are in the decline phase and then try to adapt. The most constructive and best time to change is when you do not have to—when things are going well, before a crisis occurs.

Exhibit 5.2. Sample UMMC Quality Tools for Managers.

• Mission	• Actions for Managers	• Computerized TQ Tools
• Vision	• Manager's Guide	• Management Expectations
• Values	• Quality Principles	• Total Quality Process Plan
• Team Reports	• Storyboards	• Reward and Recognition Program

When change is planned and gradually implemented, the organization can adjust more easily. Unfortunately, it is more difficult to initiate change when the need is not obvious. To create the energy necessary for change, a threshold of pain must be reached and recognized. There must be a felt need to change, or the change will not occur. To create this energy we suggest several steps. First, clearly indicate the rationale for change. Use ideas from Chapter One, and visit other quality organizations and find what stimulated them to change. Next, develop an on-site program with speakers who have implemented successful programs. Develop an executive meeting to begin the process for examination of your current situation. Leadership must ask: What elements of the quality process are evident in our organization? What are our strengths and weaknesses? Which elements will require setting up a task team for further study?

In *Transforming Healthcare Organizations*, we expressed the belief that "there is a limit to the rate of corporate change an organization can tolerate; we call this the threshold of corporate change. If the rate of change is too fast an organization can become dysfunctional, if the rate is too slow, people lose sight of the vision and enthusiasm may fizzle" (Marszalek-Gaucher and Coffey, 1990, p. 53). There should be a balanced approach, neither too fast nor too slow. While goals should provide stretch objectives that cause people to reach a little further, the organization must be able to view them as attainable. Too much change can be threatening; if people believe the change is beyond their capability, change can immobilize. The quality council should assess the environment and the readiness for change to determine the steps and the order of those steps.

Action Step: Assess the readiness for change. Is the support appropriate for the proposed rate of change? Are the goals clear? Does the plan require enough of a stretch for organizational change?

A Plan for Change

If there is not a clear, strategic plan with a step-wise approach, there will be false starts and many disappointments in your quality process. Most people cannot conceptualize building a house without a blueprint. However, when it comes to Total Quality, many, including UMMC, rushed in and began the process without one. When tools are applied to problems without a plan, chaos can ensue. Developing the plan up front, before you begin the teams, will save you much time and energy. Advance planning allows the synergy required to sustain the momentum.

The development of a quality plan should follow the guidelines for any strategic planning process. First, the executive group should develop broad organizational goals and the means to achieve them. Second, assign responsibility and create the resources to meet the responsibilities. Third, develop the educational curriculum to support the required changes and create a reward and recognition process to reinforce the new behaviors. Finally, establish an evaluation process to review performance against the goals.

Many believe the best planning approach for quality is a process called Policy Deployment (PD). Through PD, improvement activities are tied to your long-term vision. This type of planning integrates strategic direction and improvement initiatives. There is broad organizational participation in setting goals and then a process to link departmental and organizational goals. The Ernst & Young Quality Consulting Group list the following ten characteristics of PD:

- Top management is responsible for developing and communicating a vision, then building an organizationwide commitment to its achievement.
- The vision is deployed through the development and execution of annual policy statements (annual plans).
- All levels of employees actively participate in generating a strategy and action plans to attain the vision.
- At each level, progressively more detailed and concrete means to accomplish the annual plans are determined; that is, there should be a clear link to common goals in activities from the shop floor to the top floor. The plans are hierarchical, cascading downward from top management's plans.

- The Pareto principle is used at each organizational level to set priorities, to focus on areas needing significant levels of improvement, and to concentrate on activities that are the most highly related to the vision.
- Implementation responsibilities, timetables, and progress measures are determined.
- Frequent evaluation and modification based on feedback from regularly scheduled audits of the process are provided.
- Plans and actions based on analysis of the root causes of a problem/situation, rather than only on the symptoms, are developed.
- Planning has a high degree of detail, including the anticipation of possible implementation problems.
- Emphasis is on the improvement of the process, as opposed to a results-only orientation (Huge, 1990, p. 41).

In practice, PD is a way to create organizational focus on four or five top-priority goals. When each department establishes attainment plans to determine how it will help the organization achieve the key goals, there is harmony in the organization and everyone understands what is expected. In many organizations the executives have a strategic plan that is far too ambitious; there are pages of goals. This can cause paralysis because the organization cannot determine which goals have priority. There is a tendency for these organizations to have an unfocused approach and try to do too much. Consequently nothing is done well, and no one seems to understand what is wrong. When PD is used, everyone in the organization knows the critical goals and can decide the best way to meet them within their department. The level of detail of the plans increases as the plans cascade down through the organization, but the intent is to achieve a priority focus. It is also a way to create energy for change. When people know what the keys are, and how success will be measured, they are far better equipped to participate in the process.

Action Step: Consider using a Policy Deployment Process to guide your quality planning and your organization.

Summary of Critical Success Factors

The critical success factors required for smooth TQM implementation include: a clear vision, the organizational capacity for change, a managed threshold for change, and, most important, a plan for change.

Leadership for the TQ Process

Effective leadership for quality is essential. In *Transforming Healthcare Organizations*, we addressed the issue of leadership for organizational transformation in depth, including action steps to help you begin the quality process in your organization (Marszalek-Gaucher and Coffey, 1990, pp. 228–236). The thirteen leadership characteristics essential for leading a TQM effort and a brief description of each are listed below.

1. *Being a visionary.* Developing the skill to look ahead and describe a better organization in which each individual's work is optimized and quality is the number one goal of each employee.
2. *Being socially responsible.* Developing a concern about the cost effectiveness of healthcare as well as the means to provide access for all citizens of our country. Social responsibility is also about meeting the healthcare needs of our communities, truly being customer-focused rather than provider-focused.
3. *Managing uncertainty.* Becoming more flexible, capable of leading successfully in the face of increasing external challenges and ambiguity.
4. *Being a change agent.* Exhibiting a bias for action. Personally acting as a change agent and supporting other risk takers in the environment.
5. *Being people-oriented.* Believing in the collective intellectual power of people in the organization. Fostering teamwork and collaboration and empowering people so they can contribute to organizational success.
6. *Sharing information.* Sharing all types of information

broadly. Recognizing that information is a way to empower others and give them a big-picture perspective of
the organization.

7. *Being driven by your customers' values.* Learning to listen to
the customer's requirements effectively. Developing action
plans to exceed requirements and delight the customer.
Encouraging and reinforcing the customer focus at all
levels in the organization.

8. *Being committed to innovation.* Promoting innovation and
creativity throughout the organization. Teaching and
modeling creative problem-solving skills for managers
and employees.

9. *Being visible.* Management by walking around builds employee commitment and loyalty to the organization.
Providing instant recognition to those who are modeling
quality behaviors reinforces commitment. Speaking directly to customers indicates the level of personal involvement in achieving customer satisfaction goals.

10. *Being committed to education and training.* Setting the tone for
the learning organization by attending educational sessions and demonstrating the importance of knowledge.

11. *Being willing to decentralize and delegate.* Recognizing the
importance of delegation. Constantly assess how to push
power, information, and knowledge down in the organization to the people who interface with the customer.

12. *Fostering supplier relationships.* Promoting strategic partnerships with suppliers to improve products and services
jointly.

13. *Knowing yourself.* Constantly assessing personal strengths
and weaknesses and developing an action plan for improvement. Utilizing performance evaluations as a two-
way street where the boss and the subordinate each discuss
what went well, what went poorly, and what needs to be
improved. The goal is for each party to understand how to
make the other successful.

Developing an Empowering Style

Empowering leadership means an openness to the ideas of
others. It is about sharing organizational power and giving

autonomy and discretion over tasks to employees. Empowering leaders build relationships by acting as coaches and mentors. They use reward and recognition to change limiting behaviors. We know the transition to empowering leadership is difficult because we are trying to accomplish the transition ourselves. It is very easy, even when empowering skills have become part of your management style, to regress to your old style of operating. If you feel your management style needs to be adjusted to fit with the new philosophy, how can you begin? One helpful technique to begin the transition is to identify what type of leader you are today. Place your leadership styles on a continuum such as the one listed in Figure 5.4. The far left behavioral style is autocratic leadership, one where the leader tells, controls, and makes all the decisions for the subordinates. As one moves down the continuum toward a participative style, there is more involvement and interaction with others. Participative leaders are more team oriented. A participative leader seeks broad input and consults with others before decisions are made. The far right side of the continuum is empowering leadership. An empowering leader encourages those on the front lines, dealing with the customers, to make quality decisions. This type of leader provides counseling, coaching, and opportunities for growth. Where does your style fall on the continuum?

We are convinced that empowering leadership can be learned, as long as you are willing to invest the time and energy needed to develop and experiment with the behaviors required. After determining where you fit on the continuum, ask yourself: Do I push power, knowledge, information, and rewards downward in the organization to the lowest possible level, where the

Figure 5.4. Continuum of Leadership Styles.

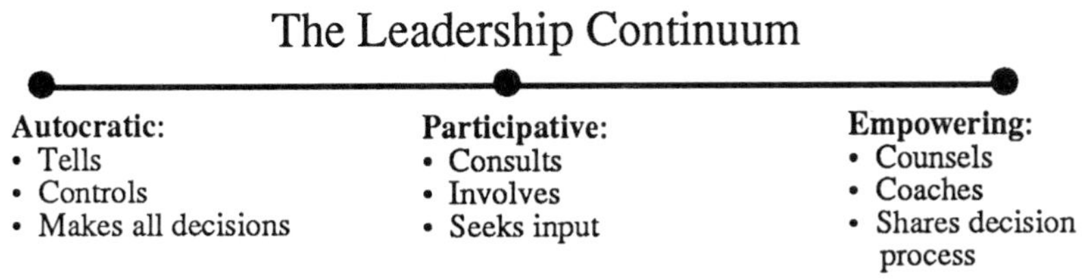

The Leadership Continuum

Autocratic:	Participative:	Empowering:
• Tells	• Consults	• Counsels
• Controls	• Involves	• Coaches
• Makes all decisions	• Seeks input	• Shares decision process

customer interface takes place? Do I challenge all employees to think for themselves and address customer issues as they occur? Or do I operate from a bureaucratic, hierarchical power perspective and expect people to follow the line process, seeking permission from many in the chain of command before any action can take place? Do I exhibit punishing or encouraging behaviors when things don't go the exact way I planned? Do I invest in education as a way to demonstrate commitment to my employees? Am I modeling the behaviors I wish to see demonstrated by supervisors and managers in the organization?

Action Step: Analyze your personal leadership style. What changes will you have to make to move toward an empowering style?

Extraordinary Leadership

Another important point on leadership is that during times of crisis, such as the crisis in healthcare today, extraordinary leadership is required. If the goal is organizational renewal, the leaders must be capable of a higher level of performance. James Kouzes and Barry Posner (1987) presented five common practices that extraordinary leaders demonstrate. These practices can serve as a leadership checklist for your organization. As you analyze your leadership style and that of other managers in your organization, think about these skills. Is this the prevailing management style in your organization? If not, how will you help executives and managers develop these skills of quality leadership?

- Challenge the process.
- Inspire a shared vision.
- Enable others to act.
- Model the way.
- Encourage the heart.

Challenge the process. Extraordinary leaders think as pioneers. They demonstrate the ability to take risks, innovate, experiment, and support creative ideas. They lead by seeking out change and new ways of doing things. They listen to, recognize, and implement good ideas from others. They believe in challenging all existing processes. They put processes and programs through a critical review, at least every three years, to determine if improvement is possible or a new process should take its place.

Inspire a shared vision. Extraordinary leaders inspire others to create a new organization. They draw a powerful picture of future potential and attract followers to sustain the vision. They build excitement about a better future.

Enable others to act. Extraordinary leaders encourage collaboration, build teams, and empower others to act. They push decision making down in the organization to the employees who interface with customers. By sharing power they create an empowered workforce.

Model the way. Extraordinary leaders stand up for what they believe in; they set the example, and their behavior follows quality values. They demonstrate their commitment to the process on a daily basis and "walk the talk." There may be times when their style reverts to a pre-TQM approach, but they recognize these deviations and get back on track. They are open and capable of sharing power.

Encourage the heart. Extraordinary leaders give the organization the heart to carry on, even when targets require a stretch or things get difficult. They give frequent feedback and celebrate success. These leaders also admit freely when they have made mistakes and are pursuing the wrong approach.

Executive leadership is an essential element of TQM implementation. Without leaders who are willing to assess their style and make the changes necessary to provide extraordinary leadership, organizational transformation is not possible.

Process and Phases of Implementation

There is no one best way to implement Total Quality. We have seen successful implementation strategies of all types. However, when we analyzed many of these successful models, we could see similar phases in the process. It is our belief that if you divide the TQ process into four phases and the tasks required at each phase, strategic planning and implementation are more manageable. Figure 5.5 illustrates these four phases of implementation.

These phases may be helpful to you as you lay out your plans. We found that each phase overlaps with the next. Also each person goes through the four phases at a different pace based on his or her background, knowledge, and openness to change. A department or organization will be defined to be in a given stage when a majority of people within that group are personally at or beyond it. For example, the senior leaders of an organization may be involved with steps in phase three, implementation, while the employees in the patient care units are in the second phase, knowledge.

Another issue related to the phases is that the vision for the process often becomes cloudy as the organization moves through the phases. As the quality champion becomes vague in communicating the plan, because the next step is not quite clear, anxiety rises first, then resistance (see Figure 5.6). When the next steps are not clear, there is concern about the process continuing. When transition from one phase to the next occurred in our organization, we could feel the resistance rise. When the organization or the process seems to stumble, the prevailing feeling seems to be, "oh, this is just a fad after all." At this point, reassurance and continued role modeling by the executives is key. Perhaps as successful healthcare models of TQM are more available, the resistance between phases will not be as dramatic.

Figure 5.5. Evolutionary Phases of TQM Implementation.

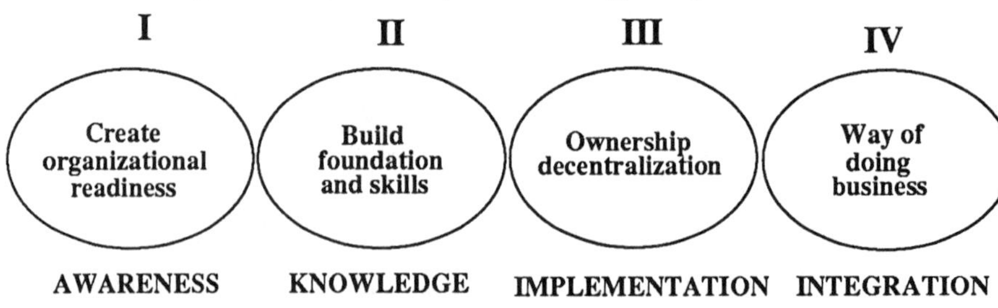

I	II	III	IV
Create organizational readiness	Build foundation and skills	Ownership decentralization	Way of doing business
AWARENESS	KNOWLEDGE	IMPLEMENTATION	INTEGRATION

Figure 5.6. Stages of QI Readiness and Resistance.

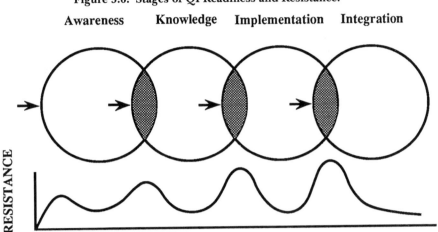

There are several ways to seek out assistance when your vision becomes cloudy. An external mentor, who has lived through an implementation process, is invaluable at these times. If such a person is not available, rereading the books of Deming, Juran, or others may help to refocus your efforts. When you read information for the first time, many of the hints do not seem relevant. However, as you learn by doing, you are ready for many of the steps you may have missed the first time around. You should also develop a network of Total Quality peers in other organizations who, during these expected transitions, can help you plan your next steps.

Action Step: Find an external mentor and/or develop a network of advisers who are further along in the implementation process and who can assist you when transitional problems occur. Continually assess readiness for change at all levels of the organization.

Another problem with implementation is that people believe the process is far easier than it is. Several times we have seen a quality champion visit an organization with a quality process in place and believe that the process is easy and can be accomplished quickly. They feel their organization will be different and the process will flow more smoothly. Typically overheard quotes include: "Oh, we can accomplish this in six months — we won't make the mistakes you did!" Perhaps this is true; however, the road will not be as smooth as you predict when you first examine the process. Nearly all persons we have talked to who are in the midst of a quality implementation tell us they didn't know as much as they thought they did. They can identify with the four phases of implementation and see that there must be an organizational readiness, but in most cases this is retrospective learning.

Another example of organizational readiness came during a consulting experience. We were in day three of a three-day seminar with an organization that thought they had the process down pat. They were feeling very secure until we began an actual case study. They had selected six pilot projects to begin the following week. The case study caused them to rethink their knowledge level and the readiness of the organization, and they decided to begin two pilot teams.

Phase One: Awareness

During this phase the organization is learning about the potential for TQ in their environment. This is where an organizational decision to implement a quality program is made and the energy is created to facilitate this change. An assessment of the current culture and a study of TQM philosophy is required. The executives and the board should be introduced to the process first. As indicated earlier, organizational members must have the question "why should we change?" answered at this phase of the process. Organizational leadership must agree on the reasons for change and then commit to the process. We have listed some of the tasks that need to be accomplished at each phase. The list is not comprehensive nor is it detailed. It is meant to serve as a guide and checklist. The details of each task are available within the text. Do the following tasks in the awareness phase:

Set up a task team to investigate TQM implementation. The purpose of this team is to begin the organizational assessment and develop the plan for the implementation decision. It is best to have senior leaders in the organization serve on this team. Those organizations that delegate this function may find they have a more difficult time achieving consensus to implement.

Arrange visits to quality organizations. Visit both healthcare organizations with a head start and industries with strong quality programs in order to learn what has been accomplished and what the elements of the process are. In our early days we visited Ford Motor Company, Detroit, Michigan; Corning Glass Works, Corning, New York; Florida Power and Light, Palm Beach, Florida; the Juran Institute, Wilton, Connecticut; Alliant Health System, Louisville, Kentucky; Rush-Presbyterian-St. Luke's Hospital, Chicago, Illinois; HCA West Paces Ferry Hospital, Atlanta, Georgia; and Hospital Corporation of America, Nashville, Tennessee. We learned many things that helped us begin to build our process. Visiting a variety of organizations points out different ways to organize and helps you decide what will work in your organization.

Develop an on-site program that features knowledgeable guest speakers. Bring your managers together for a day-long seminar on TQM in healthcare. The external speakers should have quality implementation experience so they will be prepared to answer questions from your team. We relied on our friends from Alliant Health System, Jim Stansbery and Evelyn Strange, to kick off our first program. They helped our senior managers recognize the potential of the quality process for a healthcare organization. We also utilized Dr. Donald Berwick to orient our medical staff to the physician's role in the quality process.

Circulate readings on quality. The audience should be the executive leaders, physicians, managers, board members, and other interested parties. We found so many books and articles that we asked a small panel of people to evaluate which materials were most helpful. In this way we streamlined the readings for others in the organization. We now have a standard package we share with all internal people. We update this information as new and useful information appears in the literature.

Make the decision to implement Total Quality. When the task team reports its findings, the executive management team should be ready to commit to the process. Organizational leadership is essential to successful Total Quality progress. Deming believes that "the change required is transformation, change of state, metamorphosis, in industry, education, and government. . . . The transformation must be led by top management" (Walton, 1990, p. 10).

Make the necessary leadership commitment. The leadership of the organization must make both a financial and an emotional commitment to the process. The financial commitment must exist to allocate appropriate resources for the process because it is expensive to implement; the emotional commitment is necessary because implementation can be emotionally draining for all involved. Nothing short of a full commitment will keep the process on track. The process cannot be delegated because the organizational energy will be insufficient for the transformation.

Select a Total Quality champion. The ideal administrative person to drive the process is the chief executive officer (CEO) or the chief operating officer (COO). The line management must ultimately own the TQM process. TQM requires broadscale organizational and personal change, which begins with each manager recognizing that personal change will be necessary to transform the organization. Leadership of the process cannot be delegated to a centralized quality department. The line management must integrate the quality philosophy into its everyday work and role model the skills if the process is to be successful. Quality improvement must be the goal of each manager in the organization.

Whoever emerges or is selected as the champion must have access to the CEO and a power base in the organization. If a champion does not have a strong power base, he or she will run into tremendous resistance and be unable to maintain the threshold for change. Many programs that have gone off-track chose a staff person to head up the process, and when push came to shove, the CEO and senior leaders did not support the process.

If a physician is selected, it is helpful to have a well-respected clinician. From our experience, we believe it would be helpful to have both a senior executive and a respected medical staff member serve in the role of dual leadership from the start. The responsibilities of the physician are to help plan the rollout for the medical staff and assist with the development of the physician education programs. Timing of the seminars around the busy schedules of the medical staff was a major issue for us. Since physicians tend to be conservative, skeptical, and time pressured, the educational approach may be slightly different. We have learned that each group wants to know "what's in it for me" before committing to the process. A physician leader serves as a better primary advocate when communicating to the medical staff.

Set up a Total Quality Council. The role of the council is to:

- Create the environment to support and promote continuous improvement.
- Guide and monitor the TQ process.
- Support the development of the educational curriculum.
- Sponsor and support pilot teams.
- Approve new teams.
- Monitor team progress.
- Review Requests for Proposals for consultant services and select consultants.
- Develop strategic quality plans.
- Evaluate the process and be prepared to make mid-course corrections.

Our original council at UMMC was a group of twenty-five senior leaders and interested managers who could assist with the planning and implementation and become cheerleaders for the process. As our knowledge about TQ grew, our lead team changed shape and membership. Today we would advise that the top leaders of the organization serve as the quality council.

Develop a mission statement. One of the first tasks of the TQ Council is to write a mission statement to help guide the process. The mission statement should discuss what you will do, why you do it, who you do it for, and how you will do it. The following is a mission statement from our Corporate Lead Team. "The executive leadership of UMMC formed the Corporate Lead Team to guide the Total Quality Process. Our mission is to develop policy and procedures, design quality structures, assign resources, and implement strategies to advance the quality movement in our organization. We are committed to modeling the TQ skills to facilitate employee empowerment and involvement, creating appropriate reward and recognition strategies to sustain momentum, leading by example, reviewing quality indicators to determine progress toward our goals and achievement of our vision. We will monitor our progress by evaluation and monitoring of quality indicators and by overseeing the results of teams."

Identify benefits that TQM can help you achieve. In an executive session, brainstorm the benefits of a TQM process. The list below was developed by our Quality Council and became the goals for the UMMC TQ process.

- Improve the quality of all products and services.
- Improve customer satisfaction.
- Improve cost effectiveness.
- Improve the quality of work life.
- Improve our competitive position.

Select one or more pilot teams. A pilot team can allow you to test the tools and techniques of TQ and demonstrate that it is applicable to your organization while you are laying the foundation for the process. Choose an issue where there is pain about problems, and there will be motivation and interest in finding a permanent solution. For example, our admission/discharge process was an issue no one was happy with, including our external customers. Select a team of key stakeholders, those who know the most about the process. Arrange for some on-site team training for the team. We suggest you use a case study such as the one in Chapter Thirteen or the process suggested in *The Team Handbook* (Scholtes and others, 1988).

Develop a customer focus. Your customer requirements should drive your quality process. Have you identified the major processes in your organization? Have you identified the customers these processes serve? How will you expand your customer listening potential? What skills do your managers and employees need to assess customer requirements? We tend to assume we already know how to talk to customers. Our experience proved that healthcare professionals need substantial education to begin to dialogue with customers. If you have a planning and marketing department, ask them to help you structure a series of educational programs for your employees and managers. Use these programs to develop checklists of questions to ask. The questions should allow you to gather input from customers to help you develop new customer-based quality indicators.

Appoint task teams. These institutionwide teams should work on visible organizational issues using TQM tools and techniques. For example, we set up task teams to work on developing the vision and values statements, performance planning, diversity, employee empowerment, educational curriculum, communications, and reward and recognition. These teams also serve as visible pilot teams. They should report to the Quality Council and be led by executives who serve on it. This is a visible and crucial sign of corporate buy-in.

Analyze the elements of your process. UMMC chose twelve elements of focus for the quality process. These elements were selected after visiting quality organizations and reading about quality efforts. Because task teams were effective early in our process, we decided to use the same approach to plan progress on these critical elements. Some issues were addressed immediately; others, such as supplier relationships, began as late as 1992.

1. Leadership
2. Strategic or quality planning
3. Training and development
4. Reward and recognition
5. Communication
6. Quality in operations or daily work
7. Cultural assessment
8. Empowerment
9. Supplier relationships
10. Cost of poor quality

11. Advanced Total Quality learning
12. Customer satisfaction

For each element we charged a task team to study where we were along a continuum of knowledge and practice. Each task team was led by a member of the TQ Council. Some of the questions the task teams asked about each element were:

- Were we at a beginning level? Who was involved in this issue, what plans were in place, how did we plan to improve our practice?
- Did an organizational awareness about this element exist?
- What changes would be necessary to bring this element into alignment with our quality effort?
- Did we have an educational plan in place to facilitate growth or change in this area?
- Had we reached a growing level of knowledge or practice?
- Had we advanced to a mature level where the knowledge was integrated into practice?

We used a ten-point scale to judge our progress on each element. The second step was to have the teams identify models of success for each element. Our goal was to investigate what made others successful and then benchmark to help us set priorities to advance our progress. For example, we heard Milliken, a textile firm and winner of the Malcolm Baldrige National Quality Award, had an outstanding Reward and Recognition Program. The task team was asked to find out what made the program work and what we could learn from studying their process. The task teams were also asked to advise us how we could improve our practice in each element.

There are several other planning models to consider. You might select the seven elements of the Baldrige Award to serve as your guide: Leadership, Information Systems, Quality Assurance of Products, Human Resources, Strategic Planning, Quality Results, Customer Satisfaction. Or you could use Deming's fourteen points, Juran's ten points, or Crosby's fourteen steps as a place to begin. Once you determine which elements your quality process will focus on, you have the first phase of the strategic plan in place. Next you must assess where you are on each element and what needs to happen in the organization to allow you to make continuous improvements. This is the Where are you? portion of the plan. The next step is to collect information about Where do you want to go? A graphic example, Figure 5.7, illustrates this process.

Prepare a preliminary budget. Based on the scope of the process defined at this phase, develop a budget for the quality process. As your process grows, the budget will need to be adjusted. Many decisions need to be made by the TQ Council before the budget can be finalized. Will you use consultants or internal people? How will you teach the quality tools and techniques? Will you pay overtime to facilitate team efforts?

Assess the capabilities of internal staff. Analyze the type of skills required for your process and the skills of your internal people. Is there a possibility internal people could be reassigned to begin implementation of your quality process? The more skills you bring to the process from existing resources, the better. The major push to our educational process came by utilizing our Management Systems engineers to help teach statistical mindedness and the analytical aspects of quality. We also used our Training and Development staff to teach the human dynamics and team development skills. Once we developed a cadre of people skilled in the technical and human aspects of quality, we were less dependent on our original leaders. The value of using internal people includes less time needed for orientation, less money required to begin, and usually the staff can hit the ground running due to knowledge of the people and systems in the organization. This type of analysis should also be done prior to speaking with consultants.

Determine if consultant services are required. Once your strengths and weaknesses are understood, you should decide which elements of the quality plan you will work on yourself and which you will need help with. The goal is to be self-sufficient as soon as possible. For example, some organizations need assistance with training curriculum for teams; others need assistance with a strategic planning process to get them started. The point

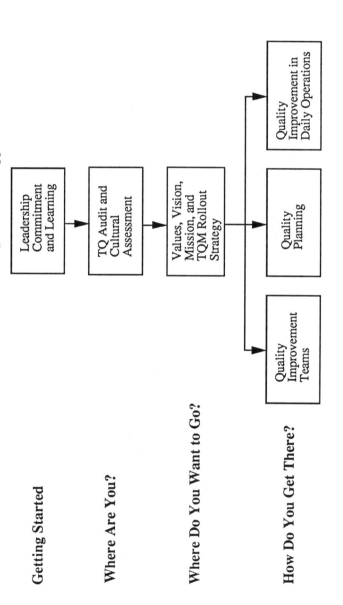

Figure 5.7. TQM Implementation Approach.

Getting Started

Where Are You?

Where Do You Want to Go?

How Do You Get There?

Leadership Commitment and Learning

TQ Audit and Cultural Assessment

Values, Vision, Mission, and TQM Rollout Strategy

Quality Improvement Teams

Quality Planning

Quality Improvement in Daily Operations

is the consulting should be tailored to your organizational needs. Be cautious of buying a consultant's prepackaged program. The "cookie cutter" approach, or one-model-fits-all, does not work well in quality implementation. Buying a standard implementation package, even if it has worked somewhere else, may mean delays and false starts. The most successful programs in business, industry, and healthcare are a flexible mix of different gurus and philsophies. Involving the executives, physicians, managers, and employees in the development of your process — Which guru seems to fit the organization best? Which problem-solving process is best for you? — is the best way to achieve buy-in and support.

Develop the quality plan and time lines to measure progress. Our first assessment of a time line for quality was this graph developed in 1987, illustrated in Figure 5.8. It was a very optimistic assessment. Today we are five years into the process and still in the third phase of implementation. Our experience parallels others in both healthcare and industry. In every organization we have interacted with, the leaders report they significantly underestimated the time and effort required to implement TQM. There are many facets that require extensive planning and mid-course corrections.

The other factor that retards progress is that various parts of the organization progress at different speeds. While we have made significant progress, there are still parts of the organization at phase two, knowledge.

How will you know when you have reached the end of the awareness phase? When the majority of the people in the executive and top management group and medical staff leadership have been oriented to the quality philosophy, attended seminars and conferences, read several books and articles on TQM, or visited quality organizations. Another key indicator is that the decision has been made to commit to a quality effort. The UMMC awareness phase lasted from September 1987 to May 1989.

Phase Two: Knowledge

This is the phase in which the foundation for quality is built. At this time the tools and techniques of the process are taught to all

Figure 5.8. UMMC Five-Year Total Quality Plan, 1987.

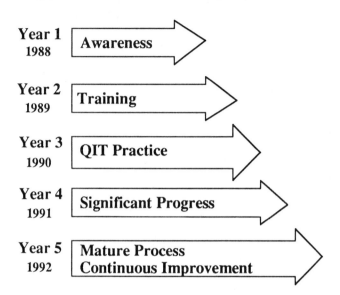

managers, physicians, and employees. The environment is assessed, and a plan to create a quality environment is in place. During this phase the first signs of the quality teamwork are visible. The organization also begins to measure and monitor quality progress through quality indicators and operational results. Chapter Nine describes the education and training programs in detail. Do the following tasks in the knowledge phase:

Develop managerial competence. Teach all managers, beginning with the senior management team, the board, and key physicians, the principles, tools, and techniques of TQM. Develop management expectations, a management education curriculum, and action plans to support the development of managerial competence.

Develop employee competence. Set up orientation sessions for all employees. Begin with teaching general philosophy and principles. A series of sessions focusing on the particulars of the process and the new efforts of teamwork and team process should follow. There must be a strong commitment to education over time. Develop a well-designed introduction to share during new employee orientations. This will allow new employees to recognize the commitment to quality and customers in your organization. The benefits of communicating the values and vision of the organization to new employees is crucial for long-term success and commitment.

Assess the culture. Select a cross section of employees to determine their perception of the current culture and what they believe is an ideal one. What are the norms that drive behavior? Develop a plan to begin to change the environment consistent with TQM values and the employees' vision. The focus of the new culture should be on the customers.

Identify customers and their requirements. Each department must identify their key processes and the customers for those processes. Customer interactions are necessary to validate that the appropriate requirements are identified. Finally, plans should be developed to first meet and then exceed these requirements. The goal of the process is to delight the customer and provide quality never imagined, through continuous improvement.

Select a problem-solving process. The method you choose for problem solving is not as important as choosing a standard, consistent process that all teams will use. See Chapter Thirteen for a full explanation of how we adapted a process to meet the unique needs of UMMC.

Develop a final budget for quality. While the first budget for TQ should be flexible, budgets in this phase need to be comprehensive. In order to perform a cost-benefit analysis of the process, all costs and benefits must be identified. While costs are relatively easy to identify, benefits are more difficult to quantify. Individual quality improvement projects have many benefits, only some of which are monetarily quantifiable. In our analysis we identified the value of increased throughput in the operating rooms, incremental admissions, and dramatic decreases in receivables, but did not attempt to attach a dollar value to significantly reduced waiting times in admitting which yielded improved customer and employee satisfaction.

Train team leaders, facilitators, and members. Select a team training methodology and train team leaders, facilitators, and members. Many organizations skimp at this phase, give a general orientation to quality, and then jump too quickly into teams. At UMMC we did just that. We found through experience that with inadequate training you will lose time rather than gain it. The teams that begin fully trained make much more substantial progress, feel less frustrated, and work better as a team than those with poor training. Spend time up-front, identify the potential training programs, select a process for your organization, and train the teams. This type of preparation will give you far better results. Training is one element of your process your director of Training and Development should research carefully before expensive training decisions are made.

Create institutional indicators. These indicators also must be based on the requirements of major customer groups. First identify your major groups. At UMMC we determined our five major customer groups to be patients and families, referring physicians, third-party payers (insurers, businesses, governments, and so on), employees/medical staff, and students.

The second step is to find out what the major requirements of these customers are. Ask the ultimate customers, the patients: "What are the key factors that would cause you to return to us for care?" Ask referring physicians: "What would cause you to continue to refer your patients to us?" Ask third-party payers: "Are we meeting your requirements, how could we work more effectively together?" Ask employees: "Are we the employer of choice? What steps do we have to take to move in that direction?" Ask students: "What are your requirements while in our organization?" Your customer surveys should be organized to determine how well you are meeting the major requirements of customers as defined by them personally.

Involve your suppliers. If you are having difficulty conceptualizing how to roll out your quality process, think of developing a relationship with your suppliers. Many suppliers implemented TQM programs in the early eighties and are interested in working with healthcare organizations for mutual benefit. These relationships can help you establish a strong beginning for the process in your organization. For example, the Baxter Healthcare Corporation has a very active Quality Improvement Program, and they are sharing what they have learned with their customers. David Auld, director of quality for Baxter Corporation, described the new customer partnerships his firm was developing in a presentation at Baxter in June 1991:

> When you work closely with your customers, you have a better idea of views and needs. Ideas can be exchanged along with information and technology. Teamwork can lead to such advances as just in time deliveries tailored to the customer's needs, which can reduce warehouse and transporting expenses for the hospital. Representatives from Baxter are also joining hospitals' materials management quality improvement teams to add their expertise to problem solving within the hospitals. A joint team with the University of Massachusetts Medical Center led to a revamped delivery and dispersal system for supplies that reduced cost. Baxter also has a strategic partnership with Hospital Corporation of America that led to the development of a computer ordering system to assure rapid turnaround on orders. Baxter enhanced its relationship as a supplier, and HCA reduced its inventory [Auld, 1991].

There are other examples of supplier relationships' creating innovation, and cost savings are occurring. Rear Admiral Robert B. Halder, commanding officer of the Naval Hospital in San Diego, California, invited a representative of Angelica Linen Corporation to sit on his Laundry Quality Improvement Team. Part of the team investigation included a visit to the laundry. Team members found the quality of linens purchased by the Naval Hospital was inferior to the quality of linen purchased by other hospitals. The team raised their purchasing standards and saved money because the higher-quality linen lasted longer and needed to be replaced less often (Halder, 1991).

At UMMC we worked closely with Blue Cross to determine their requirements for billing. We took several steps to
enhance rapid turnaround of questions that may hold up bill-
ings and payments. For example, a direct telephone line to Blue
Cross was established to enhance our communication potential
and make data available more quickly.

Patrick Shumaker, executive vice president of Cardinal
Glennon Hospital in St. Louis, set up a Transport Response
Team in 1991. The team included physicians, nurses, emergency
services personnel, and the external Ambulance Corporation
which supplies their patients.

We believe these types of partnerships are essential for
healthcare organizations. They will provide shortcuts to TQ
implementation and help us add value to the healthcare system.

Set up additional teams. Once team training has com-
menced, set up additional teams. To get the maximum benefit of
the training, avoid a time lag between training and team implementation. Team leaders and facilitators should be instructed
how to use their newly learned team tools and techniques in
their daily work until such time as they serve on a team. This will
facilitate practice and avoid anxiety when their team assignment begins. We also found that if there is a lag between training
and team work, sending a new leader or facilitator to a skilled
functioning team for one or two sessions as an observer can
make a big difference in confidence levels. Most teams feel
honored to be asked to serve as a model for learning.

Develop and publish a rollout plan. In the summer of 1990,
the UMMC Corporate Lead Team developed a document that
described the strategic plan for the "rollout" or implementation
of the TQ process throughout the Medical Center. It is an
educational tool that includes a definition of our process, existing quality tools, and techniques; a description of the organizational structures; an overview of the team concept, including
definitions and processes; a three-year outlook for training; and
planning targets for the implementation and integration of the
TQ process for the next three years. The plan was circulated to
all managers and through team leaders, to all team members.
The plan defines each activity in terms of:

- What is the action step?
- Why is it necessary?
- How will it be accomplished?
- Who is accountable for its completion?
- When must it begin and end?
- Indicators that determine and/or measure achievement.

At the Administrative Forum Meeting on December 12, 1990, the Total Quality Process Plan was first introduced to the institution. The plan is a living document, as it is revised every year or when new definitions, tools, and techniques are developed. Based on the feedback from employees and staff after the first two revisions, we are confident that the plan is an important and effective guide to the UMMC Total Quality Process.

The knowledge phase is completed when all managers and supervisors have attended quality training and are defining a new management paradigm. When knowledge is complete, you will notice a new vocabulary in use. The terms quality, customer, and requirements are a part of most discussions. All employees in the organization have been oriented and are developing quality skills. The team efforts expand from a few pilots to many quality teams.

Phase Three: Implementation

In this phase, decentralization and institutional ownership of the process must occur. The goal is to have line management take full responsibility for the process. This phase requires a difficult transition for the organization because each division and department must now have a quality plan. In our organization one problem was that people on every level watched the people in the level above for actions demonstrating commitment. It sometimes seemed as if we had become an organization of boss watchers. We watch the boss to see if he or she does what they say they'll do. At UMMC we often heard: "I believe in this quality stuff, but my boss doesn't, or can't, or won't." Sometimes this is an excuse, other times an unwarranted fear, and unfortunately sometimes it is the truth. Advise people who want to take action but believe the boss will not, to begin modeling the TQ behaviors themselves. If they begin to involve others, they will enhance their effectiveness and influence. By modeling the technical quality skills, they can teach others and gain supporters for the process. They also will be able to link across the organization with others who are committed to quality and serve on a cross-functional team. This approach of activism seems much more realistic than waiting for approval to begin.

This tendency to hang back unless the boss is demonstrating commitment is the major reason senior leadership commitment to the process is required. The concept of "walking the talk" is critical to give permission to the next level in the organization. When leadership commitment is evident, there are fewer barriers to implementation and there tend to be fewer excuses. If people are sufficiently involved with something, they will become committed. Keep this in mind as you plan executive and mid-level training. Do the following tasks in the implementation phase:

Review the organizational structure for quality. Is the organizational structure appropriate for phase three? Determine how you will drive quality throughout the organization to achieve decentralization, and then create the necessary structure. The structure will be simple to begin, for example, an implementation team or task team at phase one, which becomes a TQ Council as you progress. If your organization is large and complex, you may need a series of lead teams in order to support and sponsor adequately the growing number of teams.

Begin departmental quality planning. Each department should begin its quality processes, if not already under way. The steps required to improve processes include:

1. Identify key services and customers.
2. Develop a departmental mission statement.
3. Flowchart all critical processes.
4. Interview customers to validate requirements.
5. Identify service gaps.
6. Set up teams to improve or redesign processes to close these gaps.

7. Implement improvements.
8. Gather additional customer performance data.
9. Standardize the process.
10. Begin the cycle again.

Develop a departmental mission statement. Each department in the organization should develop a mission statement consistent with the institutional mission statement. One methodology for developing a mission statement is to divide the staff into small groups of six to eight people. Have each team answer the following questions in a few words:

- What do we do?
- Who do we do it for?
- Why do we do it?
- How do we do it?

Each small group then shares its thoughts with the entire group. Differences are discussed and consensus is formed to create one statement. When the single statement is developed, a second series of questions should be asked:

- Are the statements clear? Can all employees, customers, and suppliers understand?
- Does the statement support the organizational mission?
- Are daily activities consistent with the mission?
- Are our activities consistent with our customer requirements?

When these questions have been answered, the mission should be typed and distributed to all department members. The mission statement should be reviewed annually to make sure it remains accurate.

Gather data from customers. As you enter conversations with your customers on their requirements, your mission or service standards may change. The customer requirements should drive these documents. For example, the UMMC Material Management Department met with nursing to negotiate acceptable service standards. These are now written documents that specify roles and expectations and have driven the development of quality indicators.

Establish and monitor quality indicators. Each department should establish departmental quality indicators based on customers' needs. These should be monitored monthly to understand how performance compares to customer expectations. Begin with simple indicators to allow the staff to learn how and what to measure, and then facilitate the development of more complex measures.

When the organization has experience in developing indicators, the next step is to link the departmental indicators to the institutional indicators so that progress of the institution and the department can be monitored. This process allows departments to see the role they play in achieving organizational success and maintains a sense of alignment.

Include the concept of innovation and creativity in your process. Many organizations get caught up in the technical processes of quality and forget that not all processes should be improved; some should be totally replaced. Your employees should be trained to ask the question, is there a better way to do this? Some processes should be discarded and planning should start anew for a brand new service. To deal with the current healthcare environment, fresh new ideas should be frequently elicited through brainstorming, special promotions, employee suggestion programs, or through daily work.

Benchmarking. For many years in healthcare, each institution considered itself unique. We all seemed to track statistics in a different way, and, other than length-of-stay data or admissions, comparisons from hospital to hospital or across the country were difficult. In total, each organization is unique. However, there are components of processes in each organization that are similar to processes in other ones, and this provides an incredible opportunity for learning. Once your processes have been identified, flowcharted, and improved, select a partner and compare your processes. This is an ideal way to enhance quality learning. It is a fallacy to believe that you can learn only from an organization that is exactly like yours. See Chapter Fourteen for further information on benchmarking.

This phase of the quality process is complete when each department has created a mission, a vision, quality indicators, and a quality plan and can demonstrate progress toward customer satisfaction. At this phase there are many teams and evidence of the use of quality tools and techniques in daily work.

Phase Four: Integration

During this phase the process becomes the way of doing business. Total Quality is woven into the fabric of the organization. The people in the organization are empowered, decisions are made on the front lines, and there are many semi-autonomous teams in place. The organization is customer driven, and customer requirements are regularly exceeded. The common goals of the organization take priority over departmental and personal goals, and employees are recognized for their contributions to improvement. There is ongoing evaluation of the process and a plan to rejuvenate the change process if necessary. Many times organizations start a change process with great enthusiasm and energy, but after a while the old habits take over and the change process is stalled. Stopping and starting over again can cause problems with credibility and trust in leadership. Employees may wonder, if we couldn't do this before, what guarantee do we have now? Do the following tasks in the integration phase:

Assess progress of first three phases. Conduct a quality audit. A quality audit is a management tool to evaluate quality activities and determine if they will help the organization achieve its goals. The question to be answered is whether the quality system is functioning appropriately. Audits can be internal, within a department, or institutionwide. External audits may add a new level of objectivity. Invite external experts to assess your organization's progress and provide feedback to help your program continue to grow.

Develop updated stretch goals to sustain momentum. Assess the quality of goals and determine if they will provide the opportunity for the organization to reach a little higher. This concept of "raising the bar" can keep people energized and your customers delighted. Benchmarking other organizations and implementing best practices is a way to enhance performance.

Review educational curriculum. Base new programs on needs assessments of various internal customer groups and feedback from staff who have completed courses and applied the knowledge in their areas. Always be on the lookout for innovative educational programs to sustain the momentum.

Conduct formal assessment of the process by internal and external customers. There must be a formal assessment of the organization's progress that includes business practices, activities, and attitudes that are enhancing or inhibiting quality progress. An analysis of how well internal and external customer requirements are being satisfied is also necessary. Data should be collected, analyzed, and shared with everyone in the organization. There are several tools to help you begin the assessment. At the first audit you may wish to measure your own progress. With the second audit you may measure yourself against others. There are several ways to begin this type of quality audit. The first is completing the application for the Healthcare Forum/Witt Award. This award is given each April at the annual Healthcare Forum Conference. Information on obtaining an application from the Healthcare Forum is included in Chapter Fourteen. This application is helpful because it is designed for healthcare organizations and melds quality assurance and TQM concepts. The application requires a comprehensive review of quality efforts.

We suggest your organization conduct a self-assessment based on the criteria in the application and then ask for an assessment by an external party, such as a former winner of the award or one of the award judges. The previous winners are:

- 1992: Florida Hospital Medical Center, Orlando, Florida
- 1991: Intermountain Health Care, Salt Lake City, Utah
- 1990: University of Michigan Hospitals, Ann Arbor, Michigan

- 1989: Methodist Hospital, Houston, Texas
- 1988: Alliant Health System, Louisville, Kentucky

Preparing the application is a great learning experience. After completing this step, compare your organization's process against those of the winning organizations. Finally, set up an opportunity for the people in your organization to review the results of your analysis, review where your strengths and weaknesses are, and develop a plan for the next year's application.

Using Malcolm Baldrige Criteria to Assess Progress

In 1987 Congress passed Public Law 100-107 to establish the Malcolm Baldrige National Quality Award (MBNQA). Each year American corporations compete for this prestigious quality award. The process gives executives a means to measure their quality progress against that of others. To date, the MBNQA excludes not-for-profit healthcare organizations. However, the application can be used for self-assessment in any organization. We developed a self-audit tool based on the Baldrige Award to allow our managers to view their own departments and assess where they are on the Transformation Continuum, and to help us assess the progress of the organization. This tool can also be used by your Quality Council to assess your organization and begin the planning necessary for the quality process. The tool is included in Appendix A.

Developing the Organizational Structure

The Structure Changes as the Organization Learns

The organizational structure for the UMMC Total Quality Process changed several times. In 1987, when we began, we set up a series of task forces to help us begin to transform the organization. They were:

Vision and Values Task Force. The work of this task force was to determine what values the Medical Center should live by in the 1990s. The task force suggested hosting a series of focus groups composed of employees from every job category to determine what employees felt the key values should be. Our staff of volunteer facilitators were trained by an outside agency in the necessary techniques to conduct focus sessions. Over 350 employees participated in this exercise. The second step was to have the CEO, COO, and the director of planning and marketing review the data and create a first draft of the quality statement. The document was then circulated first to the focus group members and then to other standing committees of the Medical Center. Revisions were made, and the statement was framed and hung in all meeting rooms and public places throughout the Medical Center.

Total Quality Task Force. This task force was charged with exploring the potential for TQ in our environment. The task force consisted of twenty-five members from senior administration, medical and nursing leadership, and several enthusiastic managers who would help us study and then promote the TQ process. As we learned the quality language and process, this task force evolved into the Total Quality Council, which later evolved into the Corporate Lead Team.

Work Redesign Task Force. We also began to look at the concept of work redesign in 1987. We recognized that there were many changes necessary within the healthcare system. Like most healthcare organizations, we have become very specialized and have narrowly defined job descriptions. Our goal was to review the literature, start some pilot projects, and create the opportunity to redesign work. We felt we should be asking employees to think of how the work should be structured, what elements could be deleted, how could we best accomplish the necessary tasks. Some of the pilot projects accomplished were a flexible work schedule and redesigned functional work plan in our Finance Division. The Finance Division also experimented with semi-autonomous work teams to redesign work and to facilitate the implementation of a new patient accounting system.

Innovation and Creativity Task Force. This task force worked to identify environmental barriers to institutional creativity and innovation. They read the literature and developed a very successful pilot program aimed at enhancing the creative and innovative potential of the learners. The program has now become part of the educational curriculum for managers. As Patrick Townsend and Joan Gebhardt write: "if creativity and innovation are going to take hold and become habitual, middle managers will have to be active proponents. And for that to happen, they will have to understand their new role and what is in it for them" (1991, p. 26). The course is open to employees as well, but it is our goal to support the creative process through management action.

As these task forces began their work and we learned more about the TQ Process, it became obvious to us that three of the task forces were a subset of the fourth. Figure 5.9 illustrates the change in focus whereby Total Quality is seen as the umbrella for many other activities.

Total Quality Council. About the time our educational process began, our TQ Task Force became a TQ Council (TQC).

Figure 5.9. Total Quality as Umbrella for Other Activities.

Total Quality

Total Quality Task Forces

- Vision and Values

- Work Reorganization

- Creativity and Innovation

- Diversity

- Performance Planning

- Employee Empowerment

- Communications

- Reward and Recognition

- Training and Education

We were no longer investigating whether a TQM process was possible but how to implement the process. The role of the council also changed, and the work became more formalized. The council approved the quality curriculum, approved the sequence for training, monitored the work of teams, and developed organizational policies and procedures related to the quality effort.

Corporate Lead Team. In 1990 we realized that the TQC, as configured, did not have the appropriate organizational leadership to sustain the quality momentum and fully integrate the process into the organization. We developed a new plan to include the senior leaders of the medical school and hospital on the Corporate Lead Team. Our goal was to move quality from a hospital process to a Medical Center process and from a shadow organization to a part of line management. By creating the new lead team, we sought to emphasize that Total Quality Management was going to be the way we did our work in the future. Rather than sustaining a separate TQM department or council, we wanted to integrate TQM into each division in the organization. Figure 5.10 illustrates the structure for the UMMC Total Quality Process.

Divisional Lead Team. Because our organization is large and complex, our next step was to create a series of Divisional Lead Teams, each led by the Corporate Lead Team members. Smaller organizations would not be faced with this level of expansion. This new organization would achieve the goal of decentralizing the process and emphasize the importance of divisional leadership. The goal of TQM is to reach as many employees as possible. When the divisions and the leaders of the divison are developing their own implementation strategies, there is the best chance for achieving full employee participation. The second benefit to having the divisional leaders play a major role is that when leaders are role-modeling the behaviors, those reporting to them are likely to adopt the same behaviors. A change in behavior allows people to grasp how the process really works and what the process has the potential to yield. We agree with Pat McLagan's statement: "My belief is that you haven't implemented quality until every person in the organization has

Figure 5.10. UMMC Structure for Total Quality Process.

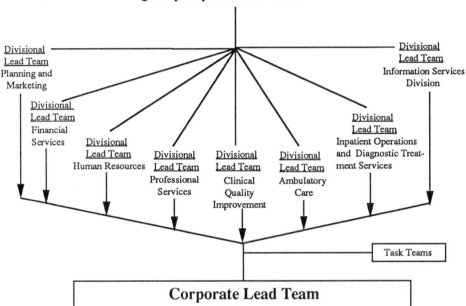

Quality Improvement Teams

Divisional Lead Team Planning and Marketing

Divisional Lead Team Financial Services

Divisional Lead Team Human Resources

Divisional Lead Team Professional Services

Divisional Lead Team Clinical Quality Improvement

Divisional Lead Team Ambulatory Care

Divisional Lead Team Inpatient Operations and Diagnostic Treatment Services

Divisional Lead Team Information Services Division

Task Teams

Corporate Lead Team

Hospital Executive Director
Senior Hospital Associate Director
Associate Director, Ambulatory Care Services
Associate Director, Inpatient Operations & Diagnostic Treatment Services
Associate Director, Professional Services
Administrator, Human Resources
Chief Information Officer
Senior Associate Dean/Chief of Clinical Affairs
Associate Dean of Clinical Affairs, Medical School
Chief of Nursing Affairs
Director, Alternate Revenue
Director, Planning & Marketing
Hospital Financial Officer
President, M-Care
Surgeon in Chief
Physician in Chief
Pediatrician in Chief

Joint Staff

Hospital Executive Director
Senior Hospital Associate Director
Hospital Financial Officer
Vice Provost Health Affairs
Chief of Clinical Affairs
Dean of Medical School
Senior Associate Dean of Clinical Affairs, Medical School
Director for Administration and Professional Services, Medical School

a major personal 'aha' experience with quality" (1991, p. 3). Decentralization and implementation of TQM at all work sites is the best method to achieve full participation.

Action Step: Decentralize your process. Build in the appropriate level of structure to allow TQ to permeate all levels of your organization.

Clinical Lead Team. Our process began as the result of the National Demonstration Project. We were taught about quality by industrial experts and, because the leaders of the UMMC process were administrative, our process took on an administrative focus. Few of our teams were dealing with clinical issues. As we evaluated our progress in 1990, we realized we needed to emphasize clinical applications. A retreat of clinical chairmen and section chiefs was held in April 1991 to discuss how to bring TQM to clinical issues. The outcome of that retreat was to establish a Clinical Quality Improvement Lead Team consisting of physicians, nursing leaders, and administrators to focus on the clinical side. Today the team is sponsoring seven teams: four are QITs following the seven-step process and three are improvement teams following an improvement methodology developed by Leon Wyszewianski, from the Michigan School of Public Health, who is working with us as a special consultant. There are also two quality projects that the lead team is sponsoring. The three different types of clinical quality improvement efforts are illustrated in Figure 5.11.

Your Organization for Quality

The involvement of the senior executives in your quality planning gives a push to the process; the increased understanding helps the leaders of the organization move from awareness to knowledge to implementation. While some organizations have had success with the use of a task force, this approach may slow down the process. The people selected to lead the effort may not have enough power or be capable of speaking for the organization, and a bureaucratic process ensues. If a task force or task team is your choice, make sure there is a leader who sees the

Figure 5.11. UMMC Clinical Quality Improvement Efforts.

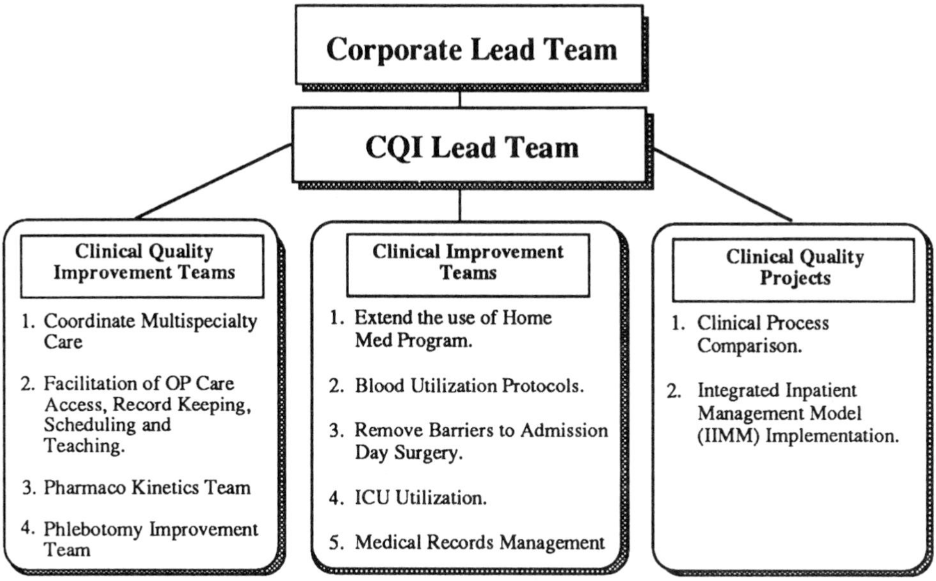

```
                    ┌─────────────────────────────────┐
                    │      Corporate Lead Team        │
                    └─────────────────────────────────┘
                    ┌─────────────────────────────────┐
                    │         CQI Lead Team           │
                    └─────────────────────────────────┘
```

Clinical Quality Improvement Teams	Clinical Improvement Teams	Clinical Quality Projects
1. Coordinate Multispecialty Care	1. Extend the use of Home Med Program.	1. Clinical Process Comparison.
2. Facilitation of OP Care Access, Record Keeping, Scheduling and Teaching.	2. Blood Utilization Protocols.	2. Integrated Inpatient Management Model (IIMM) Implementation.
3. Pharmaco Kinetics Team	3. Remove Barriers to Admission Day Surgery.	
4. Phlebotomy Improvement Team	4. ICU Utilization.	
	5. Medical Records Management	

potential for organizational transformation and is a skilled change agent. Thomas Berry (1991, p. 16) strongly recommends that "the team leader be CEO or COO and include other officers that report to him or her. This matter is far too important and far reaching to be delegated to others in the organization."

Agenda for Change of the Total Quality Council

The first task for the TQC is to write a mission statement. The elements of the statement should reflect the who, what, for whom, and how aspects of the council's role. This mission statement illustrates the first step for the TQC Major Activities:

• Study the TQM process.
• Assess the organizational readiness for change.

Exhibit 5.3. Implementation Checklist.

Plan

- Determine which group will evaluate the potential for TQ in your organization.
- Evaluate the potential elements of your quality plan.
- Assess the capabilities of internal personnel and determine consulting requirements.
- Plan the process to develop a vision statement.
- Determine how to align the organization behind the vision.
- Plan how to determine customer requirements on a department-by-department basis.
- Determine which problem-solving methodology to utilize.
- Plan how to roll out the process in your organization.
- Identify pilot teams.
- Assess where you are and where you need to go.
- Develop quality indicators, institutional as well as departmental, so you will be able to measure progress.
- Develop a five-year plan for the TQ process.
- Develop an employee empowerment plan.
- Identify the stages in a communication plan.

Do

- Arrange visits to quality organizations.
- Develop on-site quality education seminars with expert speakers.
- Circulate readings to administrative and clinical leaders and board members.
- Educate senior management.
- Achieve leadership commitment.
- Select or empower a quality champion.
- Set up a TQ Council.
- Educate all managers.
- Educate all employees.
- Establish a team to develop the management expectations for your institution.
- List major customer groups.
- Begin customer requirement analysis.
- Educate all employees in philosophy, tools, and techniques.
- Estimate the cost of poor quality.
- Measure performance against your quality indicators.
- Evaluate the culture of your organization.
- Teach all supervisors and managers the new skills. Develop an organizational structure to support process.
- Set up pilot projects.
- Select and train team leaders and facilitators.
- Involve suppliers in the process.
- Develop and publish a rollout plan.
- Promote creativity and innovation.

Exhibit 5.3. Implementation Checklist, Cont'd.

Check

- Check level of improvement achieved according to vision, goals, and customer expectations.
- Analyze the structure for the process. Is it working? Can it be streamlined?
- Analyze customer requirements. Are they being met? What progress has been made?
- Evaluate pilot teams. If successful, set up additional teams. If teams did not achieve goals, what changes need to be made?
- Evaluate training programs. Are they having the desired results? Do you need additional modules?
- Conduct a quality audit. How extensive is the commitment to quality?
- Measure progress using criteria from the Malcolm Baldrige or Healthcare Forum/Witt awards.
- Invite internal customers to evaluate your process.

Act

- Adjust all plans as necessary.
- Standardize to hold the gains.
- Begin the planning cycle again.

- Discuss the rationale for pursuing a quality approach to answer the "why" TQM question.
- Develop an educational program for the TQ Council members.
- Develop goals for the process.
- Plan a cultural assessment.
- Ensure that TQM is consistent with other institutionwide initiatives.
- Plan communications.

TQM Implementation Checklist

This checklist presented in the Plan-Do-Check-Act format (Exhibit 5.3) can help you analyze where you are and what needs to be accomplished in your organization. The checklist is not in sequential order.

Chapter Six

Organizational Culture

Organizational cultures consist of commonly held beliefs and values about work life. "A strong culture, with well-socialized members, improves organizational effectiveness because it facilitates the exchange of information and coordination of behavior" (Denison, 1990, p. 9). The actions and decisions of organizational leaders create and reinforce key values and shape the culture. Do the management practices in your organization cause anxiety, lack of trust, and self-protective behaviors? Or are there strong feelings of trust, collaboration, and practices that contribute to the development of each person's competence and self-esteem?

Employee involvement is one of the cornerstones in TQM implementation. Involvement and empowerment can thrive only where the culture is positive and the value of the individual is upheld. We and others we have worked with have found it is easy to talk about changing the culture, but actually changing strongly held beliefs is a very difficult and time-consuming task. In this chapter we will review beginning steps to help you evaluate, diagnose, and begin to redirect the culture of your organization.

Definition

Edgar Schein defined corporate culture as "the basic assumptions driving life in a given organization" (Schein, 1985, p. 1). A

148

working description of the word culture is, "the way we get things done in our organization." Every organization has a culture created by the shared beliefs, values, norms, and expectations of the workforce. Denison reported quantitative results that support the idea that corporate culture has a measurable impact on bottom-line performance. He states that "involvement, consistency, adaptability, and mission are significant elements of culture that help determine future organizational effectiveness" (1990, p. 87). Many authors support the concept that it is possible to change an organizational culture (Martin, Sitkin, and Boehm, 1985; R. E. Walton, 1986; Denison, 1990).

Many people wonder why we cannot have the type of organization we want. Why do we seem to snuff out innovation and change and revert to inertia? Robert Allen and Charlotte Kraft believe this is because there are two organizations, "one visible, articulated, expressed in stated goals, policy statements, and procedural manuals; the other the invisible, lying quietly under the surface, but actually determining what will happen in the long run. We call this unseen but powerful force the organizational unconscious" (Allen and Kraft, 1984, p. 37). If a change process is planned and the organizational unconsciousness takes over, the changes will be temporary. The trick in organizational transformation is to understand the organizational unconsciousness, involve everyone in the organization in the change process, and create effective new norms.

Positive Cultures

A positive culture is one where employees experience pride in their work, where everyone is involved and committed to continuous improvement, where people freely help each other to achieve goals and have fun during the process. In positive cultures people feel appreciated, their opinions are solicited, and action follows suggestions. Berry describes a Total Quality culture as "one where there is an attitude based on trust, teamwork, objective problem solving, and shared accountability" (Berry, 1991, p. 23). With positive cultures there is positive thinking, which is an organizational energizer. People are able to see new possibilities and are open to change. They develop confidence that they can solve problems themselves, and they need little or no supervision. They also take calculated risks and stretch their learning potential. Peak performance becomes possible in this type of environment. Bill Russell, former center for the Boston Celtics, described peak performance in this way: "Every so often a Celtic game would heat up so that it became more than a physical or even a mental game, and would be magical." Every pass would connect, every shot hit the basket, the team seemed to anticipate plays, and they could do no wrong. He described having chills run up and down his spine during these moments (Russell and Branch, 1979, p. 155). Robert Kriegel and Louis Patler wrote about their experience in *If It Ain't Broke. . . Break It.* They interviewed five hundred top performers from all areas of work, the arts, and sports. "No two were alike but the one quality they had in common was *passion.* It was their drive, their enthusiasm, their desire that distinguishes them" (Kriegel and Patler, 1991, p. 13). "Adams believes that a critical mass of individual members need to undergo personal transformation before their organizations can undergo system-wide transformation. Because organizational systems steadfastly attempt to maintain status-quo individuals must perceive and act in new, perhaps unfamiliar ways" (Allen and Kraft, 1984, p. 194). A TQM process can revitalize your organization and allow people to feel passionately about work. The experience of being on a team that is working extremely well and exceeding all expectations is very energizing. Once you have a "peak experience" at work, you'll be very motivated and find you want to recreate the experience again and again. You want the opportunity to achieve more. Fixing problems and improving processes is exhilarating.

Peak performance begins with commitment: to the team, to excellence, to changing the organization. Oakley and Krug ask us to "remember those times when you were working towards something you really wanted. The people who told you the reasons you couldn't have it or do it became motivators rather than deterrents. Your determination was so strong that nothing could convince you that you could not attain your goal" (1991, p. 136). One of the greatest motivators for employees is success.

Each successful team effort inspires future successful efforts. Judith Bardwick calls this type of success being "enriched." She says: "there are three conditions in order for employees to feel enriched:

- Challenge: To risk, learn and fulfill their potential.
- Empowerment: To be autonomous so they can be creative, make decisions and act.
- Significance: To do things that matter and create value" (Bardwick, 1991, p. 55).

Negative Cultures

If the environment is negative, there are also many visible signs. Negativity is an energy depleter. In negative organizations people spend a lot of time guarding their turf and protecting themselves. Energy is spent in attacking others, getting angry, and getting even. There is little risk taking because if a mistake is made, the boss searches for the guilty party and punishment occurs. Even if the punishment is subtle, such as an embarrassing comment made to peers, it creates the wrong tone. There is a tendency in punishing cultures for managers to crawl into a foxhole, hide out, and hope that the bad times will pass. Change is resisted, and maintaining the status quo becomes the goal. Rather than being pulled by a positive vision, the organization is driven by fear and the desire to protect oneself.

Understanding Your Culture

Why is it necessary to understand the culture within a health-care organization? The culture of an organization can affect the quality of care. "Dick Scott of Stanford University has shown in his research that patterns of internal organization within a hospital may influence morbidity and mortality rates. We would hypothesize an equally dramatic view: a strong culture can contribute to quality care in a hospital" (Deal, Kennedy, and Spiegel, 1983, p. 21).

If strong positive cultures contribute to positive performance and cultures can be shaped, managed, and changed, then an assessment of the current culture and an action plan for change can assist you in building an appropriate culture. If you wish to create a new culture, you personally must be willing to change and be capable of communicating both the desire to change and the rationale for change to your employees.

With change the only constant in healthcare, we must have organizational cultures where adaptation to change and flexibility are key skills. We must also learn how to tap the creative potential of each employee as we search for new and creative solutions to problems. Managers must understand the existing organizational culture if they expect to achieve their goals. How do you begin? Look at the values of the organization. Strong cultures begin with a well-articulated value system. Are the values of your organization well understood? Are meeting guidelines stated or implied? Do you need to begin values clarification exercises with employees, where values are discussed and agreed to? Deal and Kennedy describe it this way: "Companies that have cultivated their individual identities by shaping values, making heroes, spelling out rites and rituals, and acknowledging the cultural networks have . . edge" (Deal and Kennedy, 1982, p. 15).

Who are your organizational heroes? What kind of stories get communicated? Stories reflect the organizational values. Are your organizational stories positive or negative? Do they reflect the culture of quality? Do you need to create some new quality heroes in your organization? If the creation of teamwork is a major goal, perhaps you should create some "hero" teams. Strong cultures have visible heroes. This allows people to choose positive role models. What are the rites and rituals within your organization? Do you need to change these to reflect your renewed commitment to quality? How are you celebrating quality achievements such as goal completion or milestone achievement?

Action Step: Evaluate your culture. Ask:

- Have you completed a cultural assessment?
- Do you have a positive or negative climate?

- Do you have a values statement?
- Are the values communicated, understood, and upheld?
- Who are your heroes?
- How do you celebrate?
- Do positive or negative stories get repeated?
- What barriers hinder the development of a positive culture?

Organizational Barriers

Many of our institutions have functioned as a collection of superb departments with strong boundaries and barriers to interdepartmental cooperation. Figure 6.1 illustrates this vertical, departmental orientation within an organization.

This approach creates problems for our customers, who

Figure 6.1. Departmental Focus.

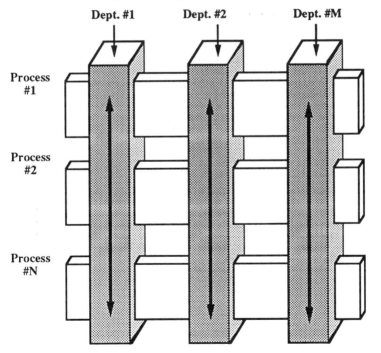

Source: Marszalek-Gaucher and Coffey, 1990, p. 97.

experience our organizations horizontally as processes that cross a series of departments, not one department at a time. For example, an outpatient is seen by admitting for registration, medicine for the visit, nursing for consultation and education, radiology for x-rays, pathology for lab tests, pharmacy for medications, patient accounts to settle the bill, and perhaps others. Although these departments may function autonomously, their independent success can be at the expense of other departments. We need to create a seamless, well-functioning system, not a series of strong departments. In many healthcare organizations, we have achieved our goals in spite of others instead of with others. A quality effort allows you to focus attention on the processes rather than the departments. Quality thinking will allow you to think about and remove turf barriers. As part of a TQM effort, the tendency to point fingers of blame at others is replaced by people trying to identify root causes for problems. Donald E. Petersen and John Hillkirk wrote of a turf-reducing strategy called the "valentines exercise," which you may wish to use to point out how departmentalized an organization can become. This exercise was utilized at a senior management seminar at Ford Motor Company: All types "were grouped by function—all the engineers in one place and the personnel people in another, for instance—and given eleven sheets of paper, one for each function. Each group then wrote a short note, or valentine, to the other eleven functions, describing 'things you do that make it difficult for us to do our job well.' After the groups talked for an hour or so about the notes they'd received, the whole crowd gathered again to report what they'd learned. This opened lines of communication that had been closed for decades" (Petersen and Hillkirk, 1991, pp. 56–57). The key is to open up the organization; allow people to learn about others' functions and to share valuable information, thus improving both communication and the organization. Figure 6.2 illustrates how a seamless organization, one that will meet the customer requirements, should look, with a focus on processes rather than departments.

Figure 6.2. Process Focus.

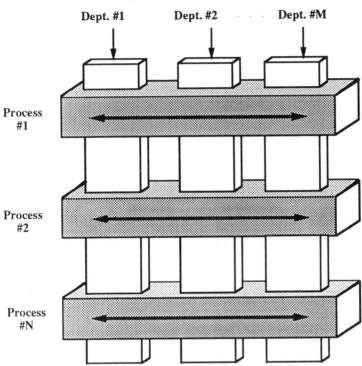

Source: Marszalek-Gaucher and Coffey, 1990, p. 98.

Steps to Cultural Change

The stronger and more established a culture is, the more difficult it will be to change it. The first step in changing a culture is an assessment of the current one. The second step is to define what people would like to see changed. Once gaps between the existing and ideal cultures are identified, plans can be developed to close the gaps and achieve the ideal.

One barrier to culture change is employee expectations. At UMMC we learned that when you begin to describe the way things can be in an organization implementing TQM, an organizational impatience for change builds up. People want to see the changes right away. Somehow when a quality process begins, people think it is a magic bullet and that change will be deep and easy. Consequently, you may actually see a decline in attitudes when you resurvey employees. Because they expect immediate change and get slow change, attitudes may be worse. Make sure you establish and communicate realistic goals for change early in the change process.

Deal and Kennedy (1982, pp. 165–166) offer five tips for those who want to manage the change process. These strategies should be the basis for your cultural plan.

- Consensus. Recognize that peer group consensus will be the major influence on acceptance or willingness to change.
- Two-way trust. Convey and emphasize two-way trust in all matters (and especially communications) related to change.
- Skill building. Think of change as skill building and concentrate on training as a part of the change process.
- Patience. Allow enough time for the change to take hold.
- Flexibility. Encourage people to adapt the basic idea for the change to fit the real world around them.

Transition Management

Understanding how people in the organization will react to change is critically important. There are predictable stages of transition that occur with any major change. One of the first people to write about this type of transition was Elisabeth Kübler-Ross, M.D. Her research was based on cancer patients coming to terms with a terminal disease. Others have found that the process described by Kübler-Ross parallels the stages of other radical changes like divorce, bereavement, alcoholism, or major organizational change (Kübler-Ross, 1969, pp. 38–138). Table 6.1 illustrates the similarities in the two models of transition.

The phases of organizational transition experienced during the implementation of TQM are analogous to Kübler-Ross's stages of transition:

Denial Stage. This stage tends to be the most difficult to

Table 6.1. Stages of Transition.

Kübler-Ross	Radical or Organizational Change
1. Denial and isolation	1. Denial
2. Anger	2. Anger
3. Bargaining	3. Resistance
4. Depression	4. Exploration
5. Acceptance	5. Commitment

manage. The initial reaction of managers and employees to the proposed change is shock. There tends to be a downturn in people's confidence levels as they react to the news of change with fear and denial. Some comments you may hear in the hallways include: "Why are they doing TQM now; we don't have a crisis? If you ask me, we'll never accomplish this; management can't change! I don't have time for this quality stuff." Denial is a temporary defense mechanism; it can best be overcome with communication and support. Keep in mind that there have been many times when employees have been excited by potential change, and the change never occurred. If this has been the case in your organization, you may have many skeptics. They will need convincing that this will not be the next fad or flavor of the month.

Action Step: Plan how you will communicate the desire to start a TQM process. What supports will be necessary to show you are serious about change?

Anger Stage. Next, people experience anger because of the change. They try to come to terms with the reality of change and experience stress. This resistance reflects an inability to accept the change. The goal of most is to maintain the status quo as long as possible and avoid personal change. You hear comments such as: "I am already a Total Quality manager, I've managed this way for years"; or "Why should I change, this is just a fad"; or "What will 'they' think of next." The best way to deal with the stress of the anger stage is to include people in the planning process. Allow open questioning and shaping of the plans; ask for employee input. Communicate the rationale supporting the change to a more participative style. Help managers evaluate the behaviors others see in them that may be barriers to TQ and give them assistance and support to change. Organizations that do not communicate effectively may find their quality process stalls before it begins. Many of their employees will not have the support to get beyond the anger stage.

Action Step: Communicate the rationale for change. Help people understand why change is necessary. Allow people to express anger, then provide appropriate support and education.

Resistance Stage. When the first two phases pass, resistance sets in. The people in the organization must go through the process of letting go of the old ways. This phase is about the loss of control and familiar ways of doing things. The focus is on the way things were! Deming calls this the period of chaos, when the old rules no longer fit and the new rules are unknown. There is fear expressed at this point. How will I learn the new ways? Can I be successful in the future? You will find people ask, "Why me?" They may be depressed or frustrated or both. They rebel against finding time to do new things, they are already too busy! They cancel places at the training sessions. "People who find it most difficult to change are first line supervisors, heads of nursing, and department chiefs, who are deeply steeped in success according to the old methods" (Scott and Jaffe, 1991, p. 34). This phase must be managed by training and support. The vision and the intentions or rationale must first be well communicated or fear will be reinforced. A strong roadmap for the change is essential for transition to the next phase. Scott and Jaffe point out that "every major and minor ailment seems to emerge in times of organizational change. Psychological stress and physical stress go hand in hand" (1991, p. 34).

Action Step: Share the plans for change and progress broadly. Provide updates, consistently allow employees to give feedback, and follow up on their recommendations. Provide emotional support by making yourself available for counseling, coaching, and mentoring.

Exploration Stage. At this phase people stop resisting change and cautiously begin to experiment with new techniques. There is a shift to more positive behaviors. They "try on" the new behaviors and experiment with the new practices and see that they work. The emphasis is on the future. They find long-standing problems are staying fixed; the results are very visible. The tools and techniques need to be available as well as the time to experiment with the new concepts. Expect mistakes to occur at this phase. Both managers and employees will make mistakes; they need to be encouraged to be persistent and stay on track.

Action Step: Be patient. Provide managers and employees the flexibility to experiment with new techniques. Encourage and support risk taking.

Commitment Stage. At this phase it becomes clear how TQ can help meet organizational and personal goals. People are excited about the process. It makes work easier. Many are aware of organizational successes. Conversations in the hallways are positive and uplifting. "An organization or team that allows people to go through all four stages, that has accepted the anger, accusations, the rumors, the grumbling, the chaos, is rewarded by a group of people who are committed and ready to help create new ways to meet the challenge" (Scott and Jaffee, 1991, p. 37). This transition curve is illustrated in Figure 6.3.

Figure 6.3. Transition Curve.

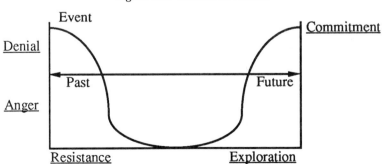

Action Step: Provide resources to support the natural transition of a cultural change and sustain the new culture.

Whatever stage your organization or department is passing through, resources must be available to smooth the way and allow progression to the next phase. Managerial encouragement and support are key elements in a successful transition. The assistance and organizational messages must be tailored to each phase. The problem is that not everyone goes through the phases at the same time. One department may be well ahead of others, or the senior officers may be at one stage while the rest of the organization may be lagging behind. Thinking about the transition model and the phases present in your organization, or where each person may be on the curve, may help you plan your strategy.

Action Step: Examine the transition model and determine which stage of the process your organization or department is in. Can you identify different phases by department? Determine what type of support is required to facilitate forward progress.

Developing the Assessment Plan

As previously pointed out, the first step is to assess your current organizational culture. The strategy we used was a formal and tested cultural assessment questionnaire. As the Total Quality Council considered how to analyze where we were and what steps needed to be taken to improve, we felt it was necessary to measure the thinking, behaviors, values, beliefs, and norms of our workforce. Since a culture is the result of practices and deeply held beliefs, it cannot be changed quickly. Change must be planned or chaos will result.

In the fall of 1990, we conducted a cultural audit to establish baseline data for the UMMC Total Quality Process. The Quality Council felt we would have more success and acceptance with a well-established and proven cultural audit tool than an internally developed one. As a result we chose a tool developed by Human Synergistics in Plymouth, Michigan.

Employees from four categories were invited to fill out questionnaires about the organizational culture. The categories included all University of Michigan Hospitals executives, all clinical chairmen, the dean of the Medical School, a large number of managers, and a random sample of 2,000 employees. Each group completed two sets of questionnaires. In the first questionnaire, participants were asked to describe the current environment, and in the second they were asked to describe the way they would like the culture to be. The survey tool asked each person to "think" about what it takes for you and people like yourself to fit in to the culture and meet expectations. They were given 120 phrases like "go along with others," "win against others," "take moderate risks," "never make a mistake." They were asked to respond on a scale from 1 to 5, from strongly agree to strongly disagree. The phrases were grouped into twelve management styles, and the totals for each management style were plotted on a graph. Separate graphs were developed for the perceived current culture and the desired culture for each group of people completing the questionnaires. Significantly, all groups described the same desired culture.

From the analysis of the survey we learned that we were a very task-driven organization. Getting things done was key, with less concern exhibited for the people doing the job. Those surveyed expressed the opinion that "you must be perfect, have the answer to everything and not make mistakes." Our data indicated that there were two subcultures at the top of the organization. One culture was competitive and power-oriented; the other was more responsive to people, values, self-actualization, and personal growth. Our consultant advised that this dichotomy was sending our employees a mixed message. Gaining this knowledge allowed us to focus our educational sessions on actions that encouraged achievement but also demonstrated high concern for employee growth and development.

Other Cultural Assessment Techniques

A simplified means of assessing your culture is to look at existing patterns of behavior. What are the existing assumptions? Are they consistent with a TQM approach? In order to change an existing culture, the current assumptions, shared beliefs, values, norms, and expectations need to be examined and challenged. Once the new goals are selected, the process can be used for goal achievement. The Total Quality Council must seek input from employees, through brainstorming exercises, to determine current cultural elements and the desired elements. It is important that the members of the council act as facilitators during the process. Their role is to listen and record the brainstormed ideas. It is critical that they be nondefensive and not interpret or debate issues as they are raised. The goal is to solicit feedback from many employee groups. The elements of the desired culture then should be described through the same brainstorming techniques. When both the existing and the desired cultures are understood, plans can be developed to create the new culture and TQM can serve as the catalyst to achieve it. Through training and planning the new norms and expectations can be laid out and supported, as illustrated in Figure 6.4.

People—Our Most Important Asset?

Many organizations say with pride that people are their most important asset. However, when you look beneath the surface there are other issues in the organization that take priority, such as capital acquisition or the pursuit of new technology. "Conven-

Figure 6.4. Comparison of Existing and New Organizational Cultures.

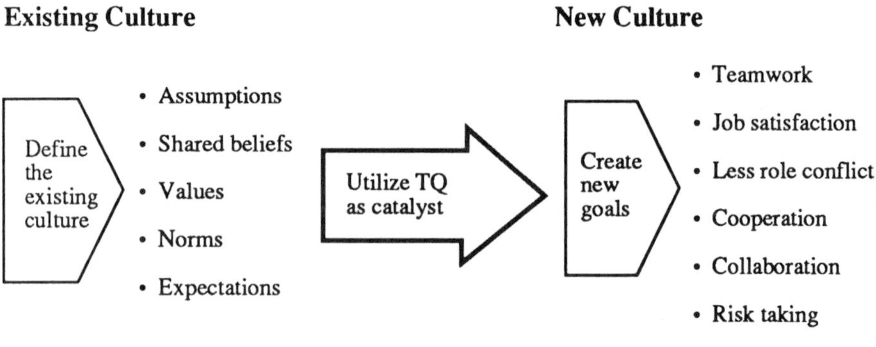

Existing Culture

Define the existing culture

- Assumptions
- Shared beliefs
- Values
- Norms
- Expectations

Utilize TQ as catalyst

New Culture

Create new goals

- Teamwork
- Job satisfaction
- Less role conflict
- Cooperation
- Collaboration
- Risk taking

tional systems of management and accounting do little to ac-knowledge the impact that effective management of human assets has on performance. People are treated as expenses rather than assets, and are managed with an eye toward reducing costs rather than increasing return on assets (Denison, 1990, p. 16). In order to implement TQM fully, the organizational leadership must increase the focus on creating a more people-oriented culture. An excellent example of a people-oriented culture exists at Federal Express. Their belief is that customer satisfaction begins with employee satisfaction. CEO Frederick W. Smith summarizes their commitment: "When people are placed first, they will provide the highest possible service, and profits will follow." He acknowledges that "putting people first in every action, every planning process, every business decision, requires an extraordinary commitment from every manager and every employee. Putting that somewhat ideal philosophy into practice means we look for a multitude of ways to replace talk with action" (Bohl, 1991, pp. 12–13).

The current environment in healthcare is heavy with uncertainty and fear. Revenues are falling behind expenses, lay-offs are becoming common, healthcare organizations are going out of business, and mergers and acquisitions are occurring at a rapid rate. The good news is that when TQM is your survival strategy, it is an uplifting process. It builds energy and excite-ment into the organization. It is a positive energy force as opposed to a fear-driven culture. Fear can cause organizational paralysis.

Empowerment and Enablement

Total Quality is a people process. To build a quality culture everyone must work together to accomplish shared organiza-tional goals. TQM requires the involvement of everyone in the organization to achieve the philosophy of continuous improve-ment. Each individual must help to improve all processes and functions in the organization. There must be personal commit-ment to the reduction of waste and rework. To accomplish this goal, each staff member must be empowered and given the tools to achieve the transformation. What is empowerment? Peter Grazier states: "Empowerment is a mechanism to involve people, at all levels of the organization in a thinking process. It sends a message of value, an understanding that all people possess some particular talent or skill. It conveys the uniqueness of every human being and celebrates the creativity that resides in each of us. It is an affirmation that we are all in this together, and no one person in the organization can ever possess more knowledge and creativity than all of us together" (Grazier, 1989, p. 165). Empowerment includes:

- Authority: the freedom to do a job the way the person thinks is the best way.
- Knowledge: the appropriate tools and information to do the job and make sound decisions.
- Importance: the tasks must accomplish something that is meaningful.
- Feedback: appropriate information about how they are doing the job is essential.

An empowered employee has the capability to solve problems with the least amount of guidance. Autonomy and the power to make decisions allow employees to contribute to organizational success. Employees that are empowered and committed to customer satisfaction build your customer base.

Warren Bennis and Bert Nanus see empowerment as a leadership responsibility: "Empowerment is the ability to generate enthusiasm and vision and communicate this to people; it is critical in any leadership role" (Bennis and Nanus, 1985, p. 19).

When your institution tries to implement an empowerment philosophy, there will be resistance. On the surface it may seem that employees are not interested. They may project a "9-to-5" mentality and show little evidence of creativity or innovation. The truth is that they may have tried to give suggestions and ideas for improvement in the past but did not see any of them implemented. The rejection of their ideas leads many employees to satisfy their need for achievement in activities outside of work. They throw themselves into hobbies, sports, church work, or community activities. If you want employees to exhibit these same creative behaviors at work, you must create the right environment. Treat your employees as if they are your most important resource. Set up opportunities for them to grow and develop.

Action Step: Set the stage for creativity and innovation. Treat employees as your most important resource. Remove barriers to innovation and empower employees to generate ideas and implement them.

The empowerment process begins with managers focusing on the type of change needed in your organization. What will the new paradigm look like, and what changes have to occur to get there? There must be significant personal changes as well as organizational ones. Richard Boyle, a Honeywell executive, described his adopting a participative management style as "wrestling with jellyfish." He commented: "Many organizations want to break out of the beat-'em up school of management and move to a participative style. But like abused children who grow up to become abusive parents, managers raised in a less enlightened manner may have difficulty operating under a new set of rules" (Boyle, 1984, p. 74).

Our Total Quality Council developed the graphic previously included as Figure 2.4 to illustrate the required paradigm shift that managers would need to make as we moved from managing to leading.

Action Step: Brainstorm the elements of the current management style in your organization. Define the paradigm you wish to create. Assess your progress at frequent intervals.

Beginning in 1991, the University of Michigan Hospitals CEO asked each of our senior managers to prepare a personal annual "paradigm report card." Each year they indicate what kind of progress they are making, on a scale of 1 to 10, in moving from a management to a leadership perspective within their division. The first year, the personal input of the managers was assessed; in successive years a written graph of responses from each senior manager's direct reports was tabulated. Our goal is to expand the number of people who use the paradigm report card to assess their bosses' management style. We believe that we have the best chance for growth through a better understanding of how our management behaviors are viewed by others.

Our goal as leaders of the process is to develop competent, motivated team players who can help us adapt to the rapidly changing demands of technology and new markets. This can occur only if our managers lead the way. Employees say that they come to work with a positive mind ready to work, but the system and leaders keep them from working as productively as they can. Many of the faulty systems can be addressed through the Total Quality approach, utilizing the workers' ideas for system redesign.

The next step was to develop a staff paradigm shift based on the management paradigm. When management is trying to change, new responses from employees are required. For example, the course instructor points out that if your manager is trying to change and express a counseling and coaching approach, he or she may ask you for ideas about a problem. What will your response be? Both managers and employees need assistance in developing the skills and required characteristics.

While employees have a major role in transformation, leadership must commit to setting the climate in order for the process to succeed. Executives in an organization shape the culture by words, actions, rewards, power, and sanctions. How do you demonstrate to people that they are your most important asset? Do you assume your employees are fully capable and work to remove the barriers that keep employees from accomplishing their goals? Bennis and Nanus (1985, p. 92) point out that "the leader operates on the *emotional and spiritual resources* of the organization, on its values, commitment, and aspirations. The manager, by contrast, operates on the *physical resources* of the organization, on its capital, human skills, raw materials, and technology."

Emphasize the importance of people in your organization. Focus on education and training; help your people grow and develop both professionally and personally. Address employees' needs to learn, and expand responsibilities by creating career paths. Make sure you keep, rather than lose to your competitor, your most talented employees. Another strategy for building loyalty is to promote from within. Allow employees to stretch and support them with the appropriate training. This builds loyalty and support. Encourage innovation, entrepreneurism, risk taking, questioning, and thinking and talking about the unthinkables. Support and encourage people to be individuals; create an environment in which people feel respected and appreciated.

The change process has been slow and difficult in most organizations. Managers and employees seem to exert tremendous energy to maintain the status quo. In the first days of the process, when the training sessions are under way, there is a tendency to think you have licked the problem, that your organization will not be like all the others and you will move full speed ahead. So far we have not met the organization fortunate enough to avoid the pitfalls. As Peter Senge points out: "An organization doesn't start out great, it learns to be great. Learning organizations are organizations where people continually expand their capacity to create the results they truly desire, where new expansive patterns of thinking are nurtured, where collective aspiration is set free, and where people are continually learning how to learn together" (Senge, 1990, p. 3). He explains further that "the organizations that will truly excel in the future will be the organizations that discover how to tap people's commitment and capacity to learn at all levels in the organization" (1990, p. 4). The question is how do we begin to excite people about the potential of learning together and mind pooling to improve the organization? To build this new type of learning organization, new skills of leadership are essential. Leaders must build the type of organization where all employees have a role in shaping it and their future.

Encourage and Support Employee Suggestions

To promote your quality process, you must solicit and support employee suggestions. Remain open to new ideas. Share both goals and organizational statistics with employees; help them to see the role they play in the organization's success. It may be helpful to see what a typical Japanese firm experiences for employee suggestions compared to what a typical American company does, as illustrated in Table 6.2.

Our employee suggestion program has grown over time, but we are still working on encouraging more suggestions through our "Preventing Waste" curriculum.

Action Step: Audit your personal response to suggestions and count how many times you say no, directly or indirectly, to employee ideas and suggestions. Keep a log and review it often. Assess your need to change in order to promote creativity in your staff.

If you want your employees to make suggestions, you must support and encourage their ideas. Even if you think the idea is poor, it is best to say, "That is an interesting idea, can you suggest a way to test it?" Support the person to conduct a low-cost, low-risk test. If the idea is poor, the employee will discover it with data and recommend against the implementation. However, the employee will feel supported and will suggest additional ideas. On the other hand, the employee may demonstrate that the idea has merit and prove your initial assessment was wrong. In this case you have both a happy employee and a beneficial idea for the organization. Both strategies will motivate the employee to explore creative opportunities in the future.

Diversity

TQM requires motivating all employees to join in a continuous improvement effort. To accomplish this the concept of manag-

Table 6.2. Comparison of Japanese and United States
Employee Involvement.

Characteristic	Japan	United States
Number of improvement ideas per employee	30.70	0.12
Percentage of workforce participating	78%	9%
Implementation rate	83%	29%
Average value of an implemented suggestion	$122	$5,126

ing and valuing diversity is important. Diversity is about race, gender, age, personal and corporate background, education, sexual orientation, management or nonmanagement, physical limitations, and other differences that exist. While diverse work groups can add vitality, new ideas, and creativity, a diverse workforce requires a greater amount of management energy to create synergy. According to the U.S. Department of Labor, within the next decade 85 percent of workforce entrants will be women, ethnic minorities, and immigrants (most of whom are ethnic minorities). Only 15 percent of new entrants will be white males (U.S. Department of Labor, 1988, p. 150). It will become more difficult to describe a typical employee; our stereotypes will no longer fit. Managerial skill building in managing diversity, or creating an environment that works for all employees, is an absolute necessity for organizational success.

Roosevelt Thomas quotes Jim Preston, CEO of Avon Products, to illustrate this point in another way:

> Some people say that by 1995, three out of four people coming into the workplace will be women or minorities. That is a fact. Well, if you are going to attract the best of those people into your organization, you'd better have a culture; you'd better have an environment in which those people feel they can prosper and flourish. If you don't they will go elsewhere and you'll be at a competitive disadvantage. This is not some type of benevolent activity on our part. There is self-interest here. We have to have a culture and environment in which these people can flourish, and that's what we are working toward [Thomas, 1991, p. 164].

How Can You Begin to Manage a More Diverse Workforce?

Education is the place to begin. Managers must have cultural awareness training to begin to explore the differences among people in the workplace. Some authors predict that the assimilation model of the past, where newcomers were expected to fit in, is dying. For example, Thomas writes: "People are saying, I am different and proud of what makes me so. I can help your team and I would like to join you, but only if I can do so without compromising my uniqueness" (Thomas, 1991, p. 8).

As we analyzed our workforce at UMMC, we found we had a very diverse population with 79 percent females and 22 percent racial or ethnic minorities. We wanted to analyze whether our climate nurtured this current pluralistic population and whether we were prepared for future changes. Did we have the requisite skills to manage effectively? Were there barriers that precluded employee contributions, and if so how could we remove them? The Total Quality Council established a task team consisting of employees from a broad cross section of the organization to look at these and other diversity issues. The task team's mission was to assess our environment and to direct resources to create and sustain one that recognizes the worth, quality, and diversity of each person. The charge of the task team was to:

1. Examine the link between the Total Quality Process and multiculturalism in the workforce.
2. Identify the impact of changing workforce demographics on the policies and practices of the Medical Center.
3. Develop a plan for enhancing sensitivity to cultural and gender differences in order to create a more supportive environment.
4. Develop models to improve interaction among management and staff of diverse backgrounds.
5. Identify ways to celebrate and recognize cultural differences among our workforce.
6. Review the recommendations, developed by a UMMC management intern, and develop an implementation plan.
7. Develop a plan to conduct an institutional diversity audit.

The task team met for a period of a year and delivered its report in October 1991. To accomplish the goals of its assignment, the team created four other task teams to address specific issues:

- Celebrating Diversity Task Team. This team was charged to suggest ways we could celebrate and acknowledge diversity at the Medical Center and recommend an implementation plan.
- The Training and Communication Task Team. This team was charged to assess training techniques and programs to develop a model for a curriculum that would encourage employees to value and manage diversity.
- The Diversity Audit Task Team. This team was charged to explore resources and develop a plan to conduct a cultural audit. They were also charged to provide recommendations on how to begin the process.
- The Policy and Practices Task Team. This team was charged to examine the link between TQ and multiculturalism, to identify the impact of the changing workforce on policies, and to review the proposal for a diversity coordinator position.

Each of the task teams successfully completed its work and presented recommendations to the organization. We celebrated their achievements at a banquet and presented each team member with a certificate of accomplishment.

The Critical Success Factors for Diversity

There are several critical success factors that need to be considered as you develop your action plan.

- Appropriate education to ensure the support and involvement of senior leadership for the process
- An organizationwide program that will generate broad employee-based participation
- A plan to conduct an organizationwide assessment of diversity issues
- A strategic plan for the change process

Action Step: Consider these six steps to enhance diversity:

Step 1: Develop a plan with senior management and appoint a diversity task team.

Step 2:   Collect data on current environment, practices, and policies.
          Develop a diversity audit to survey attitudes and practices.
Step 3:   Analyze data and present it to senior management.
Step 4:   Prioritize important issues.
Step 5:   Develop action plans to change systems and culture. Set up
          task teams.
Step 6:   Evaluate progress, communicate results to the organiza-
          tion, and begin the cycle over again.

Drive Out Fear

Many authors have pointed out that fear in the workplace is a
barrier to quality, productivity, and innovation (Deming, 1986;
Harvey, 1988; Block, 1987; Gitlow and Gitlow, 1987; Ryan and
Oestreich, 1991; Marszalek-Gaucher and Coffey, 1990). Deming
felt this concept of fear was so important he included it as point
eight in his fourteen points: "Drive out fear, so that everyone may
work effectively for the company" (Deming, 1986, p. 23). When
our senior management team first began to study the culture of
our organization, the concept of fear was foreign to us. We felt
that perhaps cultures of fear existed in manufacturing but not
in healthcare; we are, after all, a human service organization
driven by a charitable mission.

There have been many situations that have confirmed the
fact that fear does exist in our environment. Our first experience with recognizing fear in the organization occurred at a
meeting of our Administrative Forum, a group of two hundred
senior, mid-level, and first-line managers. We asked during Total
Quality training for each manager to assess their services and
identify customers and their requirements, and finally to develop departmental indicators to begin monitoring their progress toward meeting customer requirements. When the COO
asked for a show of hands to see how many people had developed their indicators, only one person half raised his hand.
When the meeting was over, people crowded around to tell the
COO that they had developed their indicators but did not want
to raise their hands because they were not sure they had done
them correctly. We learned that most of our managers are afraid
to make mistakes; they want to be perfect! This is a form of fear.

Another awakening occurred when we analyzed the results of our diversity audit. Employees reported that many times they feel they have a legitimate grievance but do not file one because they fear retaliation. We have also identified in our culture fear of speaking up, fear of making mistakes, fear of bringing bad news, fear of the boss, fear of retaliation, and fear of failure. Fear in the organization keeps people from taking risks; it inhibits creativity and innovation. We must, as Deming teaches, drive out fear if we expect to reach full implementation. Some sample fears and aids to reduce them are illustrated in Table 6.3.

Action Step: At a senior management meeting, discuss the concept of organizational fear. Brainstorm a list of possible fears, and then list aids to remove them. Communicate this list. Suggest that your managers repeat this exercise with their staff.

How Do You Begin to Reduce Fear?

"Reducing fear is an essential component of organizational transformation" (Ryan and Oestreich, 1991, p. 9). Fear keeps

Table 6.3. Sample Fears and Aids to Reduce Them.

Fear	*Aids*
Fear of making mistakes	Treat mistakes as opportunities to learn. Point out mistakes that lead to learning, not punishment. Don't kill the messenger!
Fear of speaking up	Create opportunities for employees to speak out. Encourage staff to speak at meetings. Solicit thoughts from silent people.
Fear of the boss	Talk about the fear in meetings. Ask what is the worst thing that could happen. Ask for examples of negative behavior.
Fear of retaliation	Ask for examples of retaliatory or punishing behavior. Work with the staff openly. Reinforce the management expectations; highlight management learning and new goals.

people from doing their best. It is impossible to achieve strong performance when people are anxious, resentful, and mistrustful. How do you begin to set the stage for trust building and the reduction of fear? First, the organization's leaders need to relate to people in a humanistic way; they must seek to encourage and develop people to create a trusting environment. Fear is created when employees experience or hear about blame, retaliation, reprisals, retributions, and negative consequences. One of the first steps is to create an atmosphere without blame, where mistakes are treated as opportunities to learn. Make sure employees understand it is okay to make mistakes. Mistakes should be acknowledged in a positive, nonblaming manner. Another tactic is to tell your employees they need not ask permission. Rear Admiral Robert Halder, U.S. Navy, commanding officer of the San Diego Naval Hospital, tells his staff, "proceed till apprehended." It gets the message across that he does not want employees to fall victim to the bureaucracy.

Ryan and Oestreich list four arenas that require attention to reduce fear:

- Abrasive and abusive behavior by managers and supervisors
- Ambiguous behavior by managers and supervisors
- Poorly managed personnel systems
- The culture of the organization — "how we do things here" — with special emphasis on the performance and conduct of top management (1991, p. 72).

Abrasive, Abusive Behavior. Aggressive interpersonal behavior of managers and the wrongful use of power destroy trust and two-way communication. It is difficult to establish a trusting culture when behaviors of sarcasm, verbal put-downs, insults, yelling, and other aggressive behaviors dominate daily work life. Abusive behaviors can also be more subtle such as ignoring someone, speaking down to people, blaming them for mistakes, or even displaying disapproving facial expressions. Very subtle facial expressions, comments, and actions can suppress others. Most managers are not consciously negative but are responding to the negative vibrations in the culture. They have not had positive role models. When managers are insecure and fearful, self-esteem is low and there is a tendency to be rigid. Actions show a lack of flexibility. When managers are spending time thinking of protecting themselves and their turf, there is no risk taking. There is no flexibility of thought. The game is played by the rule book, even when the rules no longer fit or people know they are wrong. Data are analyzed, debated, and reworked for fear of mistakes. Whether these behaviors are intentional or unintentional, the results are the same: fear exists, and innovation and creativity are stymied. Organizational energy is directed against the management instead of against the problems.

How can these negative climates be overcome? First, acknowledge that negativity exists. Remain open to listening to the employees; when they discuss abusive actions, try to find out what is happening. There should be opportunities for managers to discuss how they manage and what behaviors are used in good times and times of stress. Focus on creating a positive environment, giving positive recognition, and complimenting instead of criticizing. Courses and skill building in conflict management techniques may help replace old behaviors with new. Managers need to be taught how to listen to employees and instructed in involvement strategies. Define power for your managers as Rosabeth Moss Kanter does:

> Power is the ability to get things done, to mobilize resources, to get and use whatever it is that a person needs for the goals he or she is attempting to meet. In this way, a monopoly on power means that only a very few have the capacity and they prevent the majority of others from being able to act effectively. Thus the total amount of power—the total system effectiveness—is restricted, even though some people seem to have a great deal of it. However, when more people are empowered—that is, allowed to have control over the conditions that make their actions possible—then more is accomplished, more gets done [Kanter, 1977, p. 166].

Remember the best teaching occurs when the executives begin to role-model the new empowering behaviors.

Action Step: Acknowledge that negativity exists in the organization. Create forums where people can safely identify and discuss problems that require action. Model the empowering behaviors you wish to establish.

Ambiguous Behavior. When people do not understand what the rules are, confusion exists. When management behavior is inconsistent, anxiety runs high. When anxiety and confusion are the main behaviors, people are afraid to take risks, and suggestions and ideas from the employees will be nonexistent. When the leadership announces a TQM process, and all planning meetings take place with just the top executives and no employee involvement, your leadership is "not walking the talk" or practicing the principles of quality involvement. Employees experience anxiety when major organizational change occurs. They may ask: What is my role in this new culture? How will my relationship with my boss change? Leaders must clearly communicate plans for change prior to the change and model the new behaviors. Without clear and consistent leadership models, ambiguity will breed increased anxiety. Think of the messages your actions are sending.

Action Step: Evaluate your planning processes. Are there enough opportunities for employees to participate? How can you increase opportunities?

Poorly Managed Personnel Systems. Employees watch how the organization treats people. If the organization is fair and equitable in handling problems, employees will not be fearful. Is there a reasonable appeals process for employee problems, where employees get a fair hearing? Do management decisions that are faulty or do not follow process get overturned? Are the rules and regulations helpful or bureaucratic?

If there is an economic downturn, will the organization support employees that must be laid off? Is there an outplacement service? Do you have a special policy to give those who have been laid off a priority opportunity for any open positions? Do you have a fund for job retraining to keep valued employees whose positions may need to be eliminated?

What type of performance feedback do employees receive? Are employees encouraged and supported? Is feedback a mixture of positive and negative, or is only the negative performance noted? Are there clear performance standards? Are there clear, realistic goals?

Action Step: Review your personnel policies and procedures. Do they indicate the concern necessary for a people-oriented culture? Is your personnel office viewed as supporting management or the employees?

Perceptions of Top Management. How is the top management of your organization perceived by employees? Would they get a vote of confidence, or are they viewed negatively? Are they consistent, decisive, competent, team oriented? Perceptions of the management are a symbol of how people believe they will be treated by the organization. If there is a negative view held by employees, there is a good chance fear is present and will be hard to overcome unless trust can be rebuilt.

Action Step: Survey the organization to determine how top managers are viewed. When data are in hand, communicate the results and develop an action plan to address problems.

Employees and other customers want to know the results of surveys in which they participate. If results are not communicated, with an action plan, the loop remains open and no benefit to participation can be seen. If you close the loop, people receive the feedback that their participation can change the organization.

Other Strategies for Reducing Fear

To built trust, the executives also must become more visible in the organization. Spending less time in the office and more time managing by wandering around will create a more facilitative environment. Making frequent rounds, holding open forums, participating in all training sessions, stopping by to congratulate someone for a job well done — all will help employees identify names and faces of the executives. UMMC employs over ten thousand people. The opportunity to meet all of these employees is fairly remote. As a first step, we felt that we needed some help so that employees could put names and faces together. We developed an organizational chart with pictures, which is posted at the entrance to all buildings. The next step was to include photographs in the *Hospital Star*, the organization's newsletter. Our hope was that it would be easier for employees to identify the executives. We then began to utilize the management-by-walking-around approach. The first few times that executives wandered into a department unannounced it caused quite a stir. Today there is far less reaction as our executives host regular employee breakfasts and lunches; serve hot dogs, coffee, or ice cream at employee events; visit team meetings; participate in storyboard rounds; and are generally much more visible than previous executives.

Innovation and Creativity

Our organizations must become more flexible and adaptive in this time of constant change. Personal as well as organizational mind-sets must be changed. "Someone has to be brave enough to disagree with accepted ways of doing things, if changes are to occur" (Berg, 1991, p. 51). Some quality programs become very bureaucratic; they focus only on the charts, statistics, and technical side of quality. Some processes should not be improved but replaced with more effective ones. How do you create this balance? Promote and reward creativity, remove barriers to creative thinking, support risk taking, keep bureaucracy at a minimum, find new ways to seek employee input on all types of issues, communicate in every direction — up, down, and sideways. "Those organizations that do the best job of becoming highly adaptive and creative in their inner workings have the best chance of surviving, thriving, and gaining a business advantage over their competitors. Creativity, at the individual and corpo-rate level, may become one of the new weapons in the com-petitive arsenal of business" (Albrecht, 1987, p. 10).

Ask employees to explore whether they are creative or reactive thinkers, as illustrated in Table 6.4.

Teach your managers to use peripheral vision. Many times managers have difficulty observing problems in their own en-vironment. This problem has been called job blindness. A mechanism to overcome this problem is to ask managers to visit major competitors and critique what they see. For example, Marriott sends employees to visit other hotels. They check on such things as brands of soap and shampoo, special services, and registration procedures (Whiteley, 1991, p. 81). When man-

Table 6.4. Extreme Thinking Styles.

Reactive Thinkers	*Creative Thinkers*
Are resistant to change.	Are open to change.
See reasons they cannot do things.	Are "can do" oriented.
Focus on finding problems to fix.	Build on success and strength.
Are blinded by problems in a situation.	Seek the opportunity in every situation.
Avoid blame or responsibility.	Take responsibility for their actions.
Are limited by what worked in the past.	Think in terms of new possibilities.
Are poor listeners.	Are good listeners.
Run out of energy quickly.	Have a continuous supply of energy.
Find it difficult to choose and decide.	Make choices and decisions easily.
Feel they have no control of the environment.	Feel in control of the environment.
Often work very hard.	Get results without trying hard.
Are afraid of risk or major challenge.	Are driven to excel by challenge/ risk.
Suffer excessive inner stress.	Enjoy an inner calmness.
Cannot let go of the past.	Are current and future oriented.
Are devastated by failure.	Learn and grow from their mistakes.
Have low self-esteem.	Have high self-esteem.
Focus on what they want to avoid.	Focus on results they want.
Do things right.	Do the right things.

Source: Oakley and Krug, 1991, p. 40.

agers return to the home organization, many previously hidden problems are more obvious. A secondary benefit is that they may have learned valuable techniques they can apply in their departments. This approach works in almost any department — housekeeping, dietetics, materials management, and clinical units. If visits to healthcare competitors no longer provide learning experiences, have department heads visit area industries with similar processes. For example, the admitting manager could visit excellent hotels to see how the processes compare.

Action Step: Model creative problem-solving skills, such as peripheral vision, to enhance personal and organizational performance. Reward creative and innovative approaches in your managers and employees.

Conclusion

A new culture can be created by the leadership of an organization, as Edgar Schein writes: "A unique function of leadership as contrasted with management or administration is the creation and management of the culture" (1985, p. 171). The steps include a study of what exists, a vision for change, and a plan for change. The most powerful way to change the culture is for leaders to role-model and teach the new skills, and to change the reward and recognition system to reflect these behavioral changes.

Chapter Seven

Physician Involvement

Introduction

Ernest Codman (1869–1940), surgeon, Massachusetts General Hospital, Harvard Medical School, may have been the first physician Total Quality Management advocate as early as 1916: "The prevention of waste and the judgment of the proportion which each item should take, in order to be sure of a product—the satisfied and relieved patient—is the essence of good hospital management. . . . Their minds have been satisfied with treatment, not with the results of good treatment" (Donabedian, 1989, p. 246).

The principles of TQM—in particular listening to the voice of the customer, management by data, and analysis of the process of care—represent changes of emphasis in hospital management. While these concepts have produced innovation in hospital quality assurance efforts as well as restructured hospital organizations, physician resistance to these new quality efforts persists. As early as 1910, visionary thinkers such as Ernest Codman saw the benefits of applying industrial quality control methods to the analysis and methods of patient care. His revolutionary message drew sharp criticism from the medical

This chapter was contributed by Eric W. Kratochwill and L. Paul Sonda III, M.D., University of Michigan Medical Center.

181

community of the day. For aggressively advocating his "End Result System" for continuous monitoring and improvement of surgical results, Dr. Codman lost his position as surgeon and instructor at Harvard Medical School. The attitude of physicians who attacked Codman is best summarized by one of his surgeon colleagues, John Hornsby, in 1918: "We all know you cannot standardize an art. The efficiency engineers have a place with us; there is not doubt as to that, but they will have to study our problems from the standpoint of the medical profession before they can set mathematically guiding lines for us. These men are laymen; they are business people. They have not the slightest conception of what takes place in a hospital, and consequently could not possibly be the agents through which surgery could be standardized" (Reverby, 1981, p. 169).

In some ways, things have not changed. Recently healthcare leaders who had been successful in applying TQM philosophies, tools, and techniques in administrative areas began exploring strategies for gaining physician involvement in TQM efforts (Thompson, 1991, p. 1; Merry, 1990; Espinosa, 1992). This chapter describes the current pressures facing the medical community and suggests that the 1990s offer an excellent opportunity to encourage physician involvement in quality improvement efforts. Generally physicians have resisted participation in such efforts. The significant reasons that have contributed to this resistance will be discussed. Physician involvement will vary according to which physician role in healthcare delivery is addressed in quality improvement efforts. Different approaches to enhance physician involvement will be required within each physician role. This chapter offers some lessons learned from the early stages of a clinical quality improvement effort at the University of Michigan Medical Center and suggests a general approach to guide your organization toward achieving more physician participation, leadership, and support for Total Quality efforts.

Does TQM Provide Some Answers to Physician Concerns?

The traditional physician-patient relationship has undergone significant evolution. Health maintenance organizations

(HMOs), preferred provider organizations (PPOs), and other employer-controlled healthcare benefit programs increasingly restrict the freedom of patient provider choice. Armed with articles from newspapers as well as information from television programs, healthcare consumers frequently challenge physician decisions about their care. In addition, the press and regulatory agencies have charged physicians with insensitivity, poor communication, an excessive focus on money, and inadequate control of quality (Merry, 1990, p. 102).

Physicians now sense a gradual erosion of their traditional "professional dominance" in the patient care process (Freidson, 1970, pp. 127–164). In his book *Managing Doctors*, Alan Sheldon (1986) describes the inherent stress between the motivations of the individual physician and the healthcare organization in which the physician practices. Whereas physicians desire the freedom to function independently, organizations desire control and feedback because they are publicly acountable for the outcomes and particularly the costs of care. In contrast to the traditional physician-patient relationship, managed care programs and other changes in healthcare delivery systems have often shifted the control of patient care from the physician to a larger, bureaucratic organization, as illustrated in Figure 7.1. As more physicians become salaried employees of various healthcare systems, the eradication of the individual private practitioner in medicine is accelerated. The systems themselves are often chiefly concerned with the "business" of medicine. Both the physician and the employing institution may forget the ultimate goal of the system: better outcomes of care for patients.

The medical malpractice system provides additional pressure on the physician-patient relationship and the healthcare delivery system as a whole. The direct costs of malpractice are estimated to be as high as $7 billion per year, and the indirect costs (i.e., defensive medicine) may be many times the direct cost of insurance (Garnick, Hendricks, and Brennan, 1991, p. 2856). The recent establishment of the National Practitioner Data Bank encourages the healthcare system to identify and discipline those who engage in unprofessional behavior, and to restrict the ability of incompetent providers to move from state

Figure 7.1. The Shifting Doctor-Patient Relationship.

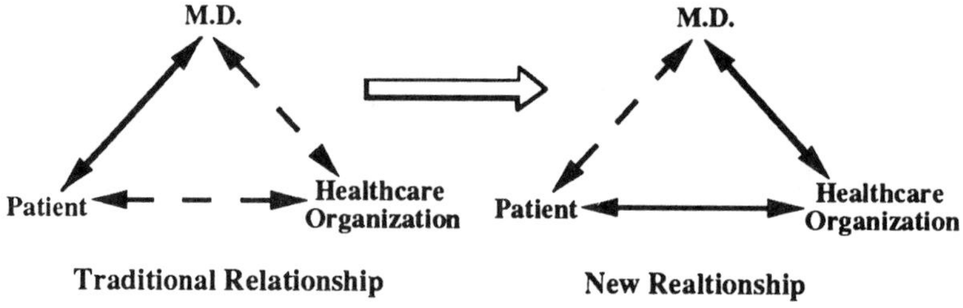

Traditional Relationship   New Realtionship

Source: Adapted from Sheldon, 1986, p. 42.

to state to avoid discovery of the practitioner's previous damaging or incompetent performance. Healthcare institutions, state licensing boards, and other entities are required to use the data bank to obtain information about practitioners they seek to license, hire, or grant clinical privileges (American Dental Association, 1990). Physicians view the establishment of the data bank as further erosion of their dominance regarding their ability to police themselves.

The ability of physicians to control their income autonomously continues to decrease. As Diagnosis Related Groups (DRGs) radically changed hospital reimbursement in the 1980s, physicians will witness dramatic changes in direct reimbursement in the 1990s. Medicare's physician payment reform plan, known as the resource-based relative value system (RBRVS), will significantly redistribute income among physician specialties and across geographic locations (Rhodes, 1991). Based on Prospective Payment Commission approaches, specialists in thoracic surgery may witness a 20 percent income drop, whereas family practice specialists may reap a 38 percent gain (Rhodes, 1991, p. 64).

Dr. Martin Merry has compared the typical physician's emotional reaction to this changing environment to Kübler-Ross's denial and anger stages of the death and dying process (Merry, 1990, p. 102). Many physicians argue that physicians should become more proactive within their environment. Through involvement in the policy decisions that produce changes in the healthcare delivery system, physicians will retain control and influence over patient care and retain the ability to practice the "art" of medicine (Merry, 1990, p. 104). Total Quality may provide the venue wherein physicians will have the opportunity to play a primary role in addressing the external pressures within their practice environment. However, many physicians remain highly skeptical of Total Quality efforts.

During the late 1980s, impressive results were achieved in the healthcare industry when Total Quality techniques were applied to administrative services or other processes which support patient care (Berwick, Godfrey, and Roessner, 1990; Kratochwill and Gaucher, 1991). However, only a few organizations, such as Intermountain Health Care in Salt Lake City, Utah, and the Harvard Community Health Plan in Brookline, Massachusetts, successfully applied quality improvement principles to clinical practices and direct patient care (Clark, 1991; Berwick, Godfrey, and Roessner, 1990, pp. 186–190). Most Total Quality initiatives have focused on either administrative processes or clinical care exclusively. Total Quality approaches span both the clinical and service components of an organization. In healthcare, administrative services that support direct patient care benefit directly from the successful application of principles learned in service industries such as overnight delivery (Federal Express) and utilities (Florida Power and Light). Viewing the actual care of patients with similar medical diagnoses as a clinical process is a relatively new concept as compared to the traditional medical model of looking at each patient as a unique clinical interaction. To reach its fullest potential, Total Quality must be an integrated, continuous process involving all employees and clinical staff in an effort to improve continuously all products, services, and transactions (GOAL/QPC, 1992). The process cannot be "total" without the involvement of everyone in the organization. The challenge, then, is to involve everyone in the organization. As clinical and service Total Quality approaches evolve in healthcare, the ultimate goal will be the simultaneous application and integration of both models. External pressures from payers, patients, and the government, and, more important, pressure to survive in an uncertain environment make this integration crucial.

Barriers to Physician Involvement

Physicians such as Paul Batalden, Donald Berwick, Brent James, and Glenn Laffel were early pioneers in the quality improvement movement in healthcare. In contrast to most of the early quality initiatives, each of these physicians led quality improvement efforts focused on clinical practice and patient care. These early physician champions were able to understand the various roles a physician assumes in healthcare delivery and were able to appeal to physicians' inherent interest in healthcare quality (Berwick, 1989, p. 56; Laffel and Blumenthal, 1989, pp. 2872–2873).

One of the most commonly asked questions at national quality conferences is, "How do you get the physicians involved?" Table 7.1 summarizes a number of techniques that have been utilized to influence physician behavior. Although physician involvement and support for quality improvement efforts initiated by administration have increased significantly over the last few years, there is still resistance to Total Quality efforts among physicians. For example, the American Medical Association recently voted down a proposal to endorse TQM principles at a July 1991 policy meeting (McCormick, 1991, p. 5).

However, many external organizations are beginning to recognize that TQM is a philosophy that will help hospitals and physicians align themselves to meet better the changing customer expectations of the 1990s. Dennis O'Leary, president of JCAHO, states that the 1993 and 1994 JCAHO standards will "require" that hospitals demonstrate continuous improvement throughout the organization (O'Leary, 1991, pp. 13–14). There is emerging recognition by professional organizations that TQM is not a program but a structured and continuous process of improvement for the entire organization (Joint Commission on Accreditation of Healthcare Organizations, 1991b).

Healthcare leaders attempting to gain physician support and involvement in quality improvement efforts have often

Table 7.1. Impact of Strategies Designed to Change Physician Behavior.

Strategy	Level of Impact on Physician Behavior (High, Medium, Low)	Degree of Intrusiveness on Clinical Autonomy (High, Medium, Low)
1. Formal Education This strategy involves department presentations, grand round presentations, outside speakers, and formal CME seminars.	Low to Medium	Low
2. Information and Decision Support Systems Development This strategy involves the development of clinical algorithms and "critical path" models of care that are clinically meaningful to physicians	Medium to High	Medium to High
3. Provider Specific Comparisons a. Patterns of resource utilization b. Outcomes comparisons	High High	Medium Medium
4. Identifying and Supporting Peer Opinion Leaders This strategy involves identifying and supporting the education of physician "peer opinion leaders." These clinicians informally encourage interest among clinical staff through their daily work.	Medium to High	Low
5. Hospital or Medical Group (HMO) Rules for Utilization of Resources.	High	High
6. Regulatory Rules a. Peer review organizations b. Licensure c. Recertification	Medium	High
7. Third-Party Payer Rules a. Policy/coverage limits b. Reimbursement levels	High	High

failed to appreciate the changing nature of the physician-patient-organizational relationship. In their fervor to achieve the successes gained in administrative areas, administrators have offered TQM as an answer to the physician's frustrations with the current healthcare system. Yet physicians have already been subjected to other quality efforts that have offered little help to the practice of the individual physician. Table 7.2 summarizes physician reactions to common administrator appeals for Total Quality based on the experience of previous efforts that were established as a result of public scrutiny of the healthcare system.

Pleas from a healthcare leader asking physicians to reduce costs have tended to fall on deaf ears. Until provided evidence to the contrary, most physicians believe they are practicing "good" medicine. Many believe cost cutting will harm patients. The best ways to gain physician attention involve the use of appropriate and clinically meaningful data collection. Attempts to collect this data by DRG, for example, normally resemble financial reports with little hint as to what clinical response might be suggested. Intermountain Health Care has addressed this problem in a pioneering approach. Dr. Brent James and his staff at Intermountain analyze procedures in terms of "units of care." A unit of care is the smallest detailed item on a patient's bill, such as a single dose of a drug, one lab test, or a minute in surgery. Patients with comorbidities or those with poor outcomes are removed from the analysis. Through this approach, a consistent and comparable patient pool is analyzed and data can be compared across physician groups to see how many units of care were required to achieve the same positive outcome (Clark, 1991). A recent book published by the American Hospital Association discusses various techniques for using data to trigger behavior change in physicians (American Hospital Association, 1991).

By taking an approach similar to Intermountain's, but modified for the individual institution, a healthcare organization can begin to identify problematic areas (e.g., wide variation in ancillaries ordered for a similar patient cohort by disease grouping and length of stay). Unfortunately, the keys to chang-

Table 7.2. Physician Reactions to Total Quality.

What Administrators Advocating TQM Say	*What Physicians Hear and How They React*
• TQM is *different* from traditional QA. It focuses on improving processes rather than a "bad apple" approach.	• TQM is QA in different clothing.
• TQM emphasizes examining and improving systems rather than focusing on outliers.	• TQM is applicable to administrative systems and industrial processes, not the clinical care of individual patients.
• TQM suggests that in controlled systems, patient care can be standardized appropriately and therefore produce higher quality and efficiency by reducing variation.	• Patient care cannot be standardized like industrial processes; TQM is a further encroachment on the individual physician-patient relationship.
• TQM uses the scientific method to improve processes.	• We have always used the scientific method—this is nothing new.
• TQM will enable physicians to take a proactive role in affecting changes that influence clinical care.	• TQM will result in more committee meetings for time-constrained physicians.
• Multidisciplinary teams of all who are involved in the process are the foundation of TQM efforts.	• TQM will wrest control of the patient care process from the physician.
• "More is *not* better." TQM is a structured process to reduce rework, duplication, and inappropriate utilization.	• TQM is another cost-cutting mechanism by administration that will limit access to resources I need for my patients.

ing physician or any other human behavior are not always straightforward. However, most physicians will respond positively to data that is accurately collected and presented in a nonthreatening, understandable way that correlates with the actual clinical decisions made. Improved methods for collecting and reporting "physician profiling" data need to evolve. Based on the experience of earlier efforts to gain active physician involvement in quality functions and administrative cost-cutting efforts, physician resistance is understandable.

Action Step: Research successful clinical information systems that focus on physician resource utilization rather than costs across relatively homogeneous patient populations. Support a physician advocate who will investigate the steps your organization must take to implement such a system and encourage the participation of the medical staff.

One of the most obvious barriers to overcome is the perception by physicians that TQM is not different from what they have been doing for years. Managing by fact based on data is the core of the quality improvement process. Physicians already use the scientific method in patient care and research. TQM emphasizes identifying root causes and practicing self-correction rather than the traditional focus on the inspection, which has been the foundation of externally mandated quality assurance. Educating physicians about the differences between quality assurance and continuous quality improvement is crucial to reducing skepticism. Pioneers at Brigham and Women's Hospital in Boston are pursuing opportunities to collaborate with the Harvard Medical School to introduce quality management theory to medical students (Laffel, 1990). Similarly, students at Case Western Reserve University in Ohio are involved in workshops that compel them to examine the costs and variation of their practice decisions and determine ways in which care can be improved (Wigton, 1992; Headrick and others, 1992).

Research suggests that although physician fees represent 20 percent of healthcare costs, their decisions impact 80 percent of the expenditures (Eisenberg, 1986, p. 3; Gibson, Waldo, and Levitt, 1983; Wilensky and Rossiter, 1983). As a result, healthcare leaders advocate that active physician involvement in an organization's quality improvement efforts will translate into immediate cost savings at the bottom line. However, many of the systems and components that contribute to the 80 percent of healthcare expenditures are *not* within the control of physicians. Physicians assume the dominant role as the decision maker in the healthcare process. Their decisions, which guide nursing care, the ordering of diagnostic tests, and ancillary services, are made at the level of the individual physician. Yet once the decision is

made, the systems and processes that produce the results desired by the physician are within the control of healthcare
management. Despite healthcare leaders' continuous improvement efforts applied to these systems and processes, physicians
control the utilization of these components. For example,
healthcare managers may improve the processes for the ordering, administration, and reporting of results for pre-operative
tests. If unnecessary tests are ordered to begin with, then the
improved system is simply providing unnecessary tests more
quickly and efficiently. Unless physicians initiate a quality improvement effort to examine the appropriate use of pre-
operative tests, then the improvement efforts in administration
will never reach their full potential. In order to establish an
integrated administrative/clinical Total Quality Process, administrators must recognize the various roles the physician assumes
in the patient care process and apply approaches properly
designed to address each role.

Total Quality and the Roles of the Physician

Just as in the TQM process a single individual functions as both
customer and supplier at different points in time, the physician
acts in more than one role in healthcare delivery, as illustrated
in Figure 7.2. Physicians frequently perform "pure" administrative duties. Examples include committee functions as well as
interactions with scheduling, admitting, and other hospital departments. While these activities certainly impact patient satisfaction (delays, etc.), they are not at the crux of the physician-
patient interaction. Physicians' objections to participation in
the Total Quality Process at this level relate mainly to the time
consumed by frequent meetings that may be required by the
process.

Another more specifically administrative physician function is administration within an individual clinical department.
The current atmosphere within clinical departments may vary
depending on whether the hospital is dominated by physicians
on a medical school faculty, hired by the hospital itself, or
completely independent private practitioners. Physician educa-

Figure 7.2. Continuum of Physician Roles in the Patient Care Process.

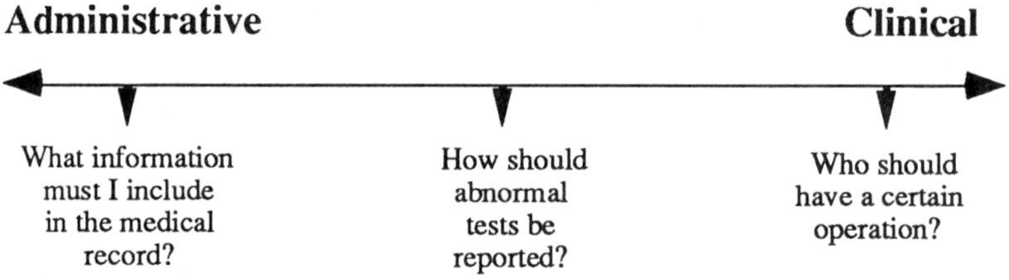

Administrative   **Clinical**

What information must I include in the medical record?	How should abnormal tests be reported?	Who should have a certain operation?

tion, training, and socialization encourage autonomy and independence. On the surface, this seems contradictory to the participative and team-oriented approaches of service-oriented quality improvement processes. To the superficial observer, an obvious hierarchy of chairman, associate chairman, section heads, president, executive committee, etc. pervades most physician working groups and organizations. However, staff physicians are not necessarily pliable and responsive to even their own administrative structure. Physicians are selected for medical school based on superior intellectual capabilities as demonstrated through undergraduate performance, medical school entrance exams, and the medical school application and interview process. They have been further trained to be independent and intellectually skeptical. Finally, they have survived an extremely competitive and emotionally challenging training program that normally provides little nurturing. However, by the very nature of their choice to enter medicine, most of these individuals wish to achieve and maintain a secure and dominant place in their society. For this reason, most physicians, while fighting fiercely for their point of view, will do so within the preexisting internal and external social and political hierarchy. From this standpoint, physician organizations, while made up of very powerful groups of individuals, are not always particularly effective at group efforts, tend toward contentiousness and defensiveness, and often lack a defined focus or consensus upon which all would agree.

TQM is composed of a balance between human dynamics or group-process skills and quantitative management tools and techniques. Physician reactions to each component of TQM may be different. Many physicians recognize their dearth of administrative training, but many are so used to assuming the dominant role that they are not by nature "team players." Physicians are trained to act as an advocate for the best interest of the patient during the process of care in order to ensure the best possible clinical outcome. Physicians are often more interested in positive outcomes gained through various diagnostic and treatment techniques rather than the efficiency of the entire process. Consequently, process-oriented thinking often seems antithetical to typical physician thinking and training. The idea of empowerment of others (decision making and problem solving by and with the people affected) is also foreign to the traditionally hierarchical and highly individualistic physician style. Physicians understand the analytical tools and techniques inherently, but have rarely been exposed to the human dynamics philosophy or found these skills applicable to their clinical work.

Perhaps the greatest challenge for those who believe that TQM should be implemented throughout the healthcare delivery system rests in the physician's role as direct care giver. In this role, the physician investigates patient complaints, physical findings, and test results in order to define better the problem and its root cause (diagnosis). The physician then determines and assigns options (treatment) and evaluates results (follow-up visits). The medical practice model is very similar to the seven-step quality improvement process, as illustrated in Figure 7.3. Note the absence of a stabilization or "Apply to Workplace" step, or a step including consideration of how improvements can be extended to other areas, in the traditional physician methodology. This comparison, based on the UMMC Quality Roadmap model, can also be drawn with Walter Shewhart's P-D-C-A cycle (see Table 7.3). The biggest issue linking the Total Quality Process with efforts to provide quality healthcare in a more cost-effective way revolves around this "stabilization" step and the extension to other areas. Research by John Wennberg suggests that the degree of variation that results among physicians treating different patients with the same diagnosis can be extreme in differing geographic areas, between specialists, by age of physi-

Figure 7.3. Medical Practice Model Compared to
Quality Improvement Process.

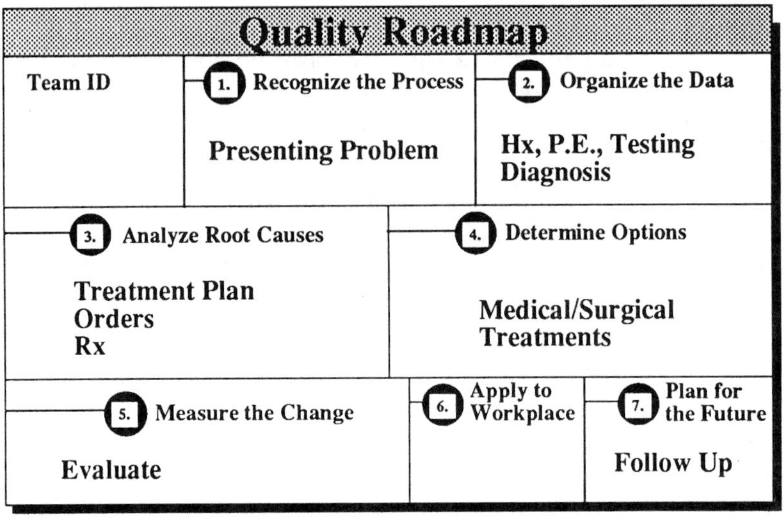

Quality Roadmap		
Team ID	**1. Recognize the Process** **Presenting Problem**	**2. Organize the Data** **Hx, P.E., Testing** **Diagnosis**
3. Analyze Root Causes **Treatment Plan** **Orders** **Rx**		**4. Determine Options** **Medical/Surgical** **Treatments**
5. Measure the Change **Evaluate**	**6. Apply to Workplace**	**7. Plan for the Future** **Follow Up**

cian, and even by the type of insurance (Wennberg, Barnes, and Zubkoff, 1982; Wennberg and Gittelsohn, 1973, 1975, 1982). The reduction in unnecessary variation is a foundation of TQM. Techniques to reduce clinical variation are evolving and are discussed later in this chapter.

TQM methodology provides an excellent vehicle for beginning the necessary standardization of care to reduce the

Table 7.3. Parallels Between P-D-C-A Cycle and Scientific Method.

Plan-Do-Check-Act Cycle	Scientific Method
• PLAN what to do. Set goals and indicators.	• OBSERVE symptoms. Generate HYPOTHESES.
• DO. Implement plans and see how they work.	• DESIGN and IMPLEMENT care plans.
• CHECK results by measurement.	• MONITOR results.
• ACT to improve the process based on the analysis of implementation results.	• OBSERVE symptoms. Generate HYPOTHESES.

Adapted from Laffel, 1990.

amount of rework and unnecessary steps in diagnosing and treating patients. Through the appropriate application of Total Quality, it is possible that billions of dollars of unnecessary medical costs could be saved (Wennerker, Weissman, and Epstein, 1990; "Better Safe Than Sorry...," 1992, p. B3).

Unfortunately, life is rarely as simple as we would like it to be. Physicians have been trained to look at each patient as an individual. In addition, diseases are biological processes with a great deal of inherent variation and uncertainty. Thus, while an idealized algorithm for care or pathway can be ascribed, attempts to standardize may be foiled by deviations from the norm required by the human condition. Many physicians are reluctant to attribute variations in length of stay, for example, to their individual clinical decisions.

Physicians have been subjected to numerous external efforts to standardize care. The two most visible are the entire malpractice system and the existing quality assurance and utilization review structures. For most physicians, these structures are associated with a great deal of pain. Most reviews of physician decisions have been attempts to cut costs under the guise of maintaining "quality." Physicians' natural skepticism and suspicion are thus aroused when the Total Quality Process seeks to look at their decisions. For physicians, the direct patient interactions and resultant decisions are sacrosanct territory. There has been no successful precedent of an external intervention that has truly resulted in physician support. Thus the challenge for advancing the Total Quality Process more into the physician arena is, first, to show that the process has something to offer and, second, to have the physicians themselves accept the idea that standardization of care and reduction of variation is a goal worthy of their attention. Finally, a proven methodology that results in consensus and then variation reduction needs more development.

John Eisenberg (1986) has analyzed physician motivation and described three broad categories: physician as self-fulfilling practitioner, as patient agent, and as guarantor of social good. Clearly, emphasizing the issues of social good such as costs, patient satisfaction, and outcomes research are consistent with

TQM. Yet the physician is often pressured to provide more rather than less care to patients. For example, patients often hear of procedures and/or tests in the media. If their physician is perceived as not knowledgeable or capable regarding the newest and latest technology or procedure, the physician may lose the patient's confidence. It is also likely that the patient may seek another physician if not satisfied (Pellegrino, 1987). In a malpractice suit, the plaintiff's attorney looks at an individual case, no matter how unusual the event, and tries to assign blame to the physician's decisions so that the case can qualify for remuneration regardless of the causes. The physician's response may be to order numerous tests on individual patients in order to protect himself or herself (that is, defensive medicine). Reducing the number of tests ordered through standardization can produce more physician anxiety. The benefits of standardization of care must be emphasized.

The issue of variation and attempts to standardize care are at the crux of TQM as it affects physicians in their role of direct care givers. Current internal monitors exist in diverse areas such as quality assurance, infection control, risk management, patient-staff relations, and utilization review. These activities are mandated and are reactive more to external regulators than reflective of potential areas of improvement identified by the physicians themselves. The techniques have emphasized the search for the "bad" doctor rather than looking at superior models of healthcare provision, juxtaposing the whole group, and seeking improvement of all physicians (Berwick, 1989). In addition, the idea that care that results in the same outcome but costs less is to be preferred has rarely been evaluated or emphasized. For physicians to seek energetically to provide more cost-effective healthcare, disincentives like malpractice, extra time consumption, and increased uncertainty must be addressed, while incentives should continue to be sought for those physicians who practice bearing costs in mind.

Classical continuous improvement models emphasize evaluating the stability of a process as a critical first step. Clearly, due to the combination of the inherent biological variation associated with a patient and his or her disease process, and the differing therapeutic and diagnostic decisions made by the physicians, much clinical care has been an unstable process. However, by separating the variation that can be ascribed to the physician's decision from the uncontrollable biological variation, one can create a stable process for analysis and improvement. Various techniques for stabilizing the processes of care have evolved. Many hospitals have analyzed such data elements as resource utilization by individual physician by DRG. This kind of information can be difficult to translate into clinically significant terms by the physician who receives it. Critical pathways show the "critical" components of care that must occur in a predictable manner to encourage timely care without waste, for example, unnecessary length of stay (Zander, 1987, p. 1; Coffey and others, 1992). The paths are generally fairly complex, noting the progression of incidents such as consults, diagnostic tests, patient activity, diet, medications, and discharge planning. While paths have been developed commercially, in most instances they require local construction or modification in order to achieve consensus. Although time-consuming to complete, when finished they result in a more stable process and coordinate care across departmental lines. The development of these pathways has evolved most frequently through departments of nursing.

A second approach toward stabilizing care utilizes clinical algorithms or guidelines against which physicians can compare their diagnostic and therapeutic decisions. Algorithms have existed for years, but little attempt to achieve consensus has ensued whether at the local hospital, regional, or national level. The Agency for Health Care Policy and Research has funded attempts to create national guidelines for the evaluation and treatment of pain, incontinence, and other conditions. However, dissemination and use at the local level remains a challenge. Getting groups of physicians to agree on "best practice" and monitoring compliance is an excellent approach to stabilizing processes to allow for further improvement.

Alternatively, the process of caring for a specific condition can be analyzed to find the "key process" or processes which, if followed *all* the time, will have major impact on quality and cost. One can then focus resources more effectively on the key areas than with the more extensive pathway or guideline. For example, at LDS Hospital in Salt Lake City, Utah, a team of physicians examined the timing of administration of prophylactic antibiotics and the risk of surgical wound infection. The team discovered wide variation in the timing of administration; some physicians administered antibiotics more than two hours prior to surgery and some greater than ten hours following the incision in surgery. Through data analysis and team consensus, the team agreed on the optimal time to administer the antibiotics. The team reduced the infection rate from 1.8 percent to 0.4 percent and saved the institution $462,000 in the first year (Classen, Evans, and Pestotnik, 1992).

Action Step: Support the development of methodologies to stabilize the processes of care within your institution. Engage the physicians in the development and approval of the selected techniques.

As physicians act to stabilize or standardize processes of care, the resultant reduction in variation can achieve major benefits. Hospital personnel will have a more clearly defined concept of what needs to be done for an individual patient. In teaching hospitals, the information acts as an educational tool for the constantly rotating physicians in training and can reduce error and the use of unnecessary resources. Patients benefit from having a better idea of exactly what will happen and when. When properly utilized, the result can be a natural patient education tool. In situations where appropriate practice parameters have been agreed upon, they provide an excellent defense against any outside review, up to and including malpractice litigation. Attention to the issue of documenting patient care situations that wander off the prescribed path must be considered. For institutions interested in clinical research, stabilized care protocols prepare "laboratories" for research regarding changes in outcome that result from altering the type of care rendered, as in new drug testing. The final anticipated benefit remains *better care for the patient*. The following is a summary of the benefits of stabilizing processes of care at an individual medical center or even physician office.

- Physicians in training learn a recommended system of care. This reduces avoidable errors that often occur during house staff rotation.
- Enhances patient education. Patients have a clearer expectation and understanding of what is happening to them.
- Improved documentation and performance when responding to outside review, including regulatory, managed care contracts, and medico-legal issues.
- Prepares a natural laboratory for potential clinical research.
- Allows for more consistent benchmarking with other organizations to share ideas to improve care.
- Consistent with efforts to establish national clinical guidelines.
- Hospital personnel have a plan of action for care, and physicians are called less frequently for routine care decisions. The entire patient care team's time is used more effectively.
- Better patient care!

Action Step: Discuss and distribute the benefits of the stabilization of care with physicians and other clinical providers.

Physician Involvement in TQM at UMMC

During 1987 Total Quality concepts were introduced at UMMC. In a comprehensive presentation to all of the clinical chairmen, industrial examples were chosen from other industries that had developed mature TQM cultures. As Ann Arbor, Michigan, is only an hour away from the auto capital of the United States, Detroit, the efforts of the Ford Motor Company were discussed. Immediately it was apparent that the physician audience was skeptical of the use of an industrial model, specifically one from the ailing auto industry based in southeast Michigan. Unfortunately, one of the most influential chairmen also shared his experiences about a "lemon" he had recently purchased from Ford.

This experience relates the first and most significant barrier we faced in efforts to encourage physician involvement — their skepticism of industrial models. No proven success stories from healthcare were available at the time. However, nearly five years after the beginning of the National Demonstration Project, Total Quality success stories in healthcare are more frequently being told throughout the country. Specifically, examples of improved direct patient care as well as the processes that directly affect patient care are beginning to emerge from places as diverse as HCA West Paces Ferry Hospital in Atlanta, Georgia, and the United States Naval Hospital in San Diego, California. In addition, evidence of successful clinical quality improvement efforts are beginning to appear more frequently in the scientific and medical literature (Joint Commission on Accreditation of Healthcare Organizations, 1991b, p. 7; Kritchevsky and Simmons, 1991; Berwick, 1989). The American Hospital Association recently published a book that summarizes the experiences of leaders who pioneered the successful application of TQM to the American healthcare system (Melum and Sinioris, 1992).

Action Step: Expose clinical staff to successful working clinical models in healthcare. Link examples of improvements in other processes with enhancements in patient care quality.

In June 1988 the Total Quality Council at UMMC was formed. The council consisted of managers and physicians who were interested in Total Quality and supported the work of the early QITs. Although physicians were involved in these early planning stages, few participated or expressed interest in pilot QITs. However, the pilot team in the operating rooms had a strong physician supporter of Total Quality at the Medical Center. This team accomplished its goal of reducing cancellations and delays and improved operating room turnaround time to allow for incremental procedures without adding capacity.

In an effort to focus institutionwide coordination of the Total Quality process, the Corporate Lead Team was formed in July 1990. Membership on the Corporate Lead Team included senior management staff, the chief of nursing affairs, the chief of

clinical affairs, the chairs of medicine, surgery, and anesthe-
siology, and an associate dean of the Medical School. Although
the physician leadership was actively involved in planning the
rollout of Total Quality throughout the institution, active physician participation in actual QITs remained minimal. Physician
leadership supported implementation in administrative and
support services areas, but clinical chairmen did not encourage
associate chairs or attending staff to attend team leader training
or participate on teams. In addition, the chairmen did not
incorporate TQM techniques into the departments they over-
saw. However, early in 1991 the leadership of the university itself,
including the university president and vice provost for health
affairs, began taking an active interest in TQM. Several of the
major academic and administrative units in the university began implementing TQM.

In April 1991 the vice provost for medical affairs, dean of
the Medical School, and hospital executive director sponsored a
chairmen's retreat on Total Quality. All of the clinical chairmen,
as well as section and division heads, attended. Along with
presentations by the vice provost and the dean, Brent James
presented clinical examples from Intermountain Health Care,
and successful QITs presented stories of their work and results.
Included in the team presentations was an example from the
operating rooms team, which demonstrated results of improved
utilization of physician time through improved scheduling. The
team also helped enhance revenue for the surgical and anesthe-
siology departments. Such examples helped demonstrate that
quality improvement efforts in administrative areas could have a
direct effect on physician practice and patient care. This retreat
enhanced the awareness of clinical chairmen and provided evidence to them that Total Quality was applicable to healthcare.

At the end of the day, the clinical chairmen brainstormed
ideas and issues for potential Quality Improvement Teams in the
clinical areas. The chairmen generated nearly one hundred
ideas. From this list, the chairmen multivoted down to three
priority issues to be pursued as pilot clinical quality improvement efforts. These teams serve as the foundation for the
Clinical Quality Improvement (CQI) initiative.

Action Step: Explore methods for identifying issues of concern among the physicians in your organization. Investigate the potential of investigating these issues through pilot *Clinical* Quality Improvement Team efforts.

The Clinical Quality Improvement Initiative

The CQI initiative at UMMC began in July 1991. It seeks to encourage the appropriate application of Total Quality tools and techniques in clinical areas. A Clinical Quality Improvement Lead Team (CQILT), analogous to a Divisional Lead Team, was formed to plan, implement, and support Total Quality efforts in the clinical areas. The mission of the CQILT is given in Exhibit 7.1.

Action Step: Establish a team of interested clinicians to encourage the appropriate application of TQM in clinical areas. Select visible and realistic pilot efforts supported by the clinical leadership for pilot clinical teams to explore. Provide appropriate administrative support to ensure the success of these efforts.

Exhibit 7.1. Mission Statement of the UMMC Clinical Quality Improvement Lead Team.

- The Clinical Quality Improvement Lead Team (CQILT) will foster the development of approaches for improving the efficiency and enhancing the quality of care at the Medical Center as part of an overall effort to achieve excellence in research, teaching, and patient care.
- The CQILT will achieve its objectives by promoting the appropriate application of the principles of Total Quality to clinical practice at the Medical Center.
- The CQILT will coordinate clinical and administrative efforts to maximize overall institutional quality and efficiency.
- The CQILT will select and prioritize team projects; establish teams; support, reward, and recognize teams; and monitor and evaluate project and team progress.
- The CQILT will strive to accomplish significant and measurable improvement over the next three years.

Source: University of Michigan Hospitals, Ann Arbor.

The pilot themes selected by the chairmen serve as a major part of the CQI initiative. These teams will utilize the UMMC seven-step quality improvement process. In addition, the CQILT selected five issues for teams to explore using a different approach. These teams will use a quality improvement process developed by Leon Wyszewianski, a professor in the Department of Health Services Management and Policy at the University of Michigan School of Public Health. Both types of teams are led by physicians and are comprised of physicians, nurses, and Total Quality facilitators and have other appropriate administrative support. Both approaches are being supported to define better a model that will be successful for teams with predominantly physician membership.

The Clinical Improvement Team process is analogous to the UMMC seven-step process described in detail in Chapter Eight yet contains some significant differences. In contrast to QITs, Clinical Improvement Teams meet less frequently, have strong staff support, and dissolve once the strategies to address the issue in question are successfully implemented. Staff assigned to the effort met with clinicians and managers who were the "owners" of the processes and systems that were affected by the issues identified. Data and information were collected in order to prevent rework of previous efforts as well as to protect against overlap with current initiatives in the departments. In most cases, these clinicians and managers became members of the team. This work served a second and more important purpose. When staff met for the first time with physicians leading the Improvement Teams, significant amounts of data and information were available to answer questions and provide a foundation for the start of the team. Prior to the first meetings of these teams, members are sent data and information with the expectation that they would be reviewed before the meeting. Through a less structured process, the team identifies a specific and solvable issue, determines clear clinical criteria and standards related to the issue in question, and designs a strategy for implementing the strategy throughout the institution (Wyszewianski, 1991). Team members also become advocates for the strategy during and following its implementation.

As physician knowledge about the Total Quality Process has progressed, a multifaceted educational approach has evolved. While some have argued that physicians should be trained like anyone else, more expeditious training sessions have been devised to supplement the more time-consuming programs. Most recently the approach has been to prepare a training session of one and a half hours that includes both philosophy and discussion of the actual management tools and process. This material is then presented to preexisting physician groups and committees, usually at their request. An education piece is also included in team training within the above-described CQI initiative. More intensive training is provided as techniques are used in the process. In addition, a newsletter emanating from the Office of Clinical Affairs under the auspices of the preexisting quality assurance program will be used to update the rest of the clinical faculty about the interaction of quality assurance with the Total Quality physician effort. These first efforts have been carefully chosen to provide a fair opportunity for the new institutional techniques.

Action Step: Develop a curriculum sensitive to physicians' unique time constraints. Shorten the training sessions to education in key concepts.

UMMC is currently exploring further strategies to encourage physician efforts in clinical quality and efficiency beyond formal team efforts. Successful critical paths have been developed in thoracic surgery, neurology, and other services. During the next year, other inpatient units will be aggressively developing critical paths in a concerted effort to establish clinically appropriate standards of care for similar patients. Additionally, clinical and administrative leadership are considering supporting a hospital-funded "small grants" program to fund clinical studies that examine innovative approaches to patient care that enhance quality and/or improve efficiency. The model being considered is analogous to one developed at Strong Memorial Hospital at the University of Rochester, Rochester, New York (Franklin, Panzer, Brideau, and Griner,

1990). Funds will cover direct costs, analytical support, and stipends for house staff or fellows, and may also be used to compensate for faculty time spent on the projects. Supporting a small grants project also provides physicians an opportunity to publish the results of their clinical studies. As a result, the hospital may enjoy increased quality and efficiency while the physician enhances professional recognition. Although this model seems most applicable to an academic medical center, experience at the University of Rochester has demonstrated that a hospital-funded small grants program can be successful in a community hospital environment as well (Panzer, Black, and Winchell, 1991, pp. 77–106).

Action Step: Establish a hospital-funded small grants program at your institution to fund innovative approaches to clinical practice. The program should have the full support of your clinical leadership. Provide necessary analytical, staff, and financial support to ensure the program's success.

Lessons Learned

The UMMC implementation of the Total Quality Process and methodologies began by reaching out from top leadership down through middle management to the employees at large. Because knowledge regarding the role of TQM in healthcare is more extensive today, we would not separate efforts along "administrative" and "clinical" areas if starting again. The distinction is arbitrary and can produce a program that focuses too heavily on success in either arena. Solving most problems in a hospital environment utilizing a TQM methodology requires the knowledge and participation of both administrative and clinical staff.

As experience with gaining the involvement of physicians at UMMC has evolved, the following observations can be made:

Leadership/support. The departmental chairmen have been engaged at the highest level of the Total Quality organizational structure, the Corporate Lead Team. Yet, of the four major physician groups represented, the amount of involvement has varied tremendously. Two of the departments are significantly committed, including training their physician managers in Team Leader training. A third department has a number of physicians leading and participating on teams, while the last has very few physicians involved or supportive of the effort. Despite this resistance, certain physicians in this department also work on teams. From an organizational standpoint, the designated physician leaders need to support the TQM effort or at least stay out of the way. However, the real work tends to be accomplished by the physicians closest to the problems, who may not be the chairmen of the departments.

The retreat concept worked well and did increase both awareness and support. Even physicians who did not attend seemed interested in finding out what occurred. Finally, trying to identify and support physician "champions" to provide leadership among the physicians has proved successful. Physicians tend to listen to another physician more than to an administrative manager or leader.

Teams. Not every problem needs to be dealt with by a team or a TQM tool. Some problems are not amenable, particularly if a quick decision must be reached. Remember that many good things were achieved before TQM arrived at the hospital. The selection of issues for physician teams to work on remains important, particularly at the outset. The UMMC physician teams evolved in three ways:

- Examples chosen at the retreat:
  - Coordination of multidisciplinary care
  - Facilitation of outpatient care: access, record keeping, scheduling, and teaching
- Examples chosen by the CQILT:
  - ICU utilization protocols
  - Extended use of home parenteral therapy
- Examples chosen because a physician came forward with his or her own ideas:
  - Pharmacokinetics: reducing inappropriate testing of therapeutic blood levels for four drugs
  - Central venous access: policy for appropriate utilization

A critique of the results achieved when the issues selected arose in these three ways reveals a number of lessons. The clinical leaders' retreat generated ideas that were so loosely defined that the teams found it difficult even to define the issue they were investigating. For example, the multidisciplinary care team struggled for the first few months to focus eventually on improving the inpatient consultation process. The other team has not gotten that far. The second group of teams has exposed different problems. While physician participation has been engaged, the teams generally have their own idea of what the issues and responses should be. The teams thus have ended up working on something very different from what was intended. The choice of a team leader has occasionally been problematic. The leader who agreed to evaluate increasing the use of outpatient and home-based parenteral therapy has acknowledged that such an increase would reduce reimbursement to that physician's department. The team has staggered rather than made rapid progress. As a result, the team will be exploring means to develop physician incentives to utilize the service as well. The teams started by physicians who came forward spontaneously with an idea of their own seemed to have progressed the most rapidly.

Action Step: Start a few clinical teams to gain visibility, then wait for physician ideas to come forward spontaneously. Avoid "world hunger" issues. Pick issues for which accessible and reliable data already exist.

Another suggestion regarding teams is to keep them small and respect physician time commitments. A group with a few committed physicians is preferable to a large group that is uninterested. Be very flexible about meeting times in order to accommodate physician members (e.g., two hours every two weeks rather than weekly). Consider having two physicians who work together act as a team and alternate their attendance. Agree on appropriate expectations to which the physicians can commit.

Training and education. We believe that specialized training material and techniques are necessary for physicians. They prefer information to be quickly dispensed, absorb concepts rapidly, and generally do well with more, rather than less, "just-in-time training." For the interested physician, the more rigorous week-long Team Leader training has been very well received. While much of the training can be accomplished through the training of team members as needed, persistent efforts are necessary to communicate the overall philosophical message across the physician groups within your organization. Remember that top-down communication does not always work with physicians. Bring information to the smaller physician groups and to their current communication structure (for example, grand rounds, departmental meetings). It is even beneficial to provide such information as readings and videotapes to individual physicians.

Develop methodology for stabilization/standardization of care processes. The whole concept of practice pattern analysis requires discussion and decisions as to the best method for the institution involved. In a community hospital, much of the approach revolves around collecting data regarding the performance of the individual physicians. At UMMC, given the interplay among the staff physicians and the rotation of the house staff, the approach has been aimed more specifically at the development of critical pathways and clinical guidelines. These efforts are more consistent with the culture and mission of an academic health center. They may be viewed as "cookbook medicine" and interfering with the individual practitioner at a community hospital. Defining a "key" process that can be improved may be more reasonable in the community setting than trying to define a whole algorithm of care that all the individual physicians will follow.

Encouraging Physician Participation, Leadership, and Support for TQ Efforts

The goal of bringing physicians actively into the Total Quality Process involves breaking down significant barriers. Many physicians are not only skeptical but simply do not feel they have the time to spend to learn new philosophies and techniques that do not appear to bear directly on patient care, research, and teaching. A clash exists between the culture that Total Quality seeks to create and that in which the physicians currently function. In application, TQM works best with the adaptation of new attitudes on the part of both the physicians and the people who work to support physician-patient interaction. The physician's decision to accept TQM principles and to change some aspect of patient care will determine the extent to which TQM will ultimately affect the healthcare system. This section will provide a summary framework of suggestions for achieving the elusive goal of gaining physician involvement.

We propose a four-step strategy to encourage the appropriate application of TQM in clinical areas through physician involvement and support. The steps are not discrete; rather, they are part of a continuous process to reinforce the benefits of TQM for improving clinical decision making, clinical care, and patient outcomes.

Step 1: Test the Environment

The first step, testing the environment, requires an organizational assessment of the readiness for TQM application in clinical areas. Most organizations initiate TQM in administrative and support services areas with the hope of integrating clinical efforts later. As mentioned earlier, we recommend that administrative and clinical TQM efforts be planned simultaneously. The points below outline some key activities to test the organization's readiness for clinical TQM efforts.

1. Assure the support of the CEO, COO, and, most important, the medical staff leaders about developing strategies for clinical TQM applications.

2. Assess the strength of the current hospital-medical staff relationship. If fundamental problems exist that are major points of contention for the medical staff, it is best to rectify

these problems prior to attempting to gain support for a new effort in the clinical areas.

3. Determine whether physicians on your staff are already proponents of TQM. Hold discussions with clinical chiefs, chairmen, or department heads to assess their interest and knowledge of TQM. Utilize interested clinical leaders to help you assess the readiness of your organization and to assist in developing strategies.

4. Brainstorm incentives that might encourage physician involvement in TQM. Finding incentives for physician involvement can be even more difficult than removing disincentives. The financial interests of the hospital and physician departments are not always mutual. Reduced length of stay for a given diagnosis may lead to hospital financial benefit but may lower physician reimbursement, such as the daily care fees collected by internists, and require that busy physicians labor harder and faster. Hospitals need to bear in mind the hardships brought on their physicians and the greater unreimbursed time commitments that may attend some cost/quality hospital efforts. Efforts that benefit both the hospital and its physicians are the best efforts. You can begin by finding out what issues are causing "pain" for your medical staff.

Step 2: Lay the Foundation

The goal of this step is to enhance the awareness of TQM's applicability to clinical care among the medical staff in your organization. As administrative and clinical leaders develop more knowledge of TQM applicability to clinical care, they must also begin to develop the strategies for the implementation of clinical teams and projects.

1. Prove it first. Several published examples of successful clinical TQM programs exist in the literature and are mentioned in this chapter. Gather these articles for use in presentations and communications to clinical staff. Useful references are

also provided at the end of this book. Avoid using outside speakers or literature until they have been screened for contents that might alienate your more vocal physicians. Meet separately with those physicians whose opinions seem to carry influence among the clinical staff and ask them to assess the appropriateness of examples to be used in your institution.

2. Identify and support physician TQM champions. Ideally you should identify one or more respected and influential physicians who support TQM efforts and who will speak informally with peers as well as conduct presentations. Most physicians are accustomed to communicating through informal channels such as brief phone conversations or discussions in the corridor rather than through formal committees or memoranda. Although a formal physician awareness or education program is necessary, informal physician-to-physician dialogue and communication create the foundation for physician involvement. Credible physicians willing to speak out in favor of TQM will carry more influence than nonphysicians among physician groups.

3. Have physician TQM champions conduct introductory presentations at grand rounds and departmental meetings. Integrate updates about TQM efforts into medical staff newsletters and communications. Most organizations have found that given physician time constraints, it is best to utilize existing channels of communication within the medical staff.

4. Hold a retreat with clinical chairmen and department heads to enhance their awareness of TQM and its applications to clinical care. Invite physician speakers who can provide some success stories from their institutions. Bring data about problems that need improvement to facilitate discussion.

5. Interview your medical staff, especially the most clinically active physicians, to identify other issues for possible investigation by clinical teams. Collect data and information to verify their statements about problems prior to establishing a

formal quality improvement team. This strategy will help you identify issues that truly cause customer pain to your physician groups. By defining specific projects as employing TQM techniques, positive outcomes that are measurable and convincing should result.

6. Where possible, involve physicians on teams that are working to improve processes that impact physicians, yet do not threaten their clinical autonomy, in order to enhance awareness of the process. For example, a team examining ways to improve the turnaround time for radiology consults to a physician's office might include a radiologist and a surgeon. Through a team approach, the two groups could agree on their requirements and develop a system that meets both their needs.

Step 3: Develop the Support Structure and Environment

This step involves the actual implementation of pilot clinical TQM efforts. It is the most crucial step in the process since the organization will commit time, money, and other resources to supporting physician-led quality efforts. It is vital that the organization fully explore the feasibility of investigating the clinical initiatives proposed by the medical staff in Step 2. The credibility of the entire effort will rest on the success of the actual implementation and support of the early pilot efforts.

1. Establish a clinical TQM lead team to guide the effort. Ideally the team should consist of voluntary members who are physicians interested in improving the quality of clinical care, and who are influential, within your institution. To encourage coordination and reduce duplication of effort, some members of the team may be the team leaders of the pilot clinical efforts. Having the team leaders of the pilot teams as members will also help the members share their experiences with new team leaders later in the process when other physicians approach the lead team for support.

2. Have the clinical TQM lead team choose the themes for pilot efforts for investigation based on ideas initiated by the clinical staff and confirmed through data, where possible. The selection of pilot projects that are likely to be visible examples of the applicability of TQM to clinical care can be guided by criteria such as those listed in Exhibit 7.2.

3. Designate staff to work closely with the physician team leaders to support the efforts of the team. Support should include data collection and analysis, preparation of meeting minutes and agendas, and overall logistical support for the team.

4. If available in your organization, designate trained facilitators to work with the team leader to encourage the use of effective group-process techniques in pilot clinical team meetings.

5. Share updates on the clinical teams and their progress along the way. It will help you answer the common question: "How are the physicians involved?"

Exhibit 7.2. Criteria for Selection of Pilot Clinical Quality Improvement Efforts at UMMC.

1. *Impact* — How large an impact is the project likely to have on the Medical Center's clinical environment and financial status?
2. *Potential Clinical Advocates* — How likely is it that at least one influential and respected clinical leader will support the project?
3. *Consensus on Clinical Practice* — How great is the clinical consensus about the desirable practice patterns in this area?
4. *Probability of Success* — How likely is it that the changes made will be successfully implemented and maintained?
5. *Availability of Relevant Data About the Issue Under Consideration* — What is the likely availability of reliable and valid data about the key elements of the process for this project?
6. *Estimated Months to Complete the Effort* — How many months will the project take to complete?

Source: University of Michigan Hospitals, Ann Arbor.

Step 4: Integrate Ongoing Clinical TQM Efforts
with Current Hospital and Medical Structure

This step involves the integration of the clinical TQM effort as an ongoing component of clinical care and practice in your organization. The pilot clinical efforts provide the foundation for additional clinical teams and initiatives. At this stage, the clinical lead team should be the recognized forum for the discussion of clinical quality issues as well as the source for support for the study of clinical care and key clinical processes.

1. Encourage physicians to initiate additional clinical team efforts and initiatives. The success of carefully selected pilot studies will help communicate to the clinical staff that TQM is applicable to clinical care and practice. You may wish to revisit the list of initial ideas that you identified through interviews and informal discussions with other clinicians. It is also important to develop a mechanism that makes submitting ideas and proposals to your lead team convenient for your clinical staff.

2. Explore a means to develop training for physician office staff members in TQM. Invite the office clerks, nurses, and other staff from physician offices to participate in TQM teams that focus on relationships with community and referring physicians. For example, a team that seeks to improve the scheduling of operating rooms would benefit from the participation of staff from the office of a surgeon who performs a high number of procedures at your institution.

3. Revitalize your quality assurance efforts to focus on quality improvement, as described in Chapter Three. If the true measure of reaching physicians with the Total Quality message will be determined by the ability to improve processes that positively affect patient care level outcomes, then mechanisms to promote and support these activities must be constructed. Hospitals have already invested resources into departments of quality assurance and utilization review, which already deal with clinical data and physician decisions and behavior.

4. Establish a methodology for providing data to physicians about their clinical activity that can be compared with their peers. Provider-specific comparisons are one such tool to stabilize clinical care. However, the techniques utilized in presenting comparative information must be considered carefully. The data must be reliable, valid, and credible from the physician's perspective. In the past, physicians have been presented DRG variance data about length of stay and costs per DRG. Many physicians are skeptical of the coding of DRGs and their sensitivity to complications. As a result, attempts to change physician behavior using such data have often proved unsuccessful. Comparative data must also be adjusted for comorbidities and complications in a manner acceptable to the physician audience. More important, attention should be directed to the positive incentives physicians have to enhance quality of care rather than to a punitive approach. In other words, the approach should emphasize the process of care that yields the optimal clinical result as perceived by the physician. Physicians can then ask: "Can the process of care be improved or can utilization of resources be reduced while still producing the optimal clinical result?" Do not immediately look for poor performers but rather the optimal performers who can then be emulated. Look for key processes to improve within the hospital or critical decisions that most greatly impact resource utilization.

5. Explore the potential for establishing a small grants program at your institution to support innovative ideas for changes in clinical practice.

Conclusion

Strategies for gaining physician involvement in quality improvement are numerous. Yet the foundation for success of any of these strategies rests on the belief within physician groups that TQM is applicable to clinical processes and care. As a result, the key strategy utilized by nearly all organizations that have successfully implemented clinical efforts has been the identification and support of physician champions. In some organizations, the TQM efforts have been initiated by physicians. Healthcare organizations, however, must be sensitive to the increasing pressures facing the physician community in the 1990s. The wise healthcare organization will be asking for help with one hand while providing help for the physician with the other.

Chapter Eight

Teamwork

While teams and teamwork are the basic building blocks of the Total Quality Process, many organizations focus solely on the teams and forget that the culture has to change to support the effort. Teamwork can be productive only if the right climate exists. To build effective teams, barriers that prevent people from working effectively together must be removed. Whether the problems take the form of a nontrusting we/they environment or a control-oriented management group that wants to change but does not know how, issues must be identified and strategies developed to facilitate change or the transition will not occur. Throughout this chapter we will address ideas to help you prepare the environment for successful teamwork.

Multiple Benefits of Teamwork

There is almost universal agreement that teamwork leads to better ideas, improved job satisfaction, and improved organizational results. The current management literature is full of examples of how teamwork can achieve superior results (Parker, 1990; Aubrey and Felkins, 1988; Larson and LaFasto, 1989; Kanter, 1989b). The complexity of business today means no one person can have the answers to organizational success. To succeed, corporations must be creative and innovative with problem solving. The best way to enhance creative decision making is

217

to increase brainpower and use the minds of many to build synergy.

There are many benefits to teamwork. Teams functioning throughout the organization provide opportunities for learning and full participation of employees. Employee teams learn how the organization functions and how to get things done. Teams can:

- Improve productivity
- Encourage creativity
- Improve communication

- Enhance involvement
- Improve relationships
- Enhance problem solving

- Develop leadership potential
- Reduce errors
- Promote personal growth

Employee Involvement Enhances Cooperation

Quality Improvement Teams are established from groups of volunteers—those workers actually responsible for doing the work. It makes sense that the people involved in a particular job know it better than anyone else. Why not seek input from them to avoid, solve, and control problems and to improve the process overall? Total Quality gives workers an ability to gain control over their jobs, an opportunity that many have never experienced before, and the ability to help the organization improve overall. Exposing employees to the difficulties of problem solving also increases their understanding of the process and reduces the time it takes to resolve major issues. Another advantage of teams is that communications between managers and workers improve dramatically. Hidden talents of team members are recognized, and managers can put their abilities to full use. When teamwork is the mode of operation, people are involved, and involved people tend to resist change less. Involving people in the planning and design of change gives them the opportunity to think and solve problems, understand the plan, and develop a sense of ownership.

Critical Success Factors. Teamwork does not simply happen. Every group of people is not a team and every team is not effective. There are several critical factors that support team formation. The right culture must be created to support the work of the teams. This means teams should have adequate resources, the ability to implement decisions, the sponsorship of managers, and an effective reward and recognition system. The appropriate training materials and time for skill building must be available during team formation. A standard problem-solving process is also required to help the team stay on track. Finally, leadership commitment to support the team effort is essential for success. Other critical success factors were discussed in Chapter Five.

Teams Within Healthcare

Within healthcare we think we know all about teams. This attitude probably springs from the fact that healthcare teams save lives. Whether in the emergency department, the intensive care units, or the operating suite, healthcare professionals come together to meet patient care crises and save many lives through their teamwork. However, when the crisis is over, the professionals tend to retreat back to their own turf, to communicate effectively again only during the next patient crisis. Healthcare professionals do not communicate well about the day-to-day issues of the workplace. By professional discipline, our language and work patterns are different. When healthcare teams learn together, a new communication link evolves. A new language is learned by all participants and joint problem solving becomes easier. The cooperative behaviors learned in teamwork become the rule throughout the organization. During 1988 one team had lapel buttons made that said, "None of us is as smart as all of us." As one team member, whose job was related to billing, reported when her team addressed the UMMC Corporate Lead Team: "prior to the development of our team we didn't even speak to the clinical people except to blame them for problems. Today our goal is to anticipate what the other person might need in order to avoid quality problems. The TQP has made my job more enjoyable" (Grostick, 1991).

Types of Teams at UMMC

As our process evolved we developed a continuum of teams and quality improvement efforts. We began by emphasizing rather formally defined Quality Improvement Teams (QITs). But our long-term goal is for managers, physicians, and other staff to use Total Quality methods as a regular part of their daily work. We found that the strong emphasis on QITs was leading to an unintended feeling among some people in the organization that if you were not part of a formal QIT that you did not count. There was never an intention to convey this feeling, but when leadership establishes a priority of time and effort, people believe this priority is key. In addition, a continuing emphasis on only QITs will not accomplish the long-term goal of integrating TQM into daily work. Consequently, we have identified a continuum of quality improvement efforts, as illustrated in Figure 8.1, to express that there are several areas we need to be successful in. We have initiated efforts in all five areas, and are beginning to recognize formally all types of quality improvement efforts.

Action Step: Support and recognize a continuum of quality improvement efforts, not just formal Quality Improvement Teams.

   Quality Improvement Teams (QITs). The most formal group efforts are Quality Improvement Teams. At UMMC we have established five criteria to be designated a QIT. The team must have a trained team leader, trained team facilitator, follow our seven-step quality improvement process, meet regularly and frequently, and be approved by a Divisional Lead Team. Most

Figure 8.1. Continuum of Quality Improvement Teams and Efforts.

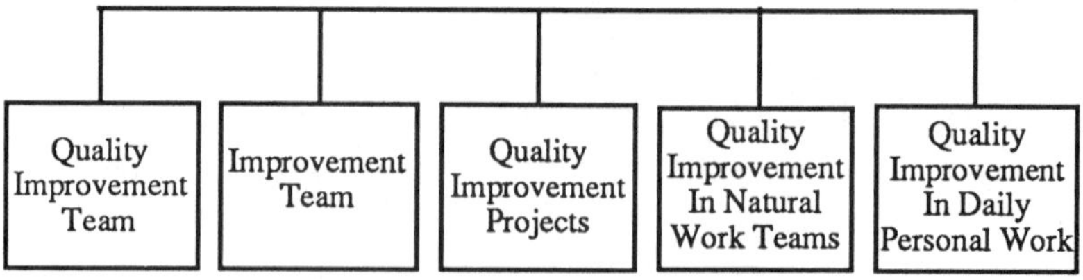

QITs meet weekly for an hour, although meeting every other week is acceptable if they meet for an hour and a half or more. We have found that teams do better if they meet frequently, especially if they are cross-functional teams. The QITs prepare their quality improvement story on storyboards or the equivalent in notebooks called story books.

Improvement Teams (ITs). Improvement Teams meet most, but not all, of the requirements for a Quality Improvement Team. The most common differences are that the teams do not use the seven-step QI process, or they lack a trained team facilitator. They tend to focus on a defined issue and disband when the problem is addressed. The same type of quality improvement process, tools, and techniques are used.

Quality Improvement Projects. A number of existing and new projects oriented to quality improvement are designated as quality improvement projects to reflect their dedication to quality improvement and their use of quality improvement tools and techniques. Sample quality improvement projects at UMMC are quality assurance projects; projects on critical path protocols of care; patient care skill-mix projects; and projects integrating clinical, utilization, and cost information to plan and evaluate clinician decisions, known as the UMMC Integrated Inpatient Management Model.

Quality Improvement in Natural Work Teams. We are evolving toward natural work teams using quality improvement methods to improve work processes and to meet customer requirements. These natural work teams may focus on processes within one department or processes that cross departments, known as cross-functional processes. A sophisticated model, called self-directed work teams, is taking place in three areas of the Medical Center. In this model the teams' employee involvement is the critical factor. Our first opportunity occurred two years ago when a manager left the organization. The nurse midwives decided to take the responsibility for staffing, scheduling, hiring, and evaluating work within their functional area. In 1992 the admitting department and activity therapy department developed models where the department director is team coordinator for a series of teams that manage the department. These teams use the tools and techniques of quality in daily work. We believe this model will continue to grow in our environment.

Quality Improvement in Daily Work. The long-term goal is that every manager, physician, and staff person thinks in terms of customers and continuous quality improvement, and uses the quality improvement vocabulary, tools, and techniques in all of his or her daily work. It will take years for this to occur, but we have seen increasing numbers of people using the vocabulary and tools and techniques in their conversations about daily work.

Within these different types of Quality Improvement Teams and efforts, there are other types of teams in our organization to differentiate the roles served by those teams:

Functional Teams. This type of team includes members from a single functional area. For example, a group of patient accounts clerks, who set up a team to look at the way telephone calls are answered, are part of a functional team. They are part of a natural work group. Membership on these teams is voluntary. Our experience has shown that it is easier to teach teams the process when they are working within a functional area. Trust levels are higher and defenses are lower. Once the tools and techniques are learned and team members understand their roles, cross-functional work is more effective. Less time is spent in turf guarding and blaming others for the problems.

Cross-Functional Teams. This type of team includes members from multiple functional areas. If a group of patient accounts employees wanted to study the process of billing end stage renal patients, they may wish to include on the team unit clerks, nurses, and physicians from the unit and patient accounts representatives internal and external to the system to look at the whole process. Membership on cross-functional teams is also voluntary.

Task Teams. Members from multiple functional areas study an improvement that cuts across departmental lines. These team members are assigned by lead teams because of their special knowledge or expertise. Their assignment is to solve a particular problem or group of problems or to find an opportunity for improvement. When the task is accomplished, the group is disbanded. For example, the development of our vision and value statement was accomplished by a task team that developed a series of focus groups to find out what type of values the organization should demonstrate in the 1990s. Task teams in our organization are also addressing such issues as how to manage a diverse workforce, how to stimulate employee involvement, and how to enhance rewards and recognition.

Lead Teams. These teams are the policy-setting teams that guide, direct, and support the quality improvement process. The key responsibilities of lead team members are to develop, review, and monitor the implementation plan for the Total Quality Process whether on a corporate or divisional basis, to support the existing teams, to sanction new teams, and to serve as role models and teachers of the quality improvement process. Multiple layers of lead teams may be necessary depending on the size of the organization. At UMMC our structure has evolved to include a Corporate Lead Team (CLT) consisting of top leadership, Divisional Lead Teams (DLTs) led by associate directors or vice presidential level executives, and Departmental and Local Lead Teams led by department heads as previously illustrated in Figure 5.10. We developed an organizational chart and then inverted it to emphasize the new focus on teams; the teams are at the top rather than at the bottom of the chart.

Selection Criteria for Teams

To be sanctioned as a Quality Improvement Team, a plan must be presented to the appropriate divisional lead team and accepted. A sample format we use is illustrated in Exhibit 8.1. This format is available on our electronic mail system, and can be pulled up, completed, and sent in a matter of minutes. If the idea is acceptable, a trained team leader and facilitator must be assigned to the team. Our model currently requires that a manager who has complete or partial responsibility for the process being studied must serve as team leader. This requirement is based on the concept that team members must see their suggestions implemented quickly, and the manager has the resources available to implement quickly without additional ap-

Exhibit 8.1. UMMC Total Quality Process Request for Initiation of QIT.

Statement of Problem(s) or Opportunity for Improvement
Data to Support Problem Exists: Yes, no, comments
Please explain how the problem impacts the process from the following
standpoints (UMMC quality goals):
- Quality of a product or service:
- Customer satisfaction:
- Working environment:
- Cost effectiveness:
- Competitive position:
Proposed Name and Title of Quality Improvement Team (QIT):
Proposed Team Leader: Name, job title, department, address, work phone.
Proposed QIT Members: For each give name, job title, department, address,
work phone.
Request Submitted by: Name, job title, department, address, work phone.
Request Endorsed by Management: For each manager supporting the pro-
posed project, give name, job title, department, address, work phone.

provals. The team leader then solicits volunteers for the team,
and the first meeting is scheduled. Many times during the beginning theme selection stage, the team may require new members.
This ensures that the key stakeholders for the process are involved. If several issues arise, new teams may be set up to deal
with the broader range of issues.

Review of the team's progress by the lead team occurs at
steps two, four, and seven in the quality improvement process
illustrated in Figure 8.2. This review allows team members the
opportunity to share what they have done and receive positive
feedback from the lead team. A note of caution before your first
management review: avoid unnecessary critique. Be sure your
senior leaders give appropriate feedback and do not focus on
finding fault during the presentation. By the time a team
reaches an information sharing point, the lead team should be
very familiar with the process the team is utilizing.

An important part of the review process is the Corporate
Lead Team (CLT) review. This review should occur when the
storyboard is complete. This is an excellent way to provide
reward and recognition to the teams. CLT members also can
learn firsthand about how the process is actually working and
some of the barriers teams are dealing with. It is hard for team

Figure 8.2. UMMC Seven-Step Quality Improvement Storyboard.

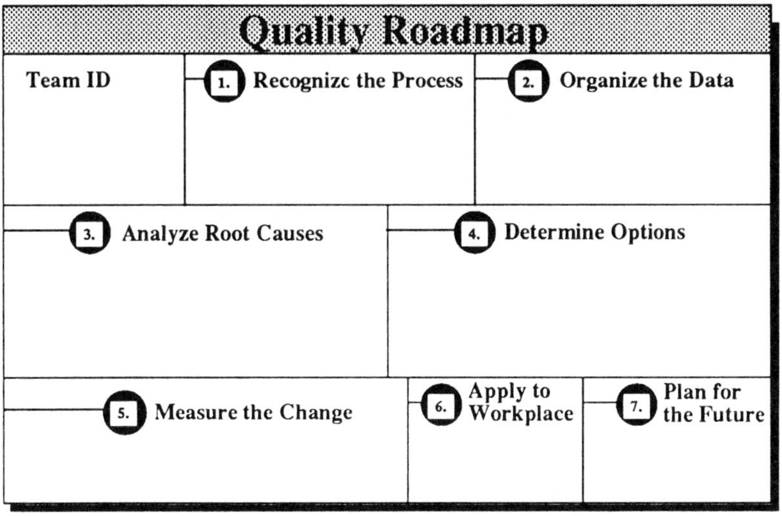

Quality Roadmap		
Team ID	①. Recognize the Process	②. Organize the Data
	③. Analyze Root Causes	④. Determine Options
	⑤. Measure the Change	⑥. Apply to Workplace ⑦. Plan for the Future

members to prepare for this CLT review. Many team members have not given presentations before, or utilized charts or other data to make a point, or for that matter, addressed the top management team. However, most team members enjoy the opportunity to share what they have learned and approach the situation with enthusiasm. The team works as a group to prepare and present their achievements. Each presentation is different, but all are both informative and interesting. After a team has completed its QI story, we develop a summary sheet that is circulated to all managers.

Other Types of Teams

No discussion of teams would be complete without referencing quality circles. This is the most common type of quality improvement team. Circles are easy to establish and require no change in the management structure. A circle is made up of volunteers, who meet once a week to improve work processes. Teams are trained in group dynamics, analysis, decision making, and statistical process control. Trained facilitators provide assistance to the teams. If there are several teams, an organizational steering committee may be formed to provide support, resources, and coordination of effort. More has been written about quality circles than any other team approach. The key to an effective employee involvement program is to have a wide range of team options to capture the majority of employees in the effort.

Techniques for Teamwork

Team efforts should be data driven; the assignment for team members is to learn how to manage by fact. Within healthcare, our old ways of problem solving can best be described as crisis management. When a problem occurs, we use the quick-fix approach, and most often the solution implemented deals only with the symptoms of the problem. The solution seems to work and the manager turns away, only to find the problem rise up again several months later. The Total Quality approach means finding root causes, implementing countermeasures, and standardizing to hold the gains. Once a team has completed its quality improvement story, the gains are monitored on a continual basis so the team knows the problem stays fixed!

Before the team can begin deliberations, a careful analysis of the current situation must occur. Using TQM tools and techniques to portray problems graphically helps team members to see and experiment with solutions rather than just talk about problems. The team training teaches people to ask *why* five times in order to get to root causes of a problem. It pushes people to examine causes beyond the obvious. Masaaki Imai shared this method of continual questioning in the book *Kaizen* (1986). Teams, managers, and staff can use this root-cause approach in their daily jobs. It helps drive a data-based culture.

Within the team, there is also an emphasis on human dynamics. The goal of the team is to make decisions by consensus, making sure everyone participates in the problem-solving process. Working with consensus is difficult and requires a time commitment. The team must find a proposal acceptable enough so that all members can support it and no member opposes the decision. The team must become skilled in listening and conflict resolution. The team experience reinforces teamwork and cooperation and the power of many minds versus one. The strategy is to unleash creativity in each of the team members as the team searches for root causes. The tools that the teams use are:

- Brainstorming, a divergent thinking style, to develop as many creative ideas as possible.
- Multivoting, a convergent thinking style, to select priority issues.
- Storyboarding, a method to tell the quality story and keep the team in process.
- Matrices, to demonstrate relationships and guide decision making.
- Seven quality tools to find root causes and make sound decisions.
- Consensus to assure ownership and buy-in to ideas and solutions.
- Seven management tools to organize and examine data.

These and other selected quality improvement methods are further explained in Chapter Twelve.

Storyboards

A storyboard is a large bulletin board used to record the progress on each step in the quality improvement process. Its purpose is to educate and communicate the quality improvement story. By having a storyboard posted in the work area, the progress can be viewed by employees and customers on the team. One useful approach is to make Post-It notes available near the storyboard, so people not on the team can ask questions and give suggestions on the storyboard to help the team.

Identification of Quality Improvement Projects

Managers and team members must learn to scan the environment for quality problems and opportunities for improvement. Some inputs we use to stimulate team development are:

- Departmental assessments of customers and their requirements that show a need for change.
- Customer surveys that point out the need for improvement.
- Quality indicators that show a gap between current performance and the desired level of quality.
- Front-line employees who are frustrated about how long it takes to accomplish a task.
- Management goals and objectives (Gaucher, 1992, pp. 148–166).

Quality improvement projects identified in both top-own and bottom-up directions are important to your organization, as illustrated in Figure 8.3. Based on departmental quality gaps and "pain" within the organization, managers and staff will identify quality improvement projects. The departmental quality gaps should be based on the departmental and corporate quality goals. An advantage of projects identified by staff is that they have high motivation to make improvements. However, unrestrained quality improvement projects identification in a bottom-up direction may not be coordinated and may not address the key corporate priorities. Hence, quality improvement projects identified in a top-down direction are also important. Based on the organization's vision, strategic plan, breakthrough strategies, corporate goals, and quality gaps, the leaders should identify quality improvement projects that address corporate priorities. These projects will be important to achieve the corporate vision. A balance of projects identified in both directions is best.

Issues Teams Face

It is often difficult for team members to learn new behaviors. Work stress and old habits and patterns tend to block learning. We have seen poor work habits formed after just a few months of operating in a crisis-oriented system. Another problem is that many employees volunteer to serve on teams expecting to play the same passive role they have played on numerous other committees. Quality teams, however, require active participa-

Figure 8.3. Top-Down and Bottom-Up Identification of Quality
Improvement Projects.

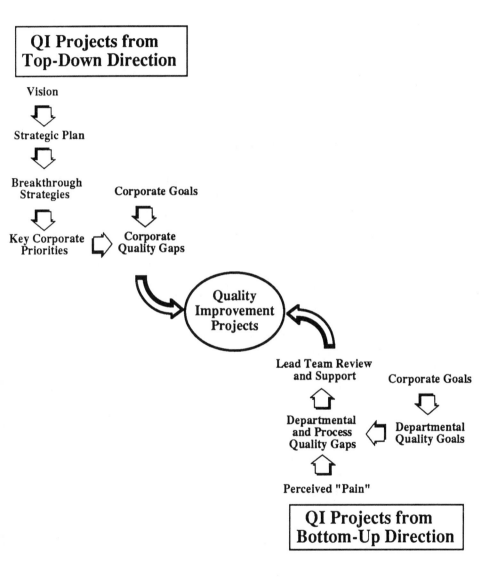

tion of all members. The team leader must reinforce the need for all to participate and both call on and assign work to those who are silent members of the team. Sometimes the team leader must schedule a one-on-one meeting with the team member to find out if there is a problem. Many times this is all that is necessary to get the participation level on the right track. The important issue is to deal with suboptimal behavior as soon as it is displayed and then give positive feedback as new behaviors replace the old.

Removing Barriers to Cooperation

We experienced much finger pointing and hostility during the early meetings of teams. This was especially true when the teams were cross-functional and cut across many departments. Turf-guarding behavior is normal along with statements such as, "Everything was fine when I handed the process to you." Efforts should focus on looking at data rather than allowing team members to assume the cause of the problem. For example, flowcharting a process allows team members and others to see exactly where problems exist. It highlights how critical informa-tion sharing is at the points of hand-off in a process. Time after time we found that, as people review the flowcharts, they learn new information that helps them understand the issues.

Another major issue is collaboration. Team members must be able to put aside their personal agendas and develop a common understanding of the problem to be effective. The team leader needs to reinforce that management by fact is the key to effective decision making and opinions not supported with fact have no place in team meetings. A quote said to be hanging on the wall at Florida Power and Light that describes the transition is, "In God we trust, all others must bring data!"

Selecting an Improvement Opportunity

Teams tend to have great difficulty in selecting the opportunity to work on. There is a tendency to select a theme that is too large, an issue too small for major impact, a theme too difficult to measure, or something outside their control. At UMMC we learned that the key to an effective team is having data to help select a reasonable theme. Guidance from skilled facilitators and team leaders can keep the teams on track and avoid pitfalls. Another problem is selecting a process no one on the team is really interested in, then there is no energy to complete the process. The most successful teams in our organization have worked on processes that cause "pain" for many people. Examples include excessive waiting times for scheduled patients in the admission lounge that caused frustrations for patients, families, physicians, nurses, and clerks; and inefficient processes in the operating suites that caused cancellations, frustrating work experiences, and extended lengths of stay. In each of these cases there was pain felt by the team members and others, providing the impetus to find a permanent solution.

Roles and Responsibilities of Team Members

Team Leader. The team leader is responsible for guiding the team through the improvement process. The team leader serves as a manager, planning the process, assessing the situation, and assigning responsibilities. The team leader must assure that the team stays in process and that evaluation becomes an ongoing part of the team process. The team leader also serves as a teacher, presenting information in a logical, clear fashion, asking appropriate questions, and checking for understanding. The leader serves as a catalyst and facilitator, listening carefully, asking questions and actively seeking participation from all participants. Finally, the team leader motivates team members by empowering and supporting all team members. The team leader and the facilitator work as a team of two to assure that the team receives appropriate support. They meet before each team meeting to discuss the team's progress and the agenda for the next meeting. The team leader must prepare a PACT for each meeting, as illustrated in Exhibit 8.2. The PACT includes a *p*urpose, *a*genda, *c*ritique, and *t*ime for the meeting. This simple planning tool can help to keep a team on track. We have adopted this methodology for all meetings within the Medical Center.

Exhibit 8.2. Sample PACT for UMMC Corporate Lead Team.

Total Quality Process
Corporate Lead Team
May 12, 1992, 12 noon–1 P.M.

Purpose: Review Material and Make Policy Decisions
Agenda:

1. Minutes—April 14, 1992 (Attachment I)	5 min.
2. Review Affinity Diagram Data (Attachment II)	20 min.
3. Updates on Lead Teams	15 min.
4. Review Goals II, III, IV (Attachment III—March 10 meeting minutes)	15 min.
Critique:	5 min.
Time:	60 min.

Our hope is to improve the process of all our meetings. The team leader and facilitator also meet following each meeting. They share the observations of the facilitator and feelings about what went well and what went wrong during the meeting. This information provides data for improvement.

An important part of each meeting for the team leader is the critique. Here team members analyze what they liked about the meeting, what they found troublesome, and, most important, how the meeting could be improved. When teams are in the beginning phases, the critique tends to be difficult. People are too polite; comments range from "we finished on time" to "we accomplished a lot." Once team members become used to the process, comments are apt to be more meaningful. Comments range from the personal, "you have been late for the last three meetings," to, "we need to plan more time for important items on the agenda." The critique uses the Plan-Do-Check-Act cycle to improve the work of the team. When the critique is combined with feedback from the facilitator, the team leader can gain insight into team problems and define an action plan to ensure team success. Several teams have found it helpful to develop a list of questions to stimulate ideas for the critique, as illustrated in Exhibit 8.3.

Carl Larson and Frank LaFasto found that "the single most distinguishing feature of the effective leaders of teams in

Exhibit 8.3. Sample Total Quality Team Meeting Evaluation Criteria.

PACE:
1. Was today's meeting well paced?
2. Was enough time allowed for agenda items?
3. Did we cover all items effectively?

AGENDA:
1. Were agenda topics pertinent?
2. Were topic leaders prepared?
3. Did we schedule agenda items in a reasonable sequence?

MEETING EFFECTIVENESS/EFFICIENCY:
1. Was team focused? Did we stick to agenda items and not digress?
2. Was the meeting productive, with good discussion?
3. Were necessary assignments given with deadlines/target dates?

ATTITUDE AND COOPERATION:
1. Are we acting as a team and trying to help one another?
2. Are all meeting attendees actively participating?
3. Do team members appear honest and candid?
4. Did I feel comfortable and trusting in today's meeting?
5. Was I able to disregard other job pressures and focus my energies on the meeting?
6. Was consensus reached where applicable?
7. Did we follow the Rules of Conduct?
8. Did I feel that questions I had were answered and that my contributions were valued?
9. Are there improvements that we can make for future meetings?

Source: Developed by teams at UMMC.

their data base was their ability to establish, and lead by, guiding principles. These principles represented day to day performance standards, essentially what the team members could expect from one another on a daily basis" (1989, p. 123). Having a standard process for teams, and spelling out the roles and expectations up front, allows the team leaders to establish a supportive climate where team members can take risks, learn, and maximize their contribution. Sample education programs are explained in Chapter Nine.

Team Facilitators. As Peter Scholtes states in *The Team Handbook*: "Most companies develop a network of individuals trained to provide technical assistance to project teams and other quality improvement efforts" (1988, pp. 1–19). Our support network started as a group of part-time facilitators from the departments of Management Systems and Training and Development. At first our facilitators were acting as team leaders by default. They were the only experts in quality concepts. As we added training for team leaders, the facilitators became counselors and coaches of leaders. They serve as technical advisors to the teams, with a primary goal of making the team leaders successful. During the meetings, they observe the process and make notations to give feedback to the team leader. They observe and flowchart such behaviors as interruptions, side conversations, silent team members, vocal members, and positive team skills. This feedback helps the team leader better understand the flow of the meeting and make adjustments for team success.

As the number of teams and the demand for facilitators grew, the Corporate Lead Team decided to invest in nine full-time facilitators, at an annual cost of $500,000. Each full-time facilitator can work with six to eleven teams, in addition to teaching quality education programs. The number of teams assigned will be determined by the experience and knowledge level of the individual facilitator. The full-time/part-time allocation allowed us to sanction many more teams. Our eventual institutional goal is to train every manager and supervisor to facilitate teams, thereby eliminating the need for full-time facilitators. Through teaching each manager how to lead and facilitate teams, we believe we will successfully integrate the new TQM managerial behaviors into daily practice.

Team Members. Team members also have responsibilities; they must participate in the development of the mission statement and then be committed to the team goals. They must listen to others with understanding and recognize and respect individual differences. They must complete any team assignments and come to meetings on time prepared to contribute ideas and suggestions. They must encourage other team members and provide feedback about team performance. Each team develops a series of items they believe will govern team behavior, and members must abide by these rules of conduct.

We have tried a variety of programs to prepare team members for teamwork. When we first began we used what we called just-in-time training. We found the teams floundered and

retraining was essential. The training model may vary for different types of teams, but frequent mini-teaches are helpful as the
team goes through the process, to provide practical knowledge
and skills with each of the methods used.

We also found that a standard process is the key to success.
It does not matter much which standardized process is used;
there are several to choose from. We found that the teams
progress faster and waste less time questioning the mission
when the tasks are spelled out.

Stages of Team Development

There are several stages of team development. Most of our early
team members described a variety of emotional ups and downs
as their teams evolved. Our early teams suffered from a lack of
effective training. There were many highs when things went
smoothly and progress was being made. There were also days
when the work seemed to stretch endlessly ahead while team
members floundered. Those who began skeptically had many
days when their skepticism was reinforced. The introduction of
the seven-step process in 1990 alleviated many of the emotional
ups and downs and has evolved into the process previously
illustrated in Figure 8.2. Now the team member who is frustrated can ask: where are we in the process, what data do we need
to collect, or what is the next step? This keeps teams from
continually asking, now what is our mission?

As each person is learning and growing through the
experience, the team is also learning and evolving. B. W.
Tuckman (1965) described the stages of team evolution. This
tool may help team leaders understand where the team is and
how to facilitate movement to a more productive phase.

Stage One: Form. Testing and dependence are the main
behaviors in this phase. The group is discussing mission, and the
member's role is unclear. The team members may wait to be told
what to do, as they have in the past. When facilitators graph what
is happening at this stage of the process, the focus of attention is
on the team leader, as illustrated in Figure 8.4. Members want
role clarification and definitions of involvement. Until auton-

omy is developed, members still expect to be told what to do and how to do it. Developing a mission or problem statement allows the team members to develop a sense of purpose, significance, and direction. Tuckman described this phase as the infancy or young child phase.

     Stage Two: Storm. Intra-team conflict occurs in this phase. As the name implies, this phase is characterized by testing, conflict, and resistance. If team interactions were graphed, they would look like those illustrated in Figure 8.5. There is free exchange of ideas but many interruptions and one-way discussions. Minimal work is accomplished. If the team leader's style prevents conflict from surfacing, the resistance may emerge in

Figure 8.4. Team Stage One: Form.

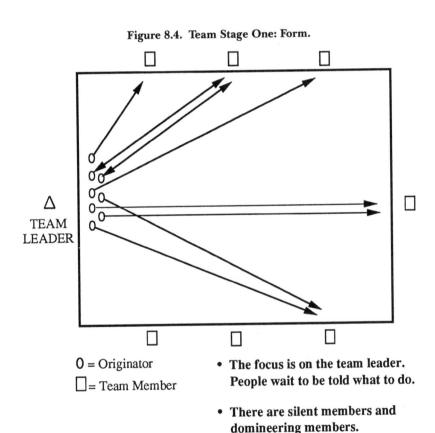

0 = Originator

☐ = Team Member

- **The focus is on the team leader. People wait to be told what to do.**

- **There are silent members and domineering members.**

Figure 8.5. Team Stage Two: Storm.

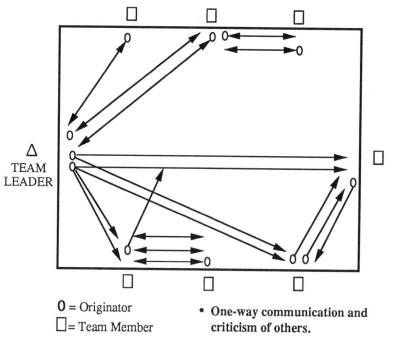

0 = Originator

☐ = Team Member

- One-way communication and criticism of others.

- There is less dependency on leader. Interruptions and side conversations occur.

the form of unproductive behaviors such as not completing assignments or missing meetings. Teams that get fixated at this level never develop the creative potential for problem solving. Tuckman compares this stage to the rebellion of a young child toward parental or school controls.

One of our teams actually started at this phase with two team members screaming at each other. To deal with the storm phase, we teach team leaders how to deal with conflict in a positive way. Conflict allows issues to be fully expressed, and if dealt with constructively, it can push teams to explore all sides of an issue. The key is that the conflict must be managed. When managed correctly, conflict can energize a team.

Stage Three: Norm. The development of team cohesion occurs in the norm phase. Conflict is reduced as team members become comfortable with the ground rules and each other. A common spirit develops, and members have much more time to spend on the project. Information is shared and acted on. Team members are open, and there is a high level of trust. Work progresses much more effectively. The team leader needs to challenge the team to reach new goals, and use new techniques and methods so that team growth continues. Tuckman compares this phase to the socialization phase of childhood. When the facilitator graphs this phase, the graph shows the relationships illustrated in Figure 8.6.

Stage Four: Perform. Functional role relatedness occurs; teams at this phase rely on facts, data, and logic. Team members make significant contributions and are gratified by the results. There is a Plan-Do-Check-Act cycle to improve the work of the

Figure 8.6. Team Stage Three: Norm.

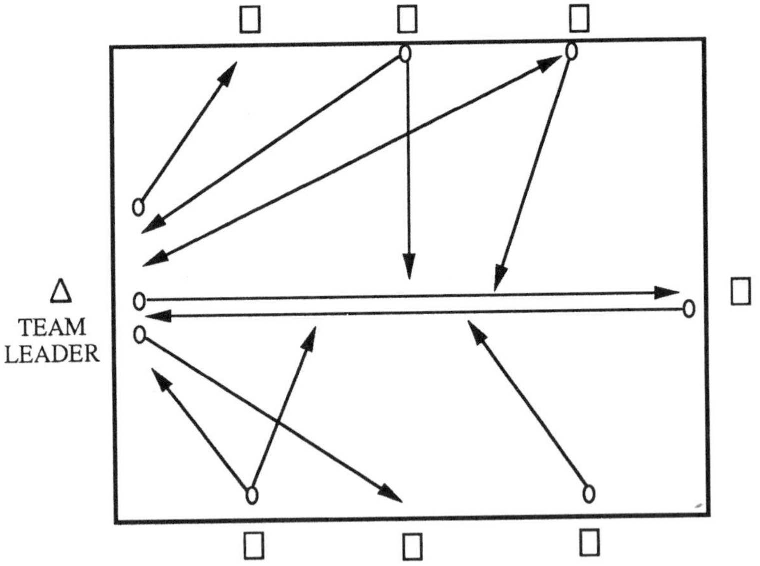

0 = Originator
□ = Team Member

• People offer suggestions freely.

• They follow the rules of conduct.

team. Utilizing the critique and feedback from the facilitator, the team leader can gain insight and adjust behavior to ensure team success. If you were to observe the team in the performing stage, you would see team members accept responsibility for sharing thoughts, feelings, doubts, and hopefulness for the future. Tuckman compared this stage to the mature phase of human development. When the facilitator graphs this phase, the graph shows all team members participating. Leadership is shared according to expertise, and much work is accomplished. Team members know what to do and how to do it. This phase is where synergy is achieved, as illustrated in Figure 8.7.

Well-Functioning Teams

Sometimes all that is necessary to determine how well a team is functioning is a few minutes of observation. When smooth-

Figure 8.7. Team Stage Four: Perform.

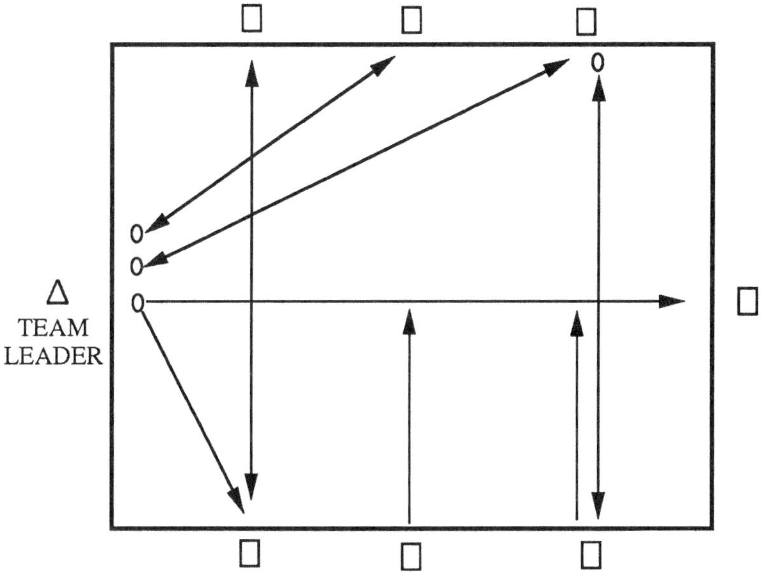

0 = Originator
□ = Team Member

• **Everyone participates.**

• **Leadership is shared according to expertise.**

functioning teams meet, the atmosphere is informal and relaxed and people are cooperative and attentive. Everyone participates in the discussion. The team leader summarizes key points and asks members for opinions, members listen to each other, and conflict is handled by the team members. During the meeting it is hard to tell who the leader is; the focus shifts depending on which team member has expertise. All decisions are made by consensus, and people leave the meetings with a sense of accomplishment.

Dysfunctional Teams

It is also easy to spot dysfunctional teams. The meetings tend to be more formal. Tension is obvious. Criticism is personal rather than focused on ideas. Team members interrupt and use the meetings to make statements or promote personal agendas. There are frequent side conversations. The team has fuzzy goals, and members are continually questioning their mission. People have a high need for safety and security, and there is no risk taking or creative idea presentation. The team does not stay in process, and decisions are made by vote. Members are often absent, and when present leave the meeting feeling something is missing. Fortunately, by following guidelines of the seven-step process and utilizing a skilled facilitator, these teams can be turned around.

Why Teams Fail

There are many reasons why teams fail. Unskilled leadership, unclear goals, an unsupportive environment, lack of reward and recognition, jumping to a desired solution instead of seeking root causes, or problem behaviors in team members can all cause teams to derail. However, in our organization the main reason for teams stumbling or failing is the lack of effective training.

Using TQ Tools and Techniques to Diagnose Team Failure

One of our team leaders was very concerned when her team stumbled and seemed unable to progress. She decided to use TQM tools and techniques to help diagnose the problem. The team began with a brainstorming session using a cause-and-effect diagram (also called a fishbone, or Ishikawa, diagram), illustrated in Figure 8.8, to find the causes for the lack of progress. The goal was to identify what help the team needed. The bones of the fish were structure, process, and people. Under structure, the causes included the fact that the structure, team role and mission, and the members' roles were all undefined. The purpose for the team was unclear. Under process, suggestions included a need for consensus on problem definition, adequate team training, a designated process, a developed theme, and a definition of customers of the process and their requirements. Under people, the team identified their size, which precluded team building, a lack of understanding of team dynamics, and inadequate knowledge of quality techniques or training. The circles at the end of each bone are called clouds and are used to point out or highlight the actionable root causes. The team continues to ask why something happens, at least five times, to get to root causes.

The next step is to take the root causes and develop an options matrix. The problems are articulated in the first column, the options in the second column, and the practical method for solution is in the third column. Each of the options can be analyzed to select the most effective solutions. The team then can address each issue on the options matrix, as illustrated in Figure 8.9. As you can see, by providing more adequate training, employing a formalized structure, the problems could be solved.

Errors in Selecting Projects

Teams can also derail because of the projects they select. If they chose a process that no one is an advocate for, they may lack the

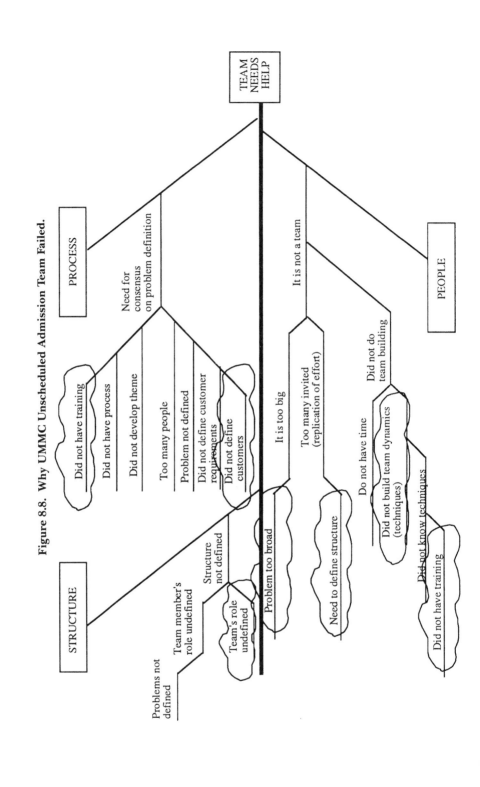

Figure 8.8. Why UMMC Unscheduled Admission Team Failed.

**Figure 8.9. Sample Options Matrix for UMMC
Unscheduled Admission Team.**

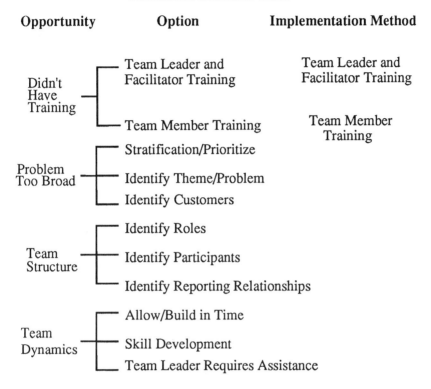

Opportunity	Option	Implementation Method
Didn't Have Training	Team Leader and Facilitator Training	Team Leader and Facilitator Training
	Team Member Training	Team Member Training
Problem Too Broad	Stratification/Prioritize	
	Identify Theme/Problem	
	Identify Customers	
Team Structure	Identify Roles	
	Identify Participants	
	Identify Reporting Relationships	
Team Dynamics	Allow/Build in Time	
	Skill Development	
	Team Leader Requires Assistance	

energy and motivation to pursue the root cause. Teams need to work on projects causing pain, where advocates want to solve the problems.

Many teams try to rush to a desired solution. With many of our teams we observed this lack of patience. The problem is that they may never get to the root cause. This approach develops solutions that may be only temporary. The role of team leader and facilitator is to keep the team in process and on track to the root cause.

Another problem is selecting a process in transition. One of our early teams was making fairly good progress with their issue when an anticipated move to a new building threw a monkey wrench into the process and progress came to a halt.

The team had to be restarted after the move, and valuable time and energy were spent with a small return on investment.

Finally, teams can select a system, not a process, to improve. This happened to the UMMC Admission/Discharge team. They did not begin to make progress until they broke the system into a group of processes and attacked them one at a time: first, the waiting times for scheduled admissions; next, waiting times for unscheduled admissions; next, discharge issues, etc.

Successful Teams

The successful teams in our organizations have had common characteristics:

1. *Clear goals.* A team must have a clear understanding of the goal to be achieved. The goal must also be perceived as "worth" achieving to team members. This can be achieved by selecting problems where there is a high level of pain and therefore motivation for problem solution.
2. *Standard process.* This helps the team stay goal-focused and on track.
3. *Trained team members.* This means members know what to expect and how to accomplish the task.
4. *External support and recognition.* Management must recognize and support the work of the teams and create the culture for effective teamwork.
5. *Effective leadership.* This is also achieved through proper training and support of teamwork.
6. *A collaborative environment.* The barriers and constraints to effective teamwork must be removed.
7. *The use of facilitators.* To provide insight and feedback to the team leader and to keep the team in process.
8. *The presence of a manager with resources to implement proposed solutions.*

Conclusion

The current situation and complexity of the problems confronting healthcare organizations require a new organization, one that inspires increased collaboration and teamwork. However, creating a supportive climate for teamwork requires extensive planning, resource allocation, and leadership. To enjoy the benefits of teamwork, the leadership must be prepared to tap the creative potential of the workforce. This means listening to the suggestions of employees performing the work, involving everyone in organizational planning to improve customer satisfaction, and recognizing and rewarding team behaviors. Develop a team-oriented structure, give people the tools and techniques, and then just stand back! As Tom Peters writes, "truly involved people can do anything!" (1987, p. 345). We believe that the effective use of teams will lead to efficiencies in healthcare never dreamed of.

Chapter Nine

Education and Training

Successful implementation of a Total Quality effort depends on strong, customer-responsive TQ education and on training programs. Without an appropriate quality curriculum, the required change cannot occur. "Long-term commitment to new learning and new philosophy is required of any management that seeks transformation. The timid and the fainthearted, and people that expect quick results, are doomed to disappointment" (Deming, 1986, p. x). Motorola, Inc., a Malcolm Baldrige quality award winner, has been the most outspoken about education and training. "In 1979, Bob Galvin, then Motorola's CEO and now chairman of the executive committee, asked the human resource department to put together a five-year training plan. He believed that all employees needed upgrading in their skills if the company was going to survive" (Wiggenhorn, 1990, p. 72). In fact, Motorola formalized its educational process to the point of forming Motorola University. Galvin believes without education his corporation could never have met the goal of the six sigma, which equates to 3.4 defects per million opportunities, or production that is 99.999966 percent defect free.

This chapter presents the reasons for investment in education and training and describes programs and lessons learned by UMMC and others. Although some make careful distinctions between the operational definitions of education and training, for our purposes the term *education* will encompass both concepts.

Customer-Responsive Education

The focus of a TQM educational program should be to increase sensitivity, knowledge, and skills to meet and exceed customer requirements. The customers in this case are the employees, managers, physicians, others within your organization, and external suppliers and customers. Education may also be extended to external suppliers and customers. While early education must focus on the principles of quality, the courses must be based on the learners' needs.

Components of TQ Educational Programs

An educational program related to Total Quality should address several components. Successful educational programs we are familiar with include the components described here. Sample educational programs from UMMC, which include these components, are explained later in this chapter.

Reason for Change. One of the first and most important issues to address is why change is needed. No one will change unless he or she sees a clear need for change. The need for change must be clearly described, with examples related to the organization and individuals, during education. But identifying a need for change during education alone does not mean the employees will agree to act on this need. Motorola, for example, admits to a number of mistakes that may be instructive to healthcare organizations. "Our first mistake was to assume that once we described the courses, the people who needed them most would sign up to take them. They didn't. . . . Since people resisted formal classes, we developed self-help material so they could pick up a package and take it home. That failed, too" (Wiggenhorn, 1990, p. 74–75). In addition to the rationale for change, you must present a positive vision for a better future if you want to motivate people to change. Several reasons why healthcare organizations must change were addressed in Chapter One. These reasons for change must be communicated broadly within your organization to overcome the natural tendency to maintain the status quo.

Action Step: Communicate the need for change broadly and frequently, in a language and context that all can understand.

TQM Philosophy. There are similar principles underlying the philosophy and techniques of W. Edwards Deming, Joseph Juran, and Philip Crosby, as illustrated in Table 9.1. However, there are differences in the way each guru recommends that change be implemented. Key concepts of TQM were described in Chapter Two. We would emphasize that successful implementation of TQM requires an integration of customer-oriented, continual-improvement philosophy, analytical skills, and people skills, within a supportive organization and structure, as in the integrated TQM model illustrated in Figure 2.1 in Chapter Two. Therefore, your educational programs should have all these elements reflected in the curriculum.

Examples. As with any new approach, specific examples of improvement achieved through a TQM approach in healthcare organizations are important. Successful examples convince participants that TQM can work. To have the greatest impact, each participant must see the examples as relevant to his or her job. Many initially resist TQM because they "believe" it is an unproven methodology or additional work. Examples are particularly important to demonstrate that customer satisfaction, quality, cost effectiveness, and working environment can all be improved simultaneously. Most people in the healthcare industry believe that quality always costs more and that increases in productivity always decrease quality. Although this position is incorrect, our experience indicates that only a series of logical and practical examples will begin to convince people that quality and cost effectiveness are not opposites.

Action Step: Use successful healthcare examples to demonstrate that TQM methods work in healthcare organizations.

Table 9.1. Alternative Approaches to Quality Improvement.

Deming's Fourteen Points for Management	*Juran's Six Steps to Quality Improvement*	*Crosby's Fourteen Steps to Quality Improvement*
1. Create constancy of purpose for improvement of product and service.	1. Identify a project. • Nominate projects. • Evaluate projects.	1. Make it clear that management is committed to quality.
2. Adopt the new philosophy.	• Select a project. • Ask: Is it quality improvement?	2. Form quality improvement teams with representatives from each department.
3. Cease dependence on inspection to achieve quality.	2. Establish a project. • Prepare a mission statement.	3. Determine where current and potential quality problems lie.
4. End the practice of awarding business on the basis of price tag alone. Instead, minimize total cost by working with a single supplier.	• Select a team. • Verify the mission. 3. Diagnose the cause. • Analyze symptoms. • Confirm or modify the mission.	4. Evaluate the cost of quality and explain its use as a management tool.
5. Improve constantly and forever every process for planning, production, and service.	• Formulate theories. • Test theories. • Identify root cause(s).	5. Raise the quality awareness and personal concern of all employees. 6. Take actions to correct problems identified through previous steps.
6. Institute training on the job. 7. Adopt and institute leadership.	4. Remedy the cause. • Evaluate alternatives. • Design remedy.	7. Establish a committee for the zero defects program. 8. Train supervisors to actively carry out their part
8. Drive out fear. 9. Break down barriers between staff areas.	• Design controls. • Design for culture. • Prove effectiveness. • Implement.	of the quality improvement program. 9. Hold a "zero defects day" to let all employees realize
10. Eliminate slogans, exhortations, and targets for the workforce.	5. Hold the gains. • Design effective quality controls.	that there has been a change. 10. Encourage individuals to
11. Eliminate numerical quotas for the workforce and numerical goals for management.	• Foolproof the remedy. • Audit the controls.	establish improvement goals for themselves and their groups. 11. Encourage employees to
12. Remove barriers that rob people of pride of workmanship. Eliminate the annual rating or merit system.	6. Replicate results and nominate projects. • Replicate the project results.	communicate to management the obstacles they face in attaining their improvement goals. 12. Recognize and appreciate
13. Institute a vigorous program of education and self-improvement for everyone.	• Nominate new projects. (See also Chapter Two, pp. 50–51.)	those who participate. 13. Establish quality councils to communicate on a regular basis.
14. Put everyone in the company to work to accomplish the transformation.		14. Do it all over again to emphasize that the quality improvement program never ends.

Sources: Compiled from Deming, 1986, pp. 23–86; Juran Institute, 1992, p. 28; Crosby, 1979, pp. 112–119.

Quality Improvement Process. Using a single problem-solving process for quality improvement projects, such as the seven-step process used by UMMC, is very important. A common process establishes a common language, approach, review process, and timeliness to assure smooth implementation. All managers and staff will need education related to this common process. Which quality improvement process you select is less important than the fact that you use a single process thoughout your organization. If you are implementing TQM within a healthcare system, a single quality improvement process used at each institution within the system will improve the communication and the ability to replicate improvements across the organization.

Analytical Tools, Techniques, and Skills. Several analytical tools are used to analyze and improve processes. Examples include flowcharts, checksheets, Pareto charts, run charts, control charts, cause-effect diagrams (also called fishbone or Ishikawa diagrams), stratification, and scatter diagrams. Your educational programs should include explanation and exercises using these tools and techniques. Case studies allow practice sessions to learn the tools and techniques and to develop the skills necessary to utilize the tools within quality improvement teams and daily work. Many people have an initial fear related to these analytical methods, feeling they require advanced mathematical knowledge. Your educational programs should focus on the concepts and simple graphical examples to overcome this fear. For most people, graphs are much easier to understand and use than numerical tables and analyses. Case studies are important to develop practical skills and confidence. Principles and examples alone will be insufficient to develop skills for most people. Analytical skills alone are not enough; they must be accompanied by people skills.

People Skills. In order to provide complex healthcare services for patients and other customers, extensive coordination of the efforts of many is required. Successful daily work and quality improvements are possible only when people work together effectively. Teaching your people to work in teams and to break down barriers is the key to success. Examples of techniques to improve the involvement and contribution of your employees are brainstorming, affinity diagrams, nominal group techniques, tree diagrams, interrelationship diagraphs, and tailored reward and recognition programs (Brassard, 1989). Again, it is best to focus on the concepts, simple examples, and practical case studies to avoid fear and develop skills related to the methods.

Case Studies and Practice. Case studies allow "hands-on" experience learning TQM philosophy, analytical tools and techniques, and people skills. Skill building in educational settings allows people to practice in a safe, risk-free environment. These skills can then be incorporated into Quality Improvement Teams and daily work. Simply knowing about the tools and techniques will not help for at least two reasons. First, without first-hand experience using the tools and techniques, you really do not fully understand their use. Second, if you demonstrate tools and techniques during team meetings and daily operations, your staff can see your visible commitment to the quality improvement process. A quality improvement case study is presented in Chapter Thirteen.

Use by Management. Although not a curriculum topic, possibly the most important characteristic of successful educational and training programs is that management regularly ask for and use the approaches taught. William Wiggenhorn, president of Motorola University, states: "Workers began to wonder why they'd taken the training. They'd learn how to keep a Pareto chart and make an Ishikawa diagram, but no one ever appeared on the floor and asked to see one. On the contrary, some of their immediate managers wanted product shipped even if it wasn't perfect" (Wiggenhorn, 1990, p. 75). The education was not being reinforced through management actions. Once again we see that management must "walk the talk" if education or any other change is to be effective.

Action Step: Use TQ methods in your own work, ask others to see how they are using the methods, and especially use the methods to make decisions.

Relation to Previous Programs. Total Quality should not be viewed or communicated as separate from other elements of your organization. To minimize confusion, TQ education should be described in relation to previous programs and management practices, as discussed in Chapter Four. To be effective, TQ must become part of your organizational and personal culture, which requires an understanding of those characteristics that are the same as and different from previous practices. Since each organization has a different history of management practices, this aspect of your TQ educational program must be tailored to your organization. In particular, you should emphasize elements of TQM that your organization is already doing well, such as customer-oriented guest relations, and show how your TQM program will build on those elements.

Action Step: List the requirements for TQ education within your organization, and compare them with characteristics of past and current management programs and practices, to define similarities and differences.

Determining Educational Requirements

Determining the requirements for educational and training programs is difficult. Directly asking managers and employees their requirements is helpful and should be done, but may miss three key issues. First, people "don't know what they don't know." If people do not understand the concepts of TQM, they would not identify the need for training related to TQM methods. Second, there must be a perceived need to change or a perceived benefit. If people do not see any need to change, few will identify training as relevant. A third, and difficult issue, is the fear, sense of intimidation, and embarrassment that people experience when they admit they do not know something. Many people fear statistics. At a different level, it is well known that people who are functionally illiterate conceal it very well. These people may be quite intelligent, but they have not learned to communicate through written language, or in some cases English is their second language. Therefore, determining educational requirements will need input from several sources. Sample types of inputs to determine educational requirements are:

- *Knowledge and skills to perform the job.* The most immediate requirements are those needed to perform the basic job functions of each person's current job. Although these requirements clearly vary widely among staff, they should be identified along with the job description. Both analytical and people skills should be included. Each person must receive education to meet these requirements, normally from the department or area in which he or she works.

- *Survey of requirements perceived by employees.* Employees should be asked what knowledge and skills they would like to develop and what education might help them achieve the knowledge and skills to improve job performance.

- *Requirements to implement TQM.* The internal or external leadership and consultants most knowledgeable about TQM should identify the knowledge and skills required to plan for quality improvement, participate in Quality Improvement Teams and projects, and continuously improve quality in daily work.

- *Basic management knowledge and skills.* UMMC, for example, has identified a set of basic management knowledge and skills that all new managers should have. Educational programs have been in place, and updated, for several years to develop new supervisors and managers. This curriculum has been modified to include TQM training also.

- *External customer expectations.* Although seldom surveyed, external customers should be asked what behaviors, knowledge, and skills they expect of different people within a healthcare organization. For example, what do patients ask of staff at the information desk or registration areas? Simply tabulating the types of requests will generate a set of educational requirements.

- *Knowledge and skills assessment.* After the required behaviors, knowledge, and skills are known, different types of assessments can provide information about current performance compared to those requirements. We are not implying that everyone should take a series of tests. Observed behaviors and actions are probably better indicators; knowledge alone is inadequate if it is not used. Good sources of the requirements for enhanced behaviors, knowledge, and skills are team leaders, team facilitators, team members, managers, and employees.

Based on the above inputs, a series of educational requirements can be developed. The priority and sequence of how those topics will be addressed by educational programs should then be determined. Several different educational programs may be required.

Action Step: Use several inputs to determine the requirements for your TQ educational programs, and repeat the assessment at least annually.

Educational Faculty

Carefully selecting faculty for educational programs is a key factor in the success of your TQM educational programs. The faculty must be knowledgeable about the curriculum content, but must also have the people skills to relax the participants and communicate the information simply. Suggested skills and characteristics for potential faculty include:

Knowledge and experience. This may seem too obvious to mention, but TQM is a complex process including diverse subject material. Personal experience implementing TQM allows faculty members to illustrate TQM concepts with specific personal examples and stories. Different faculty may be required to teach the philosophy of TQM, the analytical and statistical tools and techniques, and the people skills and techniques. When you begin, it takes substantial training and experience to be qualified to teach all of these subjects in an easy-to-understand manner. As your process progresses, more people will have the required mix of skills.

Credibility. The faculty must be credible to earn the respect of participants in your educational programs. Three barriers related to credibility of internal faculty must be overcome. First, many senior administrative and clinical leaders do not attend educational programs in their own institutions. They may feel that they cannot learn from such programs because they are too advanced, or they may be embarrassed to admit there is something they do not know. Second, managers often feel that training and development programs are for entry-level staff. Third, in some organizations training and development staff lack credibility with senior and middle management. If these issues exist, they must be addressed. Senior staff must first learn and then personally participate in TQ educational programs and quality improvement efforts to show their commitment to quality.

Strong interpersonal and teaching skills. Managers, physicians, and staff may be threatened by ideas that vary substantially from their current practice. New ideas that can change work habits are best presented by faculty who can relax the participants, communicate the reasons and methods for change in a simple manner, and excite the participants to try the strategies and techniques on their daily jobs. Faculty should be able to present fun exercises to illustrate the concepts and methods.

Senior management participation. There is nothing that communicates commitment better than to have senior administrative and clinical leaders involved as faculty. Obviously, this requires that those senior managers learn the material before presenting it. They must believe in the process to be credible. Another important role for senior managers to demonstrate commitment is to answer questions from program participants, such as: How does TQM relate to previous programs and practices? Why are we changing? How does what we are learning relate to daily practice? This approach is more effective than having questions answered by other faculty.

Action Step: To demonstrate commitment, one or more corporate leaders should introduce every TQ educational program, participate as faculty in at least part of the programs, and answer questions.

Availability. Even if knowledgeable people exist in your organization, they may not be available to teach. Making them available may require revising priorities, reallocating current staff, and possibly adding incremental resources in some areas. Adding staff and other resources should not be the first step. First, examine priorities and reassign staff if possible. With the exception of one external mentor, the design, development, and conduct of initial TQM educational programs at UMMC were accomplished by reallocating the time of existing management, management systems, training and development, and other staff. The resource requirements and use of external resources should be based on your organization's implementation plan. Today healthcare organizations move more quickly through the early stages of TQM than we did at UMMC because the approach is now better understood and there are many good TQM examples within the industry.

Principles for TQ Educational Programs

Based on experiences at UMMC, other healthcare organizations, industrial organizations, and other types of adult education, there are several useful principles for designing your TQM educational programs. The following principles are useful to guide the development and presentation of these programs.

Managers before employees. A key education strategy is that every manager should be trained before the employees who work for that manager. A manager or supervisor does not want to feel uninformed when an employee asks about a topic. If the managers are not trained before or concurrently with their employees, the managers are likely to disregard or discredit, consciously or not, the educational program and the knowledge gained in it. The strategy for rollout of the education programs begins with board, management, and clinical leadership, as illustrated in Figure 9.1. The next step may depend on the size of your organization and the level of educational effort you are willing to undertake. For a small organization, or one willing to mount a major educational effort, the strategy is to educate next all middle managers and then all employees, physicians, and others, in horizontal slices, as illustrated in Figure 9.2. However, for a large organization, or one with very limited educational

Figure 9.1. Education Begins with Leadership.

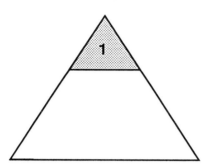

resources, a step-wise approach, training a series of vertical wedges, may be most useful, as illustrated in Figure 9.3. All supervisors and managers above the people serving on your initial quality improvement teams should be trained before the team members who report to them, so the managers will be knowledgeable and supportive of their quality improvement efforts. These managers and team members will be from all departments and organizational areas represented among the team membership. As additional quality improvement teams are chartered, those managers and team members are trained. You proceed this way, training "wedges" of managers and employees within your organization. To keep everyone informed, the strategy chosen and the plan should be widely communicated.

Figure 9.2. Education by Horizontal Slices.

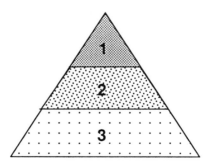

Figure 9.3. Education by Vertical Wedges.

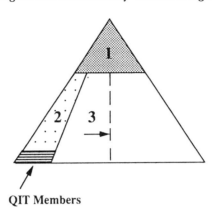

QIT Members

Comfortable environment. The environment should be comfortable for participants both physically and emotionally. There should be comfortable seating, and the room should be at a comfortable temperature. Everyone should be able to see the speaker and any displayed materials easily. If participants have handout materials or notebooks, they need a place to use those materials. Typically, round tables, which allow group discussions and exercises, are effective. For some programs, separate rooms are provided for small group break-out sessions. As an example of failing to provide an appropriate environment, last year we participated in a conference at which each participant had a large notebook containing the presentations of all speakers, but there were no tables and the chairs were so close together that people sitting next to each other could not open their notebooks at the same time. By emotionally comfortable, we mean an environment that avoids stress and conflicts. Most of the physician orientation programs and many of the employee awareness programs, for example, were provided at their respective divisional or departmental meetings, at which the people felt comfortable.

Minimal disturbances. To the extent possible, eliminate interruptions and disturbances to the educational session. This is often a problem when training programs are offered near the participants' normal work environments. They will get called away, leave on break, or not return in a timely manner. In an analogy to the Old West, "check your pagers at the door." Disturbances disrupt the agenda and all participants.

Concepts and theory. The principles, concepts, and theories should be explained to establish the basis for the education. We learn by theory and experience related to that theory. However, for most audiences the discussion of concepts and theory should be quickly followed with practical examples and experience.

Examples. Provide a number of examples, which are viewed as practical and useful by the participants. Using examples from other healthcare organizations is normally seen as relevant. Examples from your own organization are most meaningful, which is one of the reasons to begin a few TQ pilot studies early in your implementation. Industrial examples or quality improvement projects, during early learning about Total Quality, are often viewed as not applicable or irrelevant. However, the more you learn about TQM, the more you realize that examples from other industries are very relevant. Although the services and products we provide are different, the quality improvement principles and implementation issues are the same in any industry.

Action Step: Provide educational and pilot-project experiences that use vividly relevant examples, and actively involve participants in exercises, personal plans for change, and pilot projects. Then leaders should follow up to support personal changes and projects.

Experience. Hands-on exercises and experience develop detailed understanding of concepts and lead to much better questions. The "red bead" experiment developed by W. Edwards Deming, for example, provides a vivid realization that management can set any goals or say anything, but the results will not change unless the process that produces those results is changed. This is an exercise in which volunteers are asked to withdraw white beads from a box, on a paddle, but the box also contains many red beads. The exercise demonstrates that the foreman's repeated criticisms do not contribute to improvement of the process. This exercise provides a vivid realization that managers must look at the process, not just criticize employees.

Participation. To the extent practical, get every person to participate in the discussion and exercises. People learn best by active participation, which enhances their understanding and sense of belonging to the group. At all programs you should allow time for questions and answers and provide program evaluation forms so that participants can provide feedback. One method used at UMMC training programs to address questions is the "parking lot." Participants are provided notepads on which they can write questions not directly relevant to the current discussion or which they do not feel comfortable raising in the group. The faculty addresses many of the questions some-time during the program. Some of the questions are typically saved to be addressed by the organization's leaders at a final question-and-answer period. Feedback from participants is used to improve the program. If practical, it is best to communicate later the actions taken on the suggestions.

Build internal experts. An objective of your educational programs is to build internal TQM experts. It is often more timely and cost effective to use external consultants to help get a TQM process started, but there are two cautions. First, the process must be led by your leadership, not the consultant. Second, you should develop internal experts as quickly as possible to become self-sufficient rather than become dependent on external experts. These internal experts can then be developed as faculty for ongoing training programs. This approach is described later in this chapter in connection with team leader and team facilitator training programs.

Action Step: Identify internal staff who have or can develop the ability to teach analytical and people knowledge and skills, and develop a plan for your organization to become self-sufficient in providing educational programs and support for teams.

Sequence of deployment. The sequence of education is very important to successful implementation. A matrix illustrating the suggested sequence of deployment is illustrated in Table 9.2.

Table 9.2. Sequence of Deployment.

	Leadership	Managers	Physicians and Staff	Customers	Suppliers
Why?	1	2	3	4	5
What?	2	3	4	5	6
How?	3	4	5	6	7
Practice	4	5	6	7	8

There are five different general audiences: leadership, including the board, administration, and clinical leaders; managers; physicians and staff; customers; and suppliers. For effective education and implementation of TQ, each audience should address "why" issues first. Each audience must be convinced there is a need to change first, then you must answer the question, "why TQM?" Unless these and other "why" issues have been addressed, there is no reason to change. Next you should address "what" will be done. The "how" approaches, tools, and techniques have no relevance unless there is an understanding of "what" needs to be done. Finally, actual implementation and practice follow an understanding of how to implement TQ.

It is common for organizations to make a serious mistake in the sequence of deployment, especially when a consultant is hired to do education and training. Two common errors are made. First, the leaders do not go through education, review and revision of corporate values, mission, goals, and management expectations, or change their personal behaviors. If the leaders do not think TQ is important enough for commitment of their personal time, that message will be loudly communicated to managers, physicians, staff, customers, and suppliers, no matter what the leaders say. Second, it is common for organizations to jump into the middle and begin training managers and staff "how" by focusing on TQ tools and techniques, such as statistical process control, before leaders have addressed "why change?" "why TQM?" or "what is our plan for change?" This is a particular problem when a consultant sells your organization a standard training package. Therefore the managers and staff do not have a culture, environment, or context in which to apply the tools and techniques or any reason to change personal behavior. The managers and staff will be dutiful soldiers and go to the educational programs, listen quietly, and possibly even actively participate. But they then go back to their jobs and continue doing what they have always done, ignoring what they have learned. Many managers and staff in your organization have had at least some of the TQ tools and techniques in their formal education, but the organizational environment has not encouraged use or continued learning of those methods.

A suggested sequence of deployment is illustrated by the numbers in the matrix in Table 9.2. The first activity, no. 1, should involve education and debate by the board, administrative, and clinical leadership concerning "why change?" "why TQM?" and other "why" questions. Once the leadership is comfortable with "why," they can move on to "what" is planned for the organization, no. 2. At the same time, education of managers could begin addressing no. 2, "why." At the next step, no. 3, the leaders could focus on "how," managers could focus on "what," and staff could begin education about "why." The key is that each group must be at least one step further ahead in the sequence than the group in the column to the right in Table 9.2. The education and rollout of TQM are dynamic processes. Questions and issues raised by managers, staff, and others may cause the leaders to reconsider those issues and to revise the plan for the organization.

Sample Educational Programs

Education should be a lifelong process for you, your organization, and every employee. Part of the difficulty is that each person enters your organization with different knowledge and skills. Overall, healthcare organizations have a high average education and knowledge level. Yet most will have employee literacy skills ranging from a doctorate to functionally illiterate. Motorola is noted for its goal of achieving six sigma level of performance. To accomplish this, Motorola "needed a work force capable of operating and maintaining sophisticated new equipment and facilities to a zero-defect standard, and most of them could not calculate decimals, fractions, and percents" (Wiggenhorn, 1990, p. 77). One hospital noted for its work on quality improvement found, when working to improve the information system for dietetics, that some employees were functionally illiterate; they could not read the menu items. The hospitals responded by both changing the process and offering reading courses for employees. Therefore, educational programs must address a broad range of knowledge and skills to meet your employee customers' needs. Peter Senge summarizes the need for learning vividly: "The organizations that will truly excel in the future will be the organizations that discover how to tap people's commitment and capacity to learn at all levels in an organization" (Senge, 1990, p. 4).

In this section we will describe several of the TQM educational programs offered at UMMC as examples. The purpose, participants, training format, and subject material will be summarized for each program. These sample educational programs may assist you in developing TQM educational programs for your organization. We continue to develop new programs, and repeat existing educational programs, to continue learning.

Program evaluations are completed at the end of each educational and training program by the participants, and these evaluations are used to improve subsequent programs.

General Management Programs on Total Quality

The purpose of these programs was to expose managers to the concepts of Total Quality, to present the UMMC organization and approach for TQ, and to teach basic skills. When we initiated these programs in 1989, there were five one-day programs, TQ 101–105, offered for top management, selected physicians, and union leaders. As UMMC managers and staff began to learn more about TQ, and we gained more experience, the programs were shortened to four one-day programs, then to the current format of three one-day programs. Most of the programs have been offered off-site, because of facility constraints in the Medical Center, for groups of fifty to one hundred people. The rooms are set up with round tables for participants. When we initiated these programs, there were no educational programs that would meet our requirements, so we developed the programs internally with the assistance of Edward D. Rothman, professor of statistics at the University of Michigan. The initial five programs were offered over a period of eight months. The agendas have continued to change to meet our requirements. For illustration, the agendas for the current TQ 101–103 programs are illustrated in Exhibit 9.1.

The faculty includes UMMC corporate officers; the statistics professor; the director of management systems, the corporate lead facilitator, and a management specialist from training and development. All programs were opened and closed by a corporate officer, who was available to answer questions. This is very important to communicate commitment and to address the issues. We have talked with people in other organizations where the organization's leadership states that TQM is very important, but they do not attend as participants or faculty. The message is clear to everyone: "TQM isn't as important as other things the corporate leadership is working on." The same message is communicated when leaders do not have time for meetings on TQM.

At each program, participants received handouts of presentation materials. In addition, once developed, all participants received TQ lapel pins, UMMC Statement of Quality plastic wallet cards, expectations of managers, and actions for managers to begin Total Quality. Through 1991, approximately eight hundred managers, physicians, and union leaders have attended these programs.

TQ Orientation

Following the educational programs for upper and middle management, orientation programs were developed for UMMC staff and physicians. These one-and-a-half-hour programs were broadly publicized and presented on different days of the week, shifts, and times of day to allow everyone to attend them. The faculty for virtually all of these programs were UMMC corpo-

Exhibit 9.1. Sample Agendas.

Agenda for Total Quality 101:
Overview and Introduction

- Opening comments, by corporate officer. Initially all programs were opened and closed by Ellen Gaucher, the chief operating officer and corporate champion of TQ.
- What does quality mean to you?
- Why quality?
- What is quality?
- Red-bead experiment. This is an exercise developed by W. Edwards Deming to demonstrate a process, control charts, management tampering, and management behavior.
- System of profound knowledge, which is based on Deming's work.
- *Quality—The New Way.* This is a video developed by Hospital Corporation of America (HCA) relating Deming's fourteen points to hospitals (Hospital Corporation of America, 1989c).
- UMMC Total Quality Process—structure and approach.
- Question-and-answer period and closing comments, by corporate officer.

Agenda for Total Quality 102:
Learning Cycle, Measurement, and Deming's Fourteen Points

- Opening, by corporate officer.
- UMMC Operating Room quality improvement story, which describes results of a pilot study.
- Learning cycle—P-D-C-A.
- P-D-C-A exercise, which demonstrates the Plan-Do-Check-Act steps.
- Sense deceptions, which demonstrate examples in which data show perceptions are wrong.
- Measurement principles.
- Deming's fourteen points.
- Working group exercise on Deming's fourteen points.
- Question-and-answer period and closing comments, by corporate officer.

Agenda for Total Quality 103:
Tools and Techniques, Tampering, and Learning Principles

- Opening, by corporate officer.
- Tools and techniques
- Management tampering, which addresses the adverse consequences of management asking and acting on wrong questions.
- Learning principles related to quality improvement.
- Creating a Total Quality environment.
- Management actions to begin Total Quality. These are specific actions that each manager can begin immediately.
- Question-and-answer period and closing comments, by corporate officer.

rate leaders, which communicated a strong message of commitment. In addition, teaching enhances the faculty's knowledge of TQM. The programs were offered from November 1990 through March 1991, with approximately seven thousand people attending. The agenda included:

- Total Quality concepts
- UMMC Statement of Quality, including plastic wallet card for each participant
- Expectations of management
- The video *Quality— The New Way* (Hospital Corporation of America, 1989c)
- Handouts of presentation highlights and Deming's fourteen points
- TQ pins

Most employee orientation programs were given in auditorium or classroom settings to accommodate as many people as possible. All seating had space for participants to make notes. Attendance ranged from about fifty to two hundred per program.

Most physician orientation programs were given at their respective clinical section, divisional, or departmental meetings. By using this approach, it was possible to reach more physicians.

TQ Awareness Program

Although UMMC had fifty to eighty formal and informal quality improvement teams working, and included regular communications about Total Quality in several of the Medical Center's publications, many employees were unaware of progress. Therefore about six to ten months after the initial orientation program, a series of TQ awareness programs was presented late in 1991. The purpose of the awareness programs was to provide a status report on the UMMC Total Quality Process and to answer questions about it. The agenda included an update on the process, number of teams, and progress and results to date. The faculty included the UMMC corporate officers and managers. Each corporate officer gave the presentation first, then the managers and supervisors reporting to them gave the presentation at section, divisional, or departmental meetings in order to reach most employees.

Team Leader Training

Use of a standard quality improvement process throughout your organization is important. Although improvements can be made with teams using different approaches, a single approach leads to a common vocabulary, common understanding, common methodology, and much improved communications. In the spring of 1990, UMMC was experiencing a rapidly growing number of Quality Improvement Teams. With the excitement generated through our management programs on Total Quality, we had gone from five to twenty teams in four months, and many others were wanting to form teams. We were experiencing what we termed a "nuclear explosion" of interest in forming teams. It became clear that a standardized process and standardized training were necessary. Although we could have developed our own training materials for team leaders, facilitators, and members, we estimated it would take at least a year to develop, test, and refine the materials. So at that time we chose to contract with Qualtec, Inc., for the materials developed and successfully implemented at Florida Power and Light and for training our corporate leaders and training staff. We have developed our own training programs specifically for healthcare. UMMC staff now provide all training for team leaders, team facilitators, and team members, and receive excellent reviews from program participants.

The team leader program is a five-day intensive program intended for people who will lead and facilitate teams. The program has two main purposes. The first is to teach participants the seven-step quality improvement process (see Figure 8.2 in Chapter Eight) and the associated tools and techniques, which are known as task skills. The second purpose is to teach participants how to lead a team of people who will have different backgrounds and views, which are known as people skills. Each day, the participants study group dynamics, go through one or more steps of the seven-step quality improvement process in detail, and study support activities. They then gain experience as a team leader, team member, and observer. The key to the success is the balance of task skills and people knowledge and skills.

The faculty consists of two to three UMMC staff who are certified to teach the team leader program. Each trainer has gone through a one-week team leader training program, one-week team facilitator training program, and another one-week train-the-trainer program for the team leader program. The trainers are videotaped, observed teaching, critiqued, and coached to improve their knowledge and skills before certification.

Managers, supervisors, and physicians have received team leader training first. Through August 1992, more than four hundred and fifty people have been trained as team leaders. The plan is to have every UMMC manager and supervisor trained as a team leader and team facilitator by January 1994. This training is key to the paradigm shift from managing to leading. This program receives universal praise, even from very busy physicians who take a week out of their practices to participate. Some say they learned more in this program than they did in their master's degree program. In the future, experienced team members will be trained as team leaders, and the managers will support them as facilitators. We plan a continuing sequence of educational programs to enhance knowledge and skills.

Team Facilitator Training

The team facilitator program is a five-day intensive program intended for people who will facilitate quality improvement teams. Each participant must have completed the team leader program before taking the team facilitator program. The purposes of the program are to review the quality improvement process and to teach the participants how to facilitate quality improvement teams. A facilitator serves five key roles: coordinator, communicator, teacher, coach, and promoter. The agenda includes a quality improvement skills review, facilitator review, and each of the five facilitator roles. Videotapes are used to illustrate the points and techniques.

The faculty consists of two to three UMMC staff who are certified to teach the team facilitator program. As for team leader training, each trainer has gone through a one-week team leader training program, one-week team facilitator training program, and another one-week train-the-trainer program for the facilitator program, and each has been coached to improve skills before certification. Through August 1992, more than one hundred people had been trained as team facilitators.

Team Member Training

Each member of a Quality Improvement Team (QIT) needs to understand the concepts of TQ as well as the tools and techniques used for a quality improvement project. Therefore, each QIT receives approximately two days of training on the seven-step quality improvement process (see Figure 8.2 in Chapter Eight) and the associated tools and techniques. Team member training is shorter for physician teams because they have more knowledge of the scientific process and to conserve their time. We have experimented with a number of different formats and continue to use different approaches to meet the needs of each team. Two generally different approaches have been used. One approach is that the team leader and team facilitator jointly teach the five to ten team members. Some teams do the training in two full days, others in four half days, and some have tried abbreviated initial training of two to four hours with just-in-time training as the team moves through the different steps of the quality improvement process. The idea behind this approach is that team building is improved by the team going through training together. The other, more recent approach initiated in 1992 is to provide also centralized training programs for groups of approximately twenty team members from different teams. The decision to offer centralized team member training is based on the large number of QITs and the large amount of facilitator time needed to prepare the training and teach team members in small groups. Initially it is more effective to teach team members as teams, but as the number of teams increases, the centralized team member training may be more cost effective.

The agenda includes concepts of quality improvement, Quality Improvement Teams, getting started, and each of the seven steps or the quality improvement roadmap, with the associated tools and techniques.

Leadership for Total Quality

Following the cultural assessment of the organization, a series of programs was given for leaders and managers related to their personal management styles. The purpose of this two-day program was for each participant to compare personal assessment of management style with the assessment by colleagues and to develop an action plan for improvement. UMMC corporate officers and clinical chairmen participated in the program as well as other managers. Each participant completed questionnaires developed by Human Synergistics, Plymouth, Michigan, and Management Vector Analysis, Jackson, Michigan. The same questionnaires were completed before the program by five subordinates or colleagues selected by that participant. The scores were tabulated and distributed to each participant at the program. The faculty consisted of the consultant from Management Vector Analysis and a management specialist from UMMC training and development. The agenda included a description of the survey instruments; discussion of current and desired organizational culture as perceived by corporate officers, managers, clinical chairmen, and a random sample of staff; comparison of personal and colleagial perceptions of each participant's management style; and development of a personal action plan. Although each of the groups completing the cultural survey had different views of the current culture, all described the same desired cultural characteristics.

This program had a major impact on most of the participants. Most, including us, found that our employees and colleagues viewed our management style very differently from the way we did, and differently from the desired management style. This was an enlightening, and even shocking, experience but has led to a noticeable improvement in interpersonal relationships and communications. This has been determined through both subsequent formal surveys and anecdotal information.

We plan to repeat an abbreviated version of this assessment three times a year for two years to measure managers' progress, from the perceptions of the managers and their subordinates and colleagues.

Creativity and Innovation

Creativity and Innovation is a two-day program designed for supervisors and managers. The purposes of the program are to stimulate and enhance the creative process; develop creative skills such as observation, imagination, intuitive thinking, creative analysis, and problem solving; and provide the skills needed to implement creative ideas within a changing organizational climate and culture. These skills are needed to improve the environment supporting Total Quality.

The primary focus of this program is to allow managers to experience "small" creative successes and to provide assistance with those creative/innovative ideas of larger scope and/or greater impact. The agenda includes idea generation exercises, brainstorming techniques, identification and elimination of barriers to creativity, case studies illustrating critical and intuitive thinking skills, implementation strategies, and reinforcement of creativity and innovation. The faculty is from UMMC training and development.

The program has had many positive results, including the identification of all participants' creative potential and the acknowledgment of the need for creativity and innovation in an environment that typically discouraged these skills in the past. Comments from participants indicated that at the beginning of the program they did not believe they were creative, but by the end of it they were all able to identify their own creative potential. In addition, all participants have been able to leave the program with ideas they can immediately implement in their departments. There is a need for more education and reinforcement for creativity in the workplace. A short time ago a participant commented that "it is good to know that the organization (UMMC) thinks it is okay to be creative."

Managing Diversity

UMMC views the developing skills of managing a diverse workforce as an integral part of the TQ process. This led to the development of a Managing Diversity program. The purpose of this two-day program is to provide managers with a process to create a work environment that empowers and enables a diverse workforce to reach its full potential in pursuit of organizational objectives.

During the program, supervisors and managers gain knowledge and increase their sensitivity in the areas of diversity. Discussion on social interaction, raising awareness, demographics, and role-playing exercises are agenda topics. The faculty is comprised of diverse UMMC employees, coordinated by the diversity training coordinator. These employees are trained in diversity by two-person teams. During the two days, participants engage in interpersonal communication, behavioral change techniques, videotape presentations, and skill-building exercises. Participants learn how to recognize and value the contributions of their diverse workforce. "When managing diversity is integrated with total quality, the most significant implementation challenges that remain with total quality are more successfully addressed" (Thomas, 1991, p. 165).

Preventing Waste

During the fall of 1992, a program was introduced to focus manager and employee attention on preventing waste and rework as part of their daily work. The purpose of the one-hour program was to identify and eliminate/prevent at least one job activity in each department that is wasteful and to introduce Total Quality techniques that will help accomplish that. Eleven types of waste were discussed to stimulate ideas, as illustrated in Figure 9.4: ineffectively utilized people, delays and waiting time, waste of supplies, poor communication, overproduction, poor scheduling, wasted motion, unnecessary process steps, unneces-

Figure 9.4. UMMC Waste Wheel.

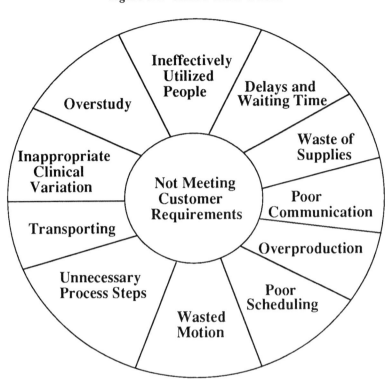

sary and delayed transporting, inappropriate clinical variation, and overstudy. The agenda included quality improvement, UMMC customer groups, an example of a process with waste, a description of the types of waste, description of brainstorming, a description of the Plan-Do-Check-Act (P-D-C-A) cycle, and an exercise to brainstorm sample wastes in participants' work areas. The faculty at first consisted of UMMC corporate officers and senior managers, then was cascaded through the organization by managers and supervisors making a standard presentation for their staff, tailored with personalized examples.

Planned Future TQM Programs

Education and training should be a continuing commitment, with an increasing set of requirements. An example of the scope of training requirements is illustrated in Table 9.3. Over time, everyone should participate in programs addressing each topic, at a level of detail appropriate to their role. We face a continuing challenge to provide training on basic methods for new staff and managers, retraining for people who have not had the opportunity to use the methods on their daily jobs, training on advanced methods, and providing training as part of cooperative efforts with our suppliers and customers. We plan to do a survey of Quality Improvement Team Leaders every six months in order to assess the tools and techniques they have used and those on which they need help.

Current plans include programs on advanced tools and techniques, benchmarking, quality function deployment, and hoshin planning, during 1992 and 1993. We have conducted one training program on quality function deployment for a team using that technique to plan the opening of a new medical procedures unit.

Lessons Learned

Several lessons have been learned through our experiences at UMMC and the experiences of our colleagues at other health-

Table 9.3. Sample Education and Training Requirements.

	Train New Staff	Train Current Staff	Retrain Current Staff	Train Suppliers	Train Customers
General Orientation	X	X	X	X	X
TQ101–103	X	X	X	X	X
Awareness	X	X	X	X	X
Team Leader	X	X	X	X	X
Team Facilitator	X	X	X	X	X
Team Member	X	X	X	X	X
Leadership for TQ	X	X	X	X	X
Managing Diversity	X	X	X	X	X
Preventing Waste	X	X	X	X	X
Advanced Tools and Techniques	X	X	X	X	X
Benchmarking	X	X	X	X	X
Quality Function Deployment	X	X	X	X	X
Hoshin Planning	X	X	X	X	X

care organizations and in other industries. These lessons may be helpful in planning and supporting your TQM educational programs.

Implementing TQM requires broad cultural change. This cultural change requires substantial education and training, but that is not enough. Behaviors, especially of administrative and clinical leaders, must change. Accomplishing those behavior changes requires practical educational experience closely linked to recognition and reinforcement for changes in behaviors on the job.

People skills delay TQM more than analytical skills. Failures and delays of TQM implementations are almost always due to a lack of education and behavioral changes related to people skills, not analytical skills. This has been reported by healthcare organizations, industrial organizations, and consultants working with those organizations. The caution is that any TQM education and implementation must have a balance of people skills and analytical or task content, with an emphasis on actual behavior change, not just knowledge.

Timing and sequence of education important. Leaders should personally go through training addressing "why," "what," and "how," and then practice TQM, before asking their staff to do so, as illustrated in Table 9.2 describing a sequence of deployment. If leaders are unwilling to do this, two things occur. First, they do not understand TQM and how it relates to the organization's values, mission, goals, and culture, in order for them to lead the TQM effort. Second, they communicate a strong message to the organization's managers, staff, customers, and suppliers that TQM is not sufficiently important for them to get personally involved. Education for each person should address in sequence "why," "what," and "how," and then the practice of TQM.

Involvement of line management. Line management must be personally and visibly involved in educational programs to communicate personal and organizational commitment to TQM.

Resources required to support plans and expectations. Resources should be made available to support education and implementation of quality improvement efforts. Experience at UMMC and other organizations has indicated the following. First, a substantial and continuing commitment of time and resources is required for education. Second, implementation of improvements takes far less resources than initially feared by the leaders. Third, in total there is a substantial benefit and return on TQ efforts. Fourth, TQ education makes a major contribution to the organization's becoming a "continuously learning" organization, which Peter Senge (1990) claims is necessary for long-term organizational survival and prosperity.

Adult education principles. TQM educational and training programs should take into account adult education principles like those previously discussed. In particular, people need to see practical examples and be involved personally in the process to fully understand and become committed to TQM.

Developing Your TQM Educational Program

You face a number of alternatives relative to Total Quality education. Selected alternatives, with advantages and disadvantages, are discussed here. Your organization may choose to implement a combination of these alternatives. The approach appropriate for your organization will be based on your requirements and the resources you have available.

Use an External Mentor

It is often helpful to have an experienced external person to serve as a mentor to senior administrative and clinical management to develop and implement TQM. Educational and training programs will be a key part of that implementation. Some advantages and disadvantages of using an external mentor are:

Advantages	*Disadvantages*
• Broad TQM expertise of mentor.	• May be incremental costs.
• Senior administrative and clinical management may heed external advice more	• May be difficult to find mentor well suited to your organization and its requirements.

readily than internal advice.

- Lower cost and resource requirements than large consulting contract.
- Can help define requirements for TQM process and training.

- May be seen as "the consultant told us to do it," which causes less internal ownership.

We recommend the use of an external mentor to assist with designing the requirements for your TQM process and educational and training requirements. The external mentor will be valuable to challenge your board and senior administrative and clinical management concerning the reasons for change, the vision and mission, and the goals and other topics that are difficult for internal staff to raise. It is much more difficult for internal staff to challenge regularly the organization's leadership practices. However, the organization should plan to phase out the external mentor over time.

At UMMC we were assigned three external mentors when we began as part of the National Demonstration Project on Quality Improvement in Health Care: Al Endres from the Juran Institute, David Groff from Corning Glass Works, and David Gustafson from the University of Wisconsin. Donald Berwick, Paul Batalden, and Blandon Godfrey also served as informal mentors to us. As we moved ahead to develop our own Total Quality Process and the associated educational and training programs, we used Edward Rothman from the University of Michigan department of statistics as a mentor. He worked regularly with us for two years to guide us as we developed our Total Quality Process, he helped develop training materials, and he served as a faculty member for several training programs.

Develop Programs Internally

TQM educational and training programs can be developed internally by your organization. Some advantages and disadvantages of internally developed educational and training programs are:

Advantages	*Disadvantages*
• Fewer incremental costs. • Customized to your organization's needs.	• Require staff knowledgeable in full range of TQM topics. • May take multiple years to develop. Can delay implementation. • Can divert resources from other continuing training and development programs.

At UMMC we developed most of our educational and training programs internally. However, we are fortunate to have talented staff in training and development, management systems, and other departments with expertise to develop a broad range of training materials.

Hire a Consultant to Assist Developing Programs

External consultants can be used to develop TQM educational and training programs and to present at those programs.

Advantages	*Disadvantages*
• External TQM expertise. • Customized to your organization's needs. • Reduces implementation time.	• Require knowledgeable training staff to work with consultant. • Can divert resources from other continuing training and development programs. • Can be costly due to daily consultant fees. • May not understand unique organizational needs.

It is important that you think very carefully about what your organization needs before hiring a consultant. In 1987, when we began working on TQM, there were only a few experienced TQM consultants, and none of them had any healthcare experience. Today virtually every management consultant claims to be an expert on TQM. Some are, some are not. If you have not thoroughly considered your requirements, some consultants will try to sell you their standard approach, whether it meets your requirements or not. It is a good idea to seek information about knowledge and previous experience of both the consulting firm and the particular individuals planned to assist your organization.

Purchase Externally Developed Training Materials

A growing supply of externally developed training materials is available on TQM. As with consultants, it is important for your organization to define its requirements before purchasing training materials. Depending on the materials and the license agreement, purchasing training materials may cost more or less. At UMMC we purchased materials to begin our team leader, team facilitator, and team member training from Qualtec, Inc. (1988, 1989a, 1989b). Some of the advantages and disadvantages of purchasing externally developed training materials are:

Advantages	Disadvantages
• Requires least time. • Low initial costs.	• May not meet your organization's requirements. • May not be able to tailor to your requirements. • Materials available from different sources are inconsistent. • May require continuing consultant support training, certification, and updating of training programs.

Use External Training Consultants and Materials

There are many consultants experienced in implementing TQM within industrial organizations, and a growing number with experience implementing TQM within healthcare organizations. These consultants offer a broad body of knowledge to help with educational and training programs. Some of the advantages and disadvantages of hiring a consultant are:

Advantages	*Disadvantages*
• External TQM expertise.	• Can have high initial cost.
• Reduces time to begin training and implementation.	• Consultant may not tailor to your requirements.

Be cautious about the subject material and experience. Because of the great interest in TQM, and the perceived consulting opportunities, virtually every major consulting company now claims to provide TQM consulting services for healthcare organizations. Some have done little more than change the title on the types of products and services they were previously selling, now relabeling them as TQM. You and your colleagues must invest enough time and energy initially to understand the principles of TQM and to define your requirements before committing to a large external consulting contract for training or other TQM assistance.

Action Step: Carefully review the credentials, experience with TQM, and experience with healthcare organizations when reviewing potential external consultants to assist with TQM education and training.

Join a Quality Network

One excellent way to learn is to join one of the several regional and national quality networks. Several of these networks are listed in Exhibit 14.1.

Chapter Ten

Reward and Recognition

To meet the demands of the current healthcare environment and compete more effectively, the people within the organization must learn to think and behave in new ways. The focus of the organization must be on meeting and exceeding customer requirements. While managers recognize that front-line employees are a valuable source of information on how the organization can improve and meet customer requirements, they are not sure how to begin or sustain the involvement of staff. While the jury is still out on the best methods to reward and recognize, current research is validating the importance of reward and recognition strategies in enhancing employee involvement. For example, a 1992 Conference Board study reported: "Recognition, ceremony, and symbol are important underpinnings to the successful functioning of a TQM process. This process both affirms employees' value to the organization and reinforces the cultural and behavioral change TQM requires" (Troy, 1992, p. 6).

The majority of healthcare organizations reward results in quantity rather than quality. Managers are rewarded for increasing admissions or operative procedures rather than improving these processes. A TQM approach requires acknowledging, recognizing, and rewarding those who are improving quality.

Monetary compensation is only one part of a reward system. Once employees feel they are fairly compensated, other factors become important. Many employees are motivated to improve by opportunities for growth, increased responsibility, recognition, and achievement. This chapter presents concepts necessary to begin a reward and recognition program that will facilitate employee growth and improved organizational performance.

Basic Concepts

It is clear that traditional reward systems are not doing what they were designed to do: recruit, retain, motivate, and satisfy competent people. In many organizations, employees believe that rewards are based on favoritism and politics rather than performance. This creates fear and suspicion about these programs. "In most organizations, reward systems are designed, implemented, and administered in a top-down authoritarian manner. As a result, the acceptance level of the reward system is often low, and fails to take into account the preferences and desires of those who fall under the system" (Lawler, 1981, p. 26).

Action Step: Set up an employee-based team to review current reward and recognition strategies and develop future plans, to overcome any existing negative perceptions. Survey employees to determine the rewards and recognition they appreciate.

A second problem is that "traditional reward systems are punitive and yield a negative return on investment" (Kanter, 1989a, p. 85). The traditional system meant here is the carrot-and-stick approach; the carrot is a positive reward, the stick is a form of fear. The stick represents fear of loss: of job, income, or self-esteem. When negative reinforcement is used, a self-fulfilling prophecy ensues; because people are expected to do poorly, they feel poorly and do poorly. This creates an atmosphere of low trust and high fear throughout the organization.

Developing a Culture That Rewards Creativity and Motivates

The first step in developing a more effective reward and recognition program is to analyze the current environment. As discussed in Chapter Six, the culture may need to be adjusted to create the appropriate climate for innovation, creativity, and teamwork. Karl Albrecht writes: "If an organization is going to be adaptive and innovative, it needs to have a culture that values, promotes, and rewards creative behavior" (1987, p. 49). What reward or recognition systems support these concepts in your organization? Are your employees satisfied, motivated, and participative? One framework for assessment is that of Michael Maccoby, who believes "employees today are motivated to work by a combination of eight value drives: survival, relatedness, pleasure, information, mastery, play, dignity, and meaning" (1988, pp. 57–76). Unlike Maslow, who described a hierarchy of needs, Maccoby believes that at certain times one drive will dominate, but one drive is not dependent on satisfaction of a lower drive.

Instead of appealing to the drives that motivate people to work, most healthcare organizations have instituted work cultures that are tightly controlled with narrowly defined job responsibilities. There are many levels of managers between the CEO and the employees. Many times employees do not have the information they need to serve customers effectively. If we expect employees to invest personally in the organization, we must demonstrate what is in it for them. How can we begin to involve people and meet the values that cause them to work? Each manager should think about the drives Maccoby described and determine whether or not his or her environment nurtures these drives.

Survival

Fear and ambiguity can reduce productivity and cause job dissatisfaction. When poor organizational performance raises the possibility of layoffs, employees are concerned about survival. As long as people are concerned about job security, they will not give their full efforts to a participative process. If you want employees to participate in a TQM effort, it is important to guarantee that no one will lose their position due to the quality effort. Early in our process at UMMC, we made the commitment that no employee would lose his or her job as a result of a Total Quality project.

Action Step: Consider an organizationwide policy to guarantee jobs that may be affected by Total Quality. If teams redesign work and cause job elimination, guarantee positions elsewhere in the organization. This allows people to get beyond the fear of survival and see that reducing the cost of poor quality is a better way to streamline an organization.

Relatedness

It is important to help employees understand how their jobs fit into the big picture and that each person in the organization is important in the pursuit of continuous improvement. The renewal of the mission statement and the creation of a vision statement, through a bottom-up approach, allows employees to participate in setting the stage for quality. This exercise helps illustrate for employees the role they play in making the vision a reality. Frequent communication about what has been accomplished also helps to create a sense of alignment and relatedness in the organization.

Action Step: Institute communication policies and practices that help employees understand the vision, mission, and goals of the organization and how their role helps achieve these goals.

Pleasure

We all perform better when we are pleased with our relationships with coworkers and feel accepted and appreciated. Don Petersen, former CEO of Ford Motor Company, said: "What we tend to forget is that human beings need positive reinforcement. We thrive on it—in a marriage, with friends, in education, and in business" (Petersen and Hillkirk, 1991, p. 108). Setting the stage for pleasurable experiences begins with developing the values to guide organizational behavior. Then you should develop management expectations based on those values. You also should personally become an active, positive role model and demonstrate the values and expectations in your daily work. Give positive feedback to those who also demonstrate positive management practices. Try to send at least one positive message or thank you for a job well done each day. Consider ways to develop teamwork and bonding of team members.

Action Step: Give frequent verbal recognition. Establish expectations of managers and rules of conduct so management can be hard on problems, not on people. Brainstorm ideas with senior management on ways to reduce job stress and avoid burnout. Spend time thinking of ways to bring "joy" back to work.

Information

If you wish to build an environment of trust, there must be effective information sharing and a chance for employees to ask questions and have them answered. In most healthcare organizations, information travels in one direction — from the top down. Survey how you communicate, and think about creating horizontal and bottom-up communication strategies. For example, one of our associate directors holds budget review sessions with all of his employees to discuss how each department individually helped the division meet the budgeted objectives and the corporate goals. The sessions are highly regarded by employees because they make their personal and departmental efforts meaningful.

Another very successful communication strategy we implemented was "CEO Breakfast Meetings." Our CEO holds breakfast meetings for twenty people once a month. These are informal sessions where employees can ask questions about anything they wish. The CEO answers as many questions as he can, and passes those he cannot answer along to the line management. The questions and answers are published in our quarterly newspaper, the *Hospital Star*. We also conduct open employee meetings on a quarterly basis in the auditorium. Separate forum meetings are held during each of the three major shifts. The CEO gives a brief update and then opens a question-and-answer period. All senior management team members attend the forums in case there are questions that pertain to their areas. Another powerful communication tool is the CEO Annual Quality Report. This report details progress with TQM achievements. It is distributed broadly in the institution with a goal of reaching every employee. In addition, the *Hospital Star* has at least one quality story in every issue.

Action Step: Develop new forums for large cross sections of employees, where they can listen, ask questions, and give input on organizational strategies and plans.

Mastery

Mastery is developing proficiency, becoming competent and adept, and being recognized for these skills. Most people want challenges and opportunities to grow. It is energizing to solve a problem no one has been able to solve or do things better or faster than they have been done before. As people master their jobs, work tends to be accomplished faster and with fewer errors. Healthcare organizations should invest in employees and help them develop new quality-oriented skills. Use performance planning techniques between employee and supervisor to teach and inspire excellent performance. TQM is a process of self-mastery. It is difficult to feel mastery in one's job when the processes consistently yield suboptimal results, there is little cooperation across departments, and complaints abound. Take action to remove barriers that preclude workers from doing a good job. Emphasize training and therefore commitment to employees. Make sure you reinforce positive behaviors by frequent compliments.

To stimulate corporate growth, consider paying employees for newly mastered skills. One example is paying extra per hour for members of autonomous teams who take on staffing and scheduling functions.

Leaders should encourage those who have mastered a task to explore ways to improve the process they work on or to seek out new challenges. The goal should be continued growth and mastery.

Action Step: Build mastery milestones into your recognition program. Remove barriers that preclude workers from performing their functions expertly. Give positive feedback and recognition for new skills and jobs well done. This will help to keep people energized and goal-oriented.

Play

People who have fun on the job tend to work better, get along better, and experience less stress. "The spirit of play is best engaged at work by the chance to experiment and innovate, to question organizational forms and practices and try out new ones" (Maccoby, 1988, p. 69). Positive climates where play is encouraged are energy-building climates. T. E. Deal and A. A. Kennedy conclude: "Play is the creative side of corporate life, it releases tension and encourages innovation. Despite the fact it has no real purpose and no rules, play in its various forms (jokes, teasing, brainstorming, and strategizing) bonds people together, reduces conflict, and creates new visions and cultural values" (1982, p. 62).

In an interesting interview, John Sculley, who had taken over the lead at Apple Computers several months earlier, talked about a return visit to his East Coast home. When friends asked how he was doing, he said: "It's great. People at Apple have this idea that work ought to be fun. My friends all looked at me like I'd lost my mind. And they said, How can it be fun? Work's supposed to be productive not fun. You must have been in the California Hot Tub too long" (*Inc.*, 1989, p. 49).

Celebration can facilitate the change process. Celebrate what you want to see more of. Organizational attention stimulates others to bring ideas forward and keeps recognition in the forefront. Attention also highlights that management considers quality important. Use informal celebration to recognize a team for success and major events to recognize organizational milestones.

One suggestion that has merit comes from Deal and Kennedy: "Strong companies create a great deal of hoopla when someone does well and exemplifies the values the company seeks to preserve. The best run firms always make certain that everyone understands why someone gets a reward whether trivial or grand ceremony" (1982, p. 72). If you are concerned about what rewards your employees consider effective, ask them. They are the customers of the reward and recognition process.

Humor is also a necessary component of play. Do employees take things too seriously? Are people encouraged and able to laugh at themselves? Many researchers have pointed out that humor can also be therapeutic, and it should play a role in the culture of the organization for patients and staff alike. Norman Cousins (1979) points out the benefits of humor in creating a therapeutic environment. To stimulate the use of humor as a therapeutic methodology, UMMC engaged a "humor therapist" who instructs the medical and nursing staff in humor techniques. We also invited Steve Allen, Jr., M.D., to address all the staff on how to use humor with patients and to reduce personal stress levels of healthcare providers. Many of his strategies were developed in conjunction with his famous father, comedian Steve Allen.

Action Step: Analyze your organization. What is the mood? Is play encouraged? Is the climate appropriate for creativity and innovation? Is humor used to enhance play and reduce stress?

Dignity

This drive is about self-worth. When employees have high self-worth, they are confident and have a positive attitude. They are more secure and apt to take risks. They grow, develop, and make many contributions to the organization. Dignity begins with respect for individuals. Without an environment of respect, there is no trust or ability to achieve mutual goals. To focus on creating an environment of respect, we developed management expectations that focus on positive human interactions and rules of conduct to help people relate positively.

Action Step: Develop a creative environment where confidence and self-esteem can be built by participative decision making, risk taking, and support. Managers should think of ways to encourage employee involvement. For example, brainstorming exercises with the staff can generate many cost-saving and improvement ideas. Implement ideas quickly and recognize and reward progress to sustain momentum.

Meaning

"Meaning is best described as the drive to integrate all other drives" (Maccoby, 1988, p. 76). People want to be able to express themselves through work and bring meaning to their lives. Studies by Yankelovich, Skelly, and White have shown that "75% of Americans no longer find it acceptable to work at a boring job as long as the pay is good; and 78% say they would refuse to leave a job they like for one that pays more" (Yankelovich, 1981, p. 152). As the values of workers are changing, what steps are you taking to understand the needs of employees to have meaningful work? The creation of an empowering environment can occur with TQM implementation. Employees learn the tools and techniques to change their processes and their work. They gain a new sense of meaning through playing a role in change that affects their work. When an organization achieves employee involvement and empowerment, personal self-esteem is enhanced, and people feel better about themselves and better about the organization. They feel appreciated and believe they can make a difference. There is a feeling of trust and a tendency to take risks.

Tom Peters and Robert Waterman point out: "We like to think of ourselves as winners. The lesson excellent companies have to teach is that there is no reason why we can't design systems that continually reinforce this notion; most of their people are made to feel like they are winners. Their populations are distributed around the normal curve, just like every other large population, but the difference is their system reinforces degrees of winning rather than degrees of losing" (1982, p. 57). Think about your organization. Are your people treated as positively as they should be? Do your employees think of themselves as winners? People tend to act according to their self-image. How do you build the self-esteem and image of your employees? Praise, appreciation, respect, supportive management, increased responsibilities, involvement, and other strategies are part of a TQM philosophy that can help your employees feel like winners and can help your organization compete more effectively. Implementing a TQM process can create a culture of pride. Employees are recognized for their competence and contributions. There is openness and a shared sense of purpose. All types of teams—quality circles, quality improvement teams, natural work teams—can be taught to use the techniques of TQM to improve work processes. Pat Townsend, author of *Commit to Quality*, suggested in a speech in Chicago on November 1, 1991, that "until everyone in the organization is on a team, you don't have Total Quality."

Action Step: Involve as many employees as possible in team efforts where they have a chance to learn how to determine root causes and permanently change the processes in their department. Communicate how these efforts are affecting the organization as a whole. This allows employees to see how their efforts relate to the larger corporate goals.

Think about these eight drives as you plan your reward and recognition system. How will you address these drives and incorporate them into your quality plan?

Customer Focus Requires New Responsiveness

The way jobs were structured in the past, with uniform job classifications and levels of bureaucracy to make decisions, will not work in the future. It is a cumbersome and slow way of operating. Our ability to compete depends on quick decisions and flexibility to meet the dynamic environment. If our goal is to stay close to the customer and meet requirements, workers must be free to solve customer problems and make decisions at the important customer interfaces. With the increasing complexity of jobs and information, it is also impossible for managers to make the best customer decisions. This activity must occur at the employee level.

Employees in healthcare suffer a unique role conflict relative to meeting customer requirements. Kate Bertrand describes this as "the perception that they cannot satisfy all the demands of the individual they must serve" (1989, p. 46). A good example of this concept is the conflicting demands of the multiple customers served by nursing. The nurses have professional standards that dictate performance as well as the requirements of the physicians, the patients, and the nursing and hospital administrations. These conflicting expectations cause anxiety. Whose needs are primary? How do these conflicts get resolved? Each department must hold sessions to define customers, primary and others, and analyze how to meet requirements to avoid role conflict situations. This concept needs to be taken into consideration when thinking of the appropriate reward and recognition program.

Key Rewards to Behavioral Change

Implementing Total Quality requires a culture that fosters trust, information sharing, and openness to change. Employees need visible signs that change will occur, and this new effort is not just designed to get the workers to work harder. It has been our experience that workers respond strangely when the organization begins to talk about empowerment. "Why would I want to be empowered?" is a frequently heard statement. We believe this feeling stems from lack of trust that the work situation actually is going to change. Ralph Kilmann's statement (1989, pp. 156–157) may help explain this phenomenon:

> It seems that a person's decision on how hard and how well to work derives from a deliberate thought process — at least until the cultural forces take over. First she surveys the situation to see if there are any rewards available that suit her needs. If there are none, she either leaves the situation or does the minimum to remain a member until she has a

better alternative. If there are rewards that suit the person's needs, she then estimates the likelihood that she can do what it takes to receive them. In essence, the individual considers what the job requires, whether she has the ability to do the job, whether she can control the tasks that lead to success, and how much time and effort she must invest to be successful. So long as she believes that the rewards will be forthcoming after she achieves a level of performance that she can control, the individual will extend all her effort and talent in the right direction—as outlined by her job and guided by her boss.

If rewards are keyed to new behaviors and are fair, meaningful, and reinforcing, it is possible to change behavior and ultimately the culture. Yet in most healthcare organizations rewards are disconnected from results. According to Ernest Huge (1990, p. 71):

> By comparison, major Japanese corporations measure and reward performance in ways consistent with quality improvement thinking. Japanese companies that are successful global competitors derive a far greater commitment to the company from a large percentage of employees, as evidenced by the following:
>
> • An astounding 20–100 suggestions per employee with over 90 percent implemented compared to less than one suggestion per employee in U.S. companies.
> • Lower absenteeism—1 percent compared to 2–4 percent for U.S. companies.

Performance measures and rewards must play a major role in a quality improvement effort.

Motivation

Motivation is a term that applies to the drives, wishes, and needs that cause people to perform. A manager's major function is to create an environment in which people are motivated to perform well. Deming has stated that all people want to perform well, but we as managers have set up artificial barriers that prevent them from reaching their goals. Many times the systems and processes prevent employees from working up to their potential. Deming explains this as the 85/15 rule. From 85 to 95 percent of the problems are related to systems and processes that are out of the employees' control, while only 5 to 15 percent are directly attributable to the employees, as illustrated in Figure 10.1. "The issue is that with the systems and processes or the 85%, the employees understand how to help permanently fix the systems problems and as managers we should invite them to do so" (Scherkenbach, 1988, pp. 100–101).

Action Step: Managers must address those systems that block effective performance. The best approach to smooth out those systems is to form improvement teams, flowchart the processes, and make the required changes. Every system and process should be evaluated.

Figure 10.1. Opportunities for Improvement.

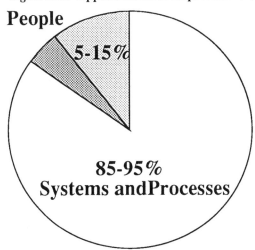

The improved processes are highly visible, and the results will spur teams and even resistant people ahead. Kathleen Ryan and Daniel Oestreich (1991, p. 243), remind us of a window of opportunity: "Most of us work in slightly schizophrenic organizations: traditional hierarchies that contain the seeds of new thinking and new energy. We may still feel the cycle of mistrust, with its low opinion of people, its distances and threats. But in the foreground there is an emerging faith and optimism." How do we maximize those positive signs of hope? What reward and recognition strategies can be implemented to create and sustain positive momentum? How do we capitalize on the positive faith and optimism without being inhibited by traditional practices and fears?

Research has shown that employee participation can enhance motivation (Locke and Latham, 1984). "Perhaps the most direct relationship between motivation and participation occurs when people participate in setting goals and commit themselves to achieving these goals. According to research, when people participate in setting goals and get information about their performance two things happen. First, they set goals that are perceived by them to be achievable. Second, their sense of self-esteem and competence becomes tied to achieving the goals and therefore they are highly motivated to achieve them" (Lawler, 1991, p. 30).

Money: A Powerful Motivator

Many people still believe money is the most powerful motivator. Managers would like to believe money is the most important motivator, because they control money and can give it or take it away. There is a wonderfully humorous line by George Bernard Shaw: "Money is indeed the most important thing in the world; and all sound and successful personal and national morality should have this fact for its basis" (Shaw, 1905).

There is no doubt that successful organizations pay their employees well. The UMMC compensation plan is based on attracting the brightest and the best employees possible. Therefore our salaries lead the market in many job categories. This was not perceived by senior management to be enough. We wanted to link our participative management approach and our reward and recognition program by allowing employees to share in the financial gain from the TQM and other efforts. An employee task force led by the manager of employee and salary administration, human resources department, was established to look at strategies to change the compensation system. The recommendations led to the development of a gainsharing approach. Gainsharing is a group incentive and reward process based on improving operating results of the organization. The practice and performance of each employee makes him or her a stakeholder in the organization. The program rewards people for working smarter, working together, and reducing costs. The goals of the process are to enhance customer satisfaction, improve institutional productivity, facilitate empowerment and teamwork, and improve communication. The gainsharing task force developed the rules and regulations for the process and the name "M-$hare." The formula provides that 50 percent of the margin from operations, beyond the agreed upon target, will be set aside and shared equally by employees.

In 1991 the CEO presented to the University of Michigan executive officers a plan to develop a gainsharing program for the hospital to begin July 1, 1991. The program was approved. The M-$hare program was developed to enhance organizational teamwork and mutual trust. It is available to all regular staff paid on hospital accounts or who contribute to hospital operations. Each employee will receive the same financial share. Our formula is as follows:

$$\frac{\text{M-\$hare Gain}/2}{\text{no. of FTE}} = \text{Gainshare}$$

The M-$hare gain excludes depreciation, interest expense, interest income, prior year settlements, and our academic enhancement fund. Fifty percent of the remaining dollars are then divided among eligible full-time equivalents (FTEs). The gains will be distributed in a special check in

October of each fiscal year. Performance measures are shared four or more times a year to allow employees to determine progress. These measures appear quarterly in the *Hospital Star* as well as in a variety of internal communications. There are several different measures of success and methods of sharing them, as illustrated in Table 10.1.

The goal is to have employees recognize the major part they play in our institution's success, and reward them for goal achievement. We believe the concept of gainsharing moves financial information and rewards to all levels of the organization. As Lawler points out: "Participation in the financial success of an organization can also have a direct, strong, impact on motivation. If money is important to the work force and there is a clear connection between pay and performance, money will be a motivator" (Lawler, 1991, p. 31).

Other Motivators

Other factors are powerful motivators as well. For example, people tend to react favorably to positive direction. When you guide a person by using suggestions, such as "you are very creative, help me think of some solutions to this problem," the person is pleased to help. This becomes a reinforcing reward when his or her suggestions are a part of the final solution.

Developing opportunities for employees that provide for

Table 10.1. Sample Measures of Success and Methods of Information Sharing.

Measures for Success	Information Sharing Method
• Revenues	• *Hospital Star* (newspaper)
• Expenses	• Medical Center Bulletin
• Admissions	• Telecare
• Clinic Visits	• Employee Letters
• Occupancy Rate	• Electronic Mail
• Length of Stay	• Posters
• Attendance	• Presentations
• Patient Satisfaction	• Quarterly Reports
• Employee Suggestions	

meaningful work, autonomy, feedback, and a chance to develop new skills and knowledge is a way to enhance motivation. Time after time we have heard what employees want over anything else is feedback on their performance and recognition for a job well done.

Regular appraisal is essential and reinforcing. It is not enough to do formal evaluations on a semiannual basis. Identifying both positive and negative behaviors and commenting on them specifically in a timely fashion is a much better way to improve performance.

Think about the behaviors you wish to enhance. For example, when the focus of your process is to enhance teamwork, the reward and recognition systems should be tailored to team rewards.

Action Step: Regularly encourage and reward team behaviors. Discuss team efforts with team members. Visit storyboards to review and comment on progress.

Understanding What Motivates Your Employees

When developing a reward system there are two types of rewards to consider—intrinsic and extrinsic. Intrinsic rewards are the positive feelings a person gets from performing the work, such as pride in doing the job well, challenge in mastering the difficult, pleasure in achievement, and fun. Extrinsic rewards are given formally by the organization, such as salary, bonuses, vacations, fringe benefits, awards, and promotions. One of the problems with developing an effective system is that rewards are perceived differently by different individuals. What is important to one group may not appeal to another group at all. The first rule is that the reward system must be flexible and capable of having broad appeal.

"Rewards—compensation, recognition, and promotion—are among the strongest statements you make to people about how you value them and their work. If you don't communicate accurately about your reward and recognition system, or if the system itself doesn't convey customer driven messages, you're missing a powerful opportunity to link people's behavior with your customer driven vision" (Whiteley, 1991, p. 100).

Recognition in Other Healthcare Organizations

Successful recognition programs find ways to expand the number of people who are acknowledged for their contributions. They use both formal and informal strategies to create a variety of incentives for staff. Showing appreciation for a job well done, saying thank you verbally or in writing, and celebrating success by planned events should be easy tasks; but many organizations have difficulty setting up recognition that employees find acceptable. "Handing out cash may be easy, but recognition is sometimes difficult for traditional American organizations. Recognition implies that top officials take the time to show appreciation for individual effort. Far too few top executives budget the time to regularly recognize and celebrate exemplary performers. That, however, is one of the easiest things to change as organizations reorient themselves in Total Quality's direction" (Dixon and Swiler, 1990, p. 7).

Alliant Health System is turning its focus to recognition by sponsoring Recognition Days once a quarter. The program is run twice; once on the day shift at a time to include both day and evening people and once on nights. A person must be nominated by coworkers to attend. The program invites outside experts to participate in an educational and fun session. Alliant also developed a celebration called the "Quality Rally" to focus on employee recognition. The process is modeled after the Milliken & Company program. Milliken, a textile company in Spartanburg, South Carolina, is a former Baldrige winner. The CEO and COO lead the events, which include QIT presentations, skits, scavenger hunts, and outside speakers.

Brent James, of Intermountain Health Care, Inc., says that it based its recognition program on the advice of Pat Townsend, author of *Commit to Quality*. The plan has four parts:

1. *Just say thank you.* The CEO visits employees in their work area and thanks them for efforts.

2. *Symbol needed.* Real quality work must occur to receive this symbol. The symbols are tie tacks, scarves, etc. One of the system's facilities, Logan Regional Hospital, used leftover silver from radiographs for mementos. These were the most popular symbol.
3. *Recognition needed.* Employee/team member's name is printed in Quality Newsletter.
4. *Reward needed.* Gift certificates good for $5 to $50 depending on the value of improvement.

According to Beverly Begovich, St. Clair Memorial Hospital in Pittsburgh, Pennsylvania, has emphasized the role of management in its recognition program. It is a basic expectation that managers will seek out opportunities to reward and recognize employees.

Inova Health System in Reston, Virginia, uses a recognition and education approach called the Quality Forum. The first forum in 1991 included one hundred members of quality teams who met at a local hotel for a half-day session. The agenda was to share experiences in the various team phases: Project Definition, Diagnostic Journey, Remedial Journey, Holding the Gains, Group Dynamics, and Storyboarding. This facilitated group learning.

After conversations with other hospitals such as Henry Ford Health System, Bethesda Hospital, Alliant Health System, Rush-Presbyterian-St. Luke's, we developed this checklist of potential reward and recognition strategies you may want to test with your employees to determine which would work the best for you and your organization.

- Saying thank you to a person or a team.
- Personal notes from managers when expectations are exceeded.
- Restructured compensation packages focusing on quality principles.
- Face-to-face interactions: visit the employees on the job, let them share their expertise.

- Bulletin boards in public places to help you share recognition broadly.
- Publications including recognition efforts, pictures of awards, and storyboards to highlight organizational progress.
- Recognition by special speeches and events to celebrate success.
- Certificates for lunch or dinner to say thank you.
- Symbolic gifts such as coffee mugs or key chains for accomplishment of milestones.
- Plaques for achievement.
- Jewelry such as quality pins. These pins can also serve as visible commitment to quality.
- Certificates to mark completion of training milestones or team milestones.
- Work-related travel to quality conferences.
- Complimentary tickets for movies or dinner for special achievement.
- Special task force assignments.
- Flexible schedules to give freedom to the employees for personal flexibility.
- New performance planning meetings that focus on the "how to" of the job.

Action Step: Set up a series of employee discussions where potential rewards are generated by brainstorming sessions, and then multivote to determine what the most important motivators are in your organization.

Table 10.2 summarizes a sample team brainstorming session to look at potential non-monetary rewards. This UMMC team chose two categories—job-related and supervisor-related rewards. The team then multivoted the three most important rewards on each list. The selections marked with an asterisk are the final multivoted, most important rewards.

Ask employee groups to brainstorm potential rewards, both monetary and non-monetary. Once you understand what is considered important to your employees, you then need to

Table 10.2. Sample of Potential Non-Monetary Rewards
from a UMMC Team.

Job-Related Rewards	Supervisor Related Rewards
Personal Growth*	Trust*
Achievement	Personal Attention
Challenge*	Information
Flexibility	Feedback*
Responsibility	Mentoring
Accountability	Coaching
Autonomy	Counseling
Professional Growth*	Education
Interesting Work	Participation
Variety	Support
Exposure to New People	Friendship
Exposure to New Ideas	Praise* (letters, notes, verbal)

* Final list, created after multivoting.

survey the organization and be certain these rewards are present. If they are not, you must build them into the system.

Action Step: Have the Total Quality Council establish a Reward and Recognition Task Team, early in the process, to develop a reward and recognition program. Audit the organization to see if the rewards listed by employees are the rewards present in your organization.

The Reward and Recognition Task Team should be cross-functional and consist of representatives from as many different job classifications as possible; include union members if there are any. Their mission is to evaluate the existing reward and recognition programs, and plan what pieces need to be added to help spread the TQM philosophy throughout the organization.

Once your plan is developed, make sure you communicate what your mission, vision, and goals are, what is considered good performance, and how it will be measured and rewarded.

Advice from corporations that have successfully implemented TQM indicates even those who used broad employee input needed to adjust their reward and recognition programs. For example: "Florida Power and Light experienced several problems with their reward and recognition process. In the beginning, there had been small monetary rewards for teams judged to be superior. FP&L discovered that people were less eager for money than appreciation. Although teams were treated to banquets with company dignitaries, the survey disclosed that what people wanted most of all was to see their solutions in place" (Walton, 1990, p. 57).

We experienced this powerful drive of wanting to see suggestions implemented as well. One of the nurses in the coronary intensive care unit wanted to come in on a vacation day in order to see a team suggestion implemented. The nurse manager agreed to postpone the implementation until the nurse's vacation was over.

Recognition Systems

Some of the successful systems that we put into place acknowledge the positive contributions of our employees. Saying "thank you" for good work makes sense. One such program UMMC implemented is "You're Super." This program provides patients, families, visitors, physicians, and employees with a mechanism to recognize employees who are performing well above expectations. The program began in 1989, in our children's hospital, the C. S. Mott Hospital. The program soon spread to other hospital units. To recognize an employee through the "You're Super" program, the nominator picks up and completes a supergram located in wall-mounted plastic containers in prominent places throughout the hospitals.

The hospital administrators sign a personal congratulatory letter to the employee and forward the letter with a cover note to the employees' direct supervisor. The supervisor then reads the letter and presents a pin that reads "I'm Super" at the next staff meeting. The manager and employee are invited to quarterly receptions that include a variety of themes and prizes. Senior-level managers are present at these events. The program is built on the recognition principles recommended by Thomas Berry in *Managing the Total Quality Transformation*; recognition should be real, relevant, and timely, have variety built in, and include direct management involvement.

Since 1989 the "You're Super" program has recognized 2,173 employees of whom 515 were recognized more than once. The program recognized eighty-one departments, and thirty-seven of these were nominated more than once. We see the program as one way to instill pride in work and to recognize committed, effective employees. Hopefully the public focus on these moments of truth will raise the overall awareness of our desire to meet both internal and external customer requirements.

We also revamped our employee suggestion program. Our goal was expanded from a cost-savings program to recognize creativity and innovation as well. Our new goals are to:

1. Allow employees to affect the work environment positively with creative ideas for improvement.
2. Earn recognition and reward for their innovative ideas.
3. Reduce costs.

We wanted to encourage employees to suggest ideas that:

- Eliminate waste or rework.
- Substitute a less costly supply item without sacrificing quality.
- Reduce, simplify, or eliminate specific activities, or paperwork, that are no longer useful.
- Improve charge capture procedures to increase net revenue.
- Modify operations to improve quality significantly.

All of these ideas qualify for financial reward. The suggestion program provides a means for employees to bring their ideas to the attention of management, convert those ideas to actual use, and at the same time earn reward and recognition for their creative and innovative ideas.

Those suggesters whose implemented suggestions are eligible for a reward will receive 10 percent of the first year's net financial benefit, up to $10,000. Quality solutions that do not generate net savings are awarded $100. Often quality improvement ideas also include financial benefits. In addition, there are annual awards of $1,000 each for the best cost-saving suggestion, revenue-increasing suggestion, and quality improvement suggestion.

Sample types of group and individual recognition and awards developed by the Reward and Recognition Task Force at UMMC are illustrated in Table 10.3. Specifically related to quality improvement teams, Table 10.4 illustrates some points of recognition for teams.

Seven Steps to an Effective Reward System

Berry describes seven steps to creating an effective reward and recognition program: determine priorities and values, identify the criteria or milestones, set a budget for recognition, determine accountability, design and describe the features, benefits, and procedures, review the program with groups of employees, modify the program based on employee feedback (Berry, 1991, pp. 166–168). The following section describes how we have implemented each of Berry's seven recommended steps.

Step 1: Determine Priorities and Values

This step requires that you determine which behaviors and values you wish to recognize and reward. Our goal was to include Maccoby's value drives, described earlier, and also to encourage celebration. Some of the behaviors we wanted to encourage in our organization were:

- Using teams and teamwork for problem solving
- Gaining new knowledge by attending training sessions
- Learning to flowchart processes
- Learning and utilizing quality tools in daily work
- Identifying and meeting customer requirements
- Developing and measuring progress on quality indicators
- Reaching consensus on departmental quality goals
- Learning the seven-step quality improvement process
- Completing a seven-step quality improvement process

Table 10.3. Sample Types of Group and Individual Recognition and Awards.

University of Michigan Medical Center
Total Quality Process, Reward and Recognition Task Force

Individual or Group	QIT or Non-QIT	Type of Recognition	Timing	Who Nominates	Who Selects
Group	Non-QIT	You're Super	Quarterly	Patient, Visitor, Staff (anyone)	Nominator
	QIT	Points of Recognition and Total Quality Expo	At each step of the QI process	(Part of Total Quality Process to recognize all QITs)	Divisional Lead Team or Corporate Lead Team for Total Quality Expo
Individual	Non-QIT	You're Super	Quarterly	Patient, Visitor, Staff (anyone)	Associate Hospital Director
	Non-QIT	Employee Suggestion Program	As submitted	Self	Suggestion Process
	Non-QIT	Employee of the Month	Monthly	Most likely staff, but could be anyone	Employee of the Month Committee
	QIT	Manager of the Month	Monthly	Anyone in the organization	Senior Associate Hospital Director

Table 10.4. Sample Points of Total Quality Team Recognition.

Points of Recognition	Team Leader and Facilitator	Divisional Lead Team	Corporate Lead Team	Supervisors and Managers	Corporate Leaders (as individuals)	Employees
Ongoing MBWA (Management by Walking Around)		V	V	V	V	
Appearing at a TQ Meeting		V	V	V	V	
TQ Expos	V	V	V	V	V	V
Visiting Storyboards		V	V	V	V	V
When One Becomes a Team Leader		V	L			
Quality Roadmap Step 1: Analyze Process*	V & RI			V		
Quality Roadmap Step 2: Measure Quality Gap*	V	V & P		V		
Quality Roadmap Step 3: Identify Root Causes*	V			V		
Quality Roadmap Step 4: Determine Options*	V & RI	V & P		V		
Quality Roadmap Step 5: Evaluate Results*	V			V		
Quality Roadmap Step 6: Maintain Gain*	V			V		
Quality Roadmap Step 7: Review and Renew*	V & RI	V & P	L	V		

* Completion of step is a milestone on Quality Roadmap.

Type of Recognition:
V = Verbal   RI = Recognition item   L = Letter   P = Presentation or report to Divisional Lead Team

Each major category required an action plan for how we would encourage these behaviors and a reward plan to reinforce the desired behaviors. The first step was to emphasize the importance of these elements in the training programs. The next step was to weave the expected mastery actions into our management expectations document so that all managers would understand the importance of the milestones. Finally, the milestones were included in each person's performance plan.

Step 2: Identify the Criteria or Milestones

At UMMC we established our major milestones as:

- Completed introductory quality course
- Completed awareness sessions
- Recognized by "You're Super" program
- Submitted an employee suggestion
- Implemented an employee suggestion
- Completed team leader training
- Completed facilitator training
- Certified as a TQM trainer
- Completed team member training
- Joined a team
- Completed a quality story, quality process, or quality project
- Presented storyboard to lead team
- Presented storyboard to the Hospital Executive Board

These milestones are consistent with several of the values Maccoby describes, including pleasure, mastery, and meaning (1988, pp. 57–76). The milestones relate to training and integrating TQM behaviors into daily work. For each training milestone we developed a formal recognition process. For example, for team leader and team facilitator training, the senior associate director or a corporate officer personally hands out the certificates on the last day of the training program. We thank each person for his or her effort and welcome him or her to the "Transformation Team." Our process includes a wrap-up on where we are organizationally in the process, what lies ahead, and how each person can help us continue to progress.

Over time we have increased recognition and celebration for all types of team efforts. Since enhanced teamwork is one of our goals, celebration of team success is very important. Many milestones relate to team presentations. When teams reach steps two, four, and seven of our seven-step quality improvement process, they give presentations to their divisional lead team. All types of teams are invited to give presentations to the corporate lead team and the Hospital Executive Board. Following the team presentation, which gives recognition to team members and their work, the team leader takes the team and its facilitator to lunch.

There also is a new annual recognition banquet, still in the planning stage, which will help us celebrate quality progress and recognize the work of teams. All senior executives and all team members and their significant others will be invited to this event to celebrate the progress of quality at our institution.

Step 3: Set a Budget for Recognition

The rule of thumb for a preliminary recognition budget, according to Berry, is $5–$10 per employee per year (1991, p. 167). Our experience was that we spent far less than this in our early years because of our lack of strategic planning. As our plans evolved and we were ready to expand to our Quality Expo and yearly recognition banquet, we spent a little more. Our per-employee budget is based on 11,000 personnel in the Medical Center. The Expo, a twenty-four-hour Total Quality exhibition, is budgeted at $1 per employee. The cost is for muffins, coffee, cheese and crackers, punch and cookies, pencils, pens, and other small items with the UMMC quality logo. The Total Quality banquet will cost about $20 per attendee. There are also decentralized expenses, determined by team leaders, for plaques, pins, lunches, dinners, certificates, and other quality mementos that average about $1 per employee. This seems to be in the ballpark with other hospitals. For example, Alliant Health System plans $25 per employee for their program. The managers and supervisors use these funds at their own discretion for reward and recognition. There are many Alliant logo items including sweatshirts, paperweights, and coffee mugs for managers to choose from.

Action Step: Develop a budget for the reward and recognition program. Consider milestones you wish to achieve, and recognize these milestones with events and rewards.

Step 4: Determine Accountability

As we entered the phase of decentralization, each Divisional Lead Team became accountable for the recognition program within its area. The budget is determined for central events, and then a proportion is shared across the divisions. This budget covers lunches, plaques, and small mementos chosen by the teams or team members. The divisional leaders also send congratulatory letters to staff after selecting/volunteering for a team, when training is completed, and when the team has completed its quality story. One lead team, Professional Services, had special plaques made for those team members who completed a storyboard. Plaques are given to team members when they present the results of their quality process at the lead team meeting.

Action Step: Determine what level in the organization will be responsible for rewards and recognition. Do you need a central and a decentralized budget? How will you communicate about rewards and recognition given?

Step 5: Design and Describe the Features, Benefits, and Procedures

Make use of the Reward and Recognition Task Team to develop feature stories for newsletters, journals, and poster sessions to share new developments and opportunities broadly. We also included the design of the recognition program in our Total Quality rollout plan, so employees would know what to expect and what the timing of the process would be. Other communications about our gainsharing, employee suggestion, and waste prevention programs are scheduled to keep employees informed and up to date. We have the use of a closed circuit television system to share videos or important quality information. Alliant Health System installed an electronic bulletin board, with TV monitors throughout the hospital, to share information about quality progress.

Action Step: Determine how to share your reward and recognition policies with all employees. Consider a special employee forum when the Reward and Recognition Task Team has completed its work in order to share the results of the policy. Also use newsletters, journals, and bulletin boards.

Step 6: Review the Program with Groups of Employees

Once the program is implemented, make sure you are soliciting feedback from employee groups. Use focus groups to gather information. This is using the Plan-Do-Check-Act cycle in daily work. Using customer input to shape your program shows significant management commitment. Use formal survey tools as well as informal discussions to find out what reward and recognition strategies will work for your unique employee population.

Action Step: Develop mechanisms for large groups of employees to give feedback on the program. Are the reward and recognition strategies meeting multiple needs? Are there other strategies that need to be added?

Step 7: Modify Your Program Based on Employee Feedback

Assess the impact of the program frequently by focus groups, surveys, and interviews. Changing the program to reflect employee concerns is another way of showing that you are committed to responding to customer requirements at all levels in the organization.

Action Step: Make use of focus groups and surveys to understand customer requirements and modify your program.

Other Achievements

Our Reward and Recognition Task Team suggested several types of programs. The first step was to look at the compensation system and determine what in the existing program was effective and what needed to change. One such suggestion was based on Deming's concepts to decrease the number of categories within the merit pay system. We decreased the number of categories from ten to three the first year. The previous categories required that you place a person on a scale of ten steps, from zero to maximum. We changed the categories to three: did not meet objectives, met objectives, and exceeded objectives. This modification was a first step in revamping our compensation program. Our Reward and Recognition Team suggested that we develop a gainsharing program, which was implemented in July 1991.

We implemented a Total Quality Manager-of-the-Month award program in 1987. This program is in addition to the Employee-of-the-Month program that has been in place since the 1970s. Anyone in the organization can recommend a manager for this award. The only rule is that he or she must demonstrate how the manager is using the TQM philosophy to manage. The senior associate director takes the winner to lunch and devotes two hours listening to the manager and discussing how they are implementing TQM in his or her area. The manager is also given a certificate of award.

Our Total Quality Expo, mentioned earlier, is a full twenty-four-hour demonstration of TQM progress. Teams are invited by their lead team to display their quality storyboard and be available to answer any questions attendees may have. A resource table is also set up to share books, articles, and other important information on TQM. Senior administrators and our chief of clinical affairs manned a table to answer questions anyone might have relative to the TQM process. Employees took full advantage of this opportunity to quiz institutional leaders. A videotape featuring employees of the Medical Center talking about how they were involved in the process ran continuously. We were surprised how many people stood for the full twenty minutes of the film to listen to experienced team members talk about their experiences. A slide-and-tape show of team meetings, set to music, was also a popular exhibit.

UMMC Employee Appreciation Week is held the first week of June each year. We began displaying storyboards and asking teams to discuss their QI Story with fellow employees in 1991. The teams and their fellow employees all seemed to enjoy this event, and it will occur on an annual basis.

For the month of October 1991, "National Quality Month," we held several reward and recognition opportunities. We rented a movie theater for 1,600 people, 800 employees and guests, for a special showing of "The Doctor," starring William Hurt. The purpose in choosing this movie was to illustrate a customer focus. The tickets were given by a drawing held each Friday during the month. We also held an essay contest for all employees to tell us in one hundred words or less why they should represent UMMC at the Healthcare Forum's Power of Quality Conference during June 1992 in San Diego. The winners, a third-year house officer and a unit clerk, were selected by the Corporate Lead Team. The prizes, two all-expense-paid trips to the conference, were announced in December. We are grateful to our friends at St. Clair Hospital, Pittsburgh, Pennsylvania, for suggesting this idea to us. It created great organizational excitement and interest.

Leadership's Role in Reward and Recognition

Just as with other elements of TQM, the role of leadership is critical. Your ability to role-model the behaviors that you want the reward and recognition process to reinforce is essential. Your personal commitment can make all the difference in the success of the program. Visibility of the leadership is a crucial variable. "Woody Allen put it best: Eighty percent of success is showing up. Pay attention in big ways, rallies, recognition, ceremonies, and attendance at five day training sessions. Also in small ways: the questions you ask at the start of every meeting;

the consistent theme of notes penned informally on memos; the five minute detour that you invariably make while you're on the inspection site; showing up at midnight on the loading dock to say thanks for a record breaking day; et cetera" (Peters, 1990, p. 7).

As you make rounds, ask questions about the mission of each department, ask to see copies of their customer analyses, review the departmental quality indicators and quality plans. Ask to see the flowcharts and storyboards their teams have developed. Make a quality audit part of each visit, and show employees quality is important to you. Asking appropriate questions relating to TQM principles and the use of tools and techniques is one of the best ways for leaders to demonstrate support.

Many quality-oriented institutions are guiding management to increase reward and recognition potential. For example, Dave Miller noted that Alliant Health System has a new recognition policy that articulates the manager's role in recognition: "Recognizing and rewarding employees when they have done a good job is part of the quality policy." Others stress role modeling. Trish Stoltz, from the Henry Ford Health System, reported that Gail Warden, the system CEO, holds the people who report to him responsible for dedicating at least 25 percent of their time to quality efforts. These types of directives and standards allow visible commitment to quality.

Visit Team Meetings

Ask existing teams, through the team leader, if they would mind a visitor. Attend a meeting and watch the dynamics. Let the staff know you appreciate what they are doing. We guarantee you will be pleased with what you see.

At every employee meeting, ask how many people are serving on teams, how many have completed a quality story, what people are learning, and what changes are happening in the hospital as a result of TQM implementation.

Personally kick off each training session. This demonstrates your commitment better than anything else. If you are unable to make it because of a scheduling problem, assign a senior officer to fill in for you. As each class of team leaders and facilitators completes the course work, personally hand out certificates, thank them for their efforts, and welcome them to an advanced role in the quality transformation. Try to point out TQM behaviors that you have observed in the learners; say something personal about each attendee. Be sure to communicate your expectations that they are adding to the ranks of trained quality leaders, and encourage them to seek out team opportunities.

Storyboard Rounds

We had great difficulty getting storyboards posted in public places. There were many excuses given and few results. Storyboards are important communication and educational tools, and we were concerned about our lack of progress. The CEO and COO decided to begin making Storyboard Rounds with the corporate officers from the areas visited. The lead teams selected areas to visit, and rounds began in October 1991. It was our belief that if leadership showed how important the storyboards were to us, they would get more attention. We found most of the resistance was due to the fear of not having perfect storyboards. Some people worried that their data analysis would not measure up. It is important to emphasize that the process is about solving problems and continuously improving, not about perfection. Reinforce that it is the identification of root causes rather than the treatment of symptoms that is important, not the quality of data presentation. As the CEO and COO make rounds, they congratulate team members personally on their efforts. They write personal Post-It notes to teams to encourage their work. They also hand out tee shirts that say "Together Everyone Achieves More."

Action Step: Make rounds to identify and recognize quality improvement storyboards and other quality improvement efforts.

Conclusion

There are few if any healthcare organizations that are comfortable with their reward and recognition programs. This is an area of quality implementation that requires experimentation with techniques and tracking of results. To develop a successful program, visit or talk to other organizations, share possible programs with employees, and experiment with strategies designed for your organization. As you develop successful strategies, share the concepts with your peer institutions.

The first step in building a comprehensive program is to invite a broad group of customers to participate in the planning process. Make sure this group extends participation to an even larger group of employees. They should use focus groups and surveys to determine which rewards and recognition strategies are seen as positive in your organization. Frequent assessment of the process is also key. Reward and recognition implementation must be viewed as a dynamic process.

PART THREE

Analytical Methods for TQM

Chapter Eleven

TQM Actions
in Daily Operations

A critically important part of a TQM process is the integration of the approach and techniques into the daily work of everyone in the organization. There are three key types of activities included in a TQM process: quality planning, quality improvement teams, and quality operations (Juran, 1988, pp. 11–12; Qualtec, Inc., 1989b). This chapter describes the need for integration of TQM into daily management and operations and provides examples of integration strategies.

Quality Perceived at Point of Service

Although an organization consists of a hierarchy with levels of positions, quality is provided and perceived at the point of service. Some call this the "moment of truth." A patient judges the quality of his or her service based on outcomes and direct, personal interaction with the physician, nurse, clerk, housekeeper, phlebotomist, transporter, dietitian, physical therapist, patient accounts representative, and many others. A physician who refers a patient to your organization may judge quality based on interaction with the telephone operator, physician's secretary, physician, house officer or resident, medical records clerk, and others. A staff physician may judge quality based on interaction with the admitting clerk, operating room scheduling clerk, nurse, pathology secretary, radiologist, and others.

Your organization's quality is judged by the timeliness, accuracy, courtesy, and outcomes of the service, product, or information provided to each customer with whom staff directly interact. Managers seldom interact directly with patients, referring physicians, staff physicians, or other external customers, unless there has been a problem. Therefore, the delivery and perception of quality are dependent on integrating TQM principles, behaviors, and methods into the daily operations of everyone in the organization. The employees who most closely interface with customers must utilize TQM methods and techniques. The role of those providing services directly to external customers is to meet and exceed their expectations. The role of other staff who do not directly interface with external customers is to provide the supportive services and information for the direct providers. The role of managers is to develop the systems and create the environment to enable the direct providers to meet and exceed customers' requirements.

Reasons for TQM in Daily Operations

There are many reasons why TQM approaches and methods should be incorporated into daily operations. Examples are to:

- Demonstrate commitment of managers by taking actions to improve quality.
- Improve all aspects of daily operations: the quality of all services, products, and information; customer satisfaction; cost effectiveness; and working environment.
- Change the role and management style of people in managerial positions from controlling to leading.
- Promote a culture in which everyone's ideas are sought and used to improve quality.
- Disperse quality improvement efforts to every person in the organization, not just those on formal Quality Improvement Teams.
- Incorporate Total Quality approach and methods into daily operations as the way of doing business.

Alternatives

Each organization faces the question of how to roll out the TQM effort. The two extreme approaches are to put all emphasis on formal Quality Improvement Teams working on top-down prioritized issues, or to involve all employees in a broad-scale, relatively uncontrolled, bottom-up approach. These approaches will be discussed to provide information for your decisions.

Emphasize Formal Quality Improvement Teams. For Quality Improvement Teams, you want each team to follow a common, specific quality improvement process. Sample standard processes are described in Chapters Two, Twelve, and Thirteen. At UMMC, for example, this requires the team meet the following criteria:

- Team leader has completed one-week team leader training, in addition to other educational programs.
- Team facilitator is used, and the facilitator has completed both the one-week team leader and the one-week team facilitator training.
- Team follows the seven-step quality improvement process (Figure 8.2).
- Team meets regularly, for approximately an average of one hour per week.
- Team is approved by, and reports results to, a divisional lead team.

The projects are often selected based on priorities established by top management. This process is very effective but imposes substantial formal structure. Some advantages and disadvantages of heavy emphasis on formal Quality Improvement Teams are listed below.

- Advantages of Emphasis on Formal QI Teams:
  — Assurance that standard process is used.
  — Assurance that team leader has formal training.
  — A trained facilitator is available to coach the team leader and improve the likelihood of team success.

- —Priority of project has been reviewed by a lead team.
- —Results formally communicated to lead teams, which can then communicate to others.
- • Disadvantages of Emphasis on Formal QI Teams:
  - —May impose unnecessary structure, effort, costs, and time delays to make improvements. This is especially true when a formal process is used for relatively simple or insignificant problems and opportunities for improvement.
  - —Some people may feel left out or disenfranchised, if they are not part of a formal QI team.
  - —Some groups may not need to or want to follow a standard process.
  - —Prevents managers who have not completed team leader training from forming a team to make improvements.
  - —Prevents a team forming if there is no trained facilitator available to facilitate the process.

It should be noted that it is difficult for QI teams to be successful without support of supervisors and managers, even if the staff are interested and involved.

Emphasize Broad-Scale, Relatively Uncontrolled Expansion of QI. Another very different approach is to emphasize widespread action by every employee, work group, and informal team to improve quality, without any specified standard quality improvement process. In his book *Commit to Quality*, Pat Townsend (1990) advocates nonvoluntary inclusion of every employee from the first day a quality improvement process is initiated. This approach represents an organizationwide effort to involve all employees to improve service quality. The approach is similar to an employee suggestion program, but with more top management emphasis and participation of all employees. Some advantages and disadvantages of this approach are listed below.

- • Advantages of Emphasis on Broad Expansion:
  - —Everyone is involved, so no one feels left out.
  - —Demonstrates personal involvement of all managers.

- — Achieves improvements quickly, by collecting what some call the "low-hanging fruit."
- — Requires less initial training and investment.
- Disadvantages of Emphasis on Broad Expansion:
  - — Everyone approaches the quality improvement effort differently.
  - — Lacks a standard process for quality improvement.
  - — Initial surge of results can slow when obvious quick improvements are accomplished and more involved process improvements require a more analytical approach.
  - — Uncoordinated quality improvement efforts can lead to duplication and unnecessary use of resources.

Tailored Approach. Each organization should tailor the approach to best meet its circumstances and environment. Most organizations and consultants agree that the long-term goal is to have everyone involved and to use a standardized quality improvement process when appropriate. As an example, UMMC took the approach of first developing rather formalized Quality Improvement Teams with trained team leaders and team facilitators. Our goal is that each manager will complete team leader and team facilitator training by January 1994. We then expanded this to a continuum of quality improvement efforts, including wide-scale employee involvement (see Figure 8.1). Managers can begin encouraging the broad understanding and application of QI through the actions listed in the next section.

Actions for Managers

Managers and supervisors are key to the rollout of TQM within your organization. Their actions establish the environment in which their employees will accept or reject its implementation. Managers can begin taking many actions consistent with QI, even before they form or join a Quality Improvement Team. In this section we summarize fifteen actions every manager/supervisor can take on his or her own job to improve both the quality and cost effectiveness of daily operations. The term *department* is

defined here in a general sense to include one or more departments, work units, or areas being managed.

This is an iterative process; after each step you should
review the impact on previous steps and revise them as necessary. For example, after defining the department's goals, functions, processes, and customers, you then determine the customers' requirements. This may lead to a redefinition of the goals,
functions, and processes.

Action Step 1: Understand and live by values, vision, mission, goals,
and management expectations.

Virtually all organizations have written statements related
to values, vision, mission, and goals. Yet few employees know,
understand, or relate to those statements. Mission statements
tend to be very general and difficult to relate to an employee's
daily job. Sample actions to accomplish an understanding and
communication of a common purpose are illustrated in Table
11.1. The first step is to review the written statements related to
values, vision, mission, goals, and other statements of common
direction, and to ask questions like the following. When were the
statements last updated? Are they understandable by all staff?
Are they pertinent? Give copies of statements to a sample of staff
from all levels of your organization, and ask them questions like:
Have you ever seen these? If so, which ones, when, and in what
context? What do these mean to you in your own words? If
employees cannot relate to the statements in their own words,
with a sense of common direction for the organization, then the
statements need to be revised. Ask employees to give examples
of work actions in their job that would not be consistent with the
statements. In revising the statements, broad input from employees, customers, and possibly suppliers and others will be
helpful. At UMMC, for example, we used focus groups involving
a total of over three hundred employees, physicians, and others
to develop our statements of quality and values. The principle
used throughout TQM is that people will strongly support
something they have developed. Therefore, in addition to gaining more ideas, involvement develops critical support. If there

Table 11.1. Sample Actions to Develop Common Direction.

Action 1: Sample Manager/Team Actions	Sample Tools and Techniques
• Review and understand your organization's: — Mission — Statement of quality — Vision — Guiding principles — Goals — Customers and quality indicators • Revise the statements as necessary, with input from customers, employees, and others. Then communicate broadly. • Read and distribute current literature on Total Quality. • Demonstrate support of common direction and Management Expectations by your daily actions. • Discuss quality at staff meetings and individually with staff. • Listen to staff for ideas related to common direction. • Incorporate expectations of management into performance plans. • Get feedback from staff on how well you personally meet Management Expectations.	• Group discussion • Brainstorming • Employee surveys • Manager's Guide • Focus groups • Management by walking around (MBWA)

are inconsistencies among the documents—and there often are—these should be discussed to determine appropriate questions for senior mangement. Once revised, the statements should be broadly communicated to employees, customers, and suppliers. Only if each person knows the organization's common direction, can he or she perform and improve in that direction.

Many managers do not have a clear understanding of what is expected of them by their organization. Communication is improved by preparing written expectations of managers and distributing them to all managers. As an example, the expectations of managers developed by UMMC are illustrated in Exhibit 11.1.

One approach to communicate the importance of the

Exhibit 11.1. UMMC Expectations of Management.

Purpose:

The underlying premise of the Total Quality Process is that we need to change to and sustain a culture of continuous improvement. *The University of Michigan Medical Center Expectations of Management* are behaviorally oriented statements that provide a framework toward achieving our *Mission* and *Statement of Quality*. Understanding and learning to live by the *Expectations of Management* is the critical step leadership must take to demonstrate a commitment to quality in pursuit of organizational excellence.

Each of us will live the Total Quality Process by constantly making improvements, preventing errors, and providing the leadership to:

I. **Develop and support a work environment where every employee's capability is improved.**
   — Emphasize and demonstrate to each employee the value of their contribution to the organization.
   — Invest in employees so that they are prepared for ongoing changes in the workplace.
   — Select, transfer and promote based on individual strengths, knowledge, competence, leadership skills and ability to work as part of a team.
   — Motivate and empower employees to achieve their potential.
   — Provide a complete orientation to employees and continuous training to accomplish their jobs and improve skills. Ensure they are familiar and act in accordance with the *Guest Relations House Rules* and *Standard Practice Guide*.
   — Ensure that employees understand their responsibilities.
   — Give employees continual feedback regarding assessment of job performance. Maintain and enhance self-esteem. Identify and compliment individuals on strengths. Problem solve with employees to improve their work.
   — Set challenging but realistic performance planning goals.
   — Achieve performance planning targets in an efficient and timely manner.
   — Identify and remove barriers that prevent employees from initiating quality improvement.
II. **Promote an environment of open communication, trust, loyalty and pride.**
   — Provide information to employees which allows them to perform their jobs.
   — Collect and share information with employees to give them a macro-view about:
   > Health care trends
   > Organizational trends
   > Internal and external customer expectations
   > Financial data
   > Departmental goals, achievements, and overall performance

Exhibit 11.1. UMMC Expectations of Management, Cont'd.

- Promote the extension of knowledge and share contributions with employees and peers to encourage education and growth.
- Cooperate with other departments in pursuing opportunities for improvement to provide the best system of patient care and customer service.
- Maintain pride in the facility. Support and maintain a safe and clean working environment for patients, visitors, customers and employees.
- Facilitate compromise and problem resolution. Emphasize that teamwork produces quality.
- Delegate and prioritize assignments in relation to employee's capability. Clarify goals and objectives, performance measures, communication expectations, and scope of authority.
- Conduct regular forums to identify opportunities for improvement.
- Utilize effective listening skills and encourage your employees to do the same.

III. **Create an atmosphere that promotes excellence through innovation and creativity.**
- Solicit and utilize employee input; recognize that employees possess the expertise to make decisions about their jobs.
- Share and give authority to individuals to resolve problems.
- Encourage employees to act on their ideas by promoting and sponsoring quality improvement ideas.
- Develop a climate where risk taking is rewarded and accept mistakes as a normal part of trying something new. Respond to errors with constructive criticism. Allow the message of past mistakes to guide future actions.
- Reward suggestions for improvement and celebrate successful implementation of ideas.
- Be futuristic and examine opportunities to expand market share.

IV. **Foster an environment which values human diversity and sustains respect for multi-culturalism.**
- Examine our own cultural background to understand how differing perspectives may lead to misunderstanding and miscommunication with others.
- Learn more about the culture of diverse groups in order to understand and respect their cultural values, customs and viewpoint.
- Avoid stereotyping and passing value judgments on others.
- Promote respect and utilize the work group diversity to create new ideas.

V. **Coordinate resources and activities to meet society's expectations as well as our own objectives of quality and efficiency.**
- Prudently allocate and utilize institutional resources based on priorities.
- Meet budget objectives. Develop and implement strategies to reduce expenses and increase revenues.
- Evaluate programs based on quality, customer benefit, profitability, and value added.

Exhibit 11.1. UMMC Expectations of Management, Cont'd.

— Ensure that budget problems are identified early and that responsible
actions are taken.
— Work with employees to create departmental mission statements.
— Continuously follow the Plan-Do-Check-Act cycle:

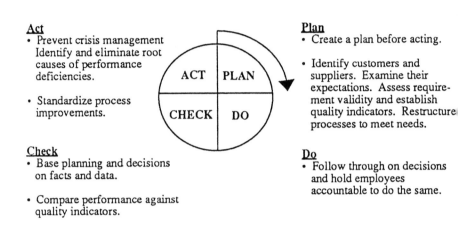

Act
• Prevent crisis management
  Identify and eliminate root
  causes of performance
  deficiencies.

• Standardize process
  improvements.

Check
• Base planning and decisions
  on facts and data.

• Compare performance against
  quality indicators.

Plan
• Create a plan before acting.

• Identify customers and
  suppliers. Examine their
  expectations. Assess requirement validity and establish
  quality indicators. Restructure
  processes to meet needs.

Do
• Follow through on decisions
  and hold employees
  accountable to do the same.

Source: University of Michigan Medical Center, "Expectations of Management." Reprinted with permission.

expected management behaviors is to incorporate them into the
performance plans for all managers and supervisors. This will
cause a review of performance compared to expectations of
management at least annually.

Some sample approaches to improve communication
and understanding of your organization's statements of mission,
vision, goals, and quality are to:

• Distribute copies of all appropriate statements to each staff
  member.
• Prepare a two-column table with organizational statements
  in left column, and blank spaces at right for staff to enter
  their own words of what the statements mean.
• Conduct group discussion on the relationship of organiza-

tional mission and goals to those for the department (see Action Step 3 below).

- Conduct surveys of staff to determine their understanding of the organizational mission and goals.
- Post statements in prominent locations: lobbies, waiting rooms, employee lounges, elevator lobbies, conference rooms, and offices.

Action Step 2: Demonstrate commitment, sponsorship, participation, and common understanding for improvement of quality and cost effectiveness.

As stated several times in this book, actions speak louder than words. Everyone is watching to see whether there is active participation and personal involvement to demonstrate real commitment. Sample actions to demonstrate commitment are illustrated in Table 11.2.

The responses on evaluation forms during our initial Total Quality education programs provided information that

Table 11.2. Sample Actions to Demonstrate Commitment.

Action 2: Sample Manager/Team Actions	*Sample Tools and Techniques*
• Read and distribute current literature on Total Quality. • Include quality and cost effectiveness as regular agenda items for meetings. • Participate in education and training sessions as a participant and as faculty. • Ensure staff availability to participate in education and training sessions. • Fill in for staff, so they can attend education programs and QI team meetings. • Manage by walking around—visit and compliment staff in work areas. • Watch and listen, don't tell, while observing. Communication is key. • Demonstrate and encourage Total Quality upward, laterally, and downward in organization.	• Group discussion • Management by walking around (MBWA) • Active listening • Read literature on quality and pass on to others

employees at each level in the organization were skeptical that the managers above them were really committed. Many employees entered comments like, "TQM makes sense to me, but my supervisor will never change." Several supervisors entered comments like, "TQM makes sense to me, but my manager will never change." Several managers entered comments like, "TQM makes sense to me, but the administrators and corporate officers will not change." Even the administrators and corporate officers were questioning where the CEO and clinical chairmen stood on their ability to change. Each group was looking for visible actions to indicate real commitment.

Action Step 3: Develop mission and goals for your department(s).

Workload, performance, and productivity are relevant only if they contribute to the goals of the department and the organization to meet the customers' requirements. For employees to identify with the organization and to contribute, with the least rework and waste and their greatest creative ideas, they must understand the organizational and departmental goals and how they contribute to those goals. Sample actions to develop and communicate a departmental mission are illustrated in Table 11.3.

Action Step 4: Identify and understand functions and processes within your department(s) and involving other departments.

It is important to focus quality improvement efforts on the functions and processes as your customers see them, rather than to focus simply on your departmental borders. Many managers, employees, and physicians focus too narrowly on their departments. Sample actions to identify and understand processes are illustrated in Table 11.4.

Based on the experiences at UMMC and several other organizations, one of the most important tools is flowcharting processes from their beginning to their end. Flowcharting is further explained and illustrated in Chapters Twelve and Thirteen. It is best to begin with a general flowchart, then develop

Table 11.3. Sample Actions to Develop Departmental Mission.

Action 3: Sample Manager/Team Actions	Sample Tools and Techniques
• Read and understand organization's values, vision, mission, etc. • Listen to customers and staff to gain input for departmental mission. • Prepare brief departmental mission and goal statements based on: 　− Organizational mission 　− Statement of quality 　− Vision 　− Guiding principles 　− Goals 　− Customers and quality indicators • Communicate mission and goals to all involved staff, customers, and suppliers.	• Group discussion • Set aside time in departmental meetings for discussion • Brainstorming • Affinity diagram • Multivoting • Nominal group technique

more detailed flowcharts as appropriate. To create an accurate flowchart of a process, all categories of employees performing activities in the process should be involved as either team members or consultants to the team. Our experience indicates that, by the time a detailed process flowchart is completed, each team member:

- Realizes that he or she does not understand all phases of the process in detail
- Develops an improved understanding and respect for other team members and people involved with the process
- Understands the whole process much better than before
- Identifies steps that do not add value and identifies opportunities for improvement as the flowchart is being prepared

Although hand-drawn flowcharts are perfectly acceptable, it is often easier to update them later if they are prepared using commercially available computer software like MacFlow for Macintosh microcomputers, or Easyflow, RF Flow, or ABC Flow for IBM-compatible microcomputers.

Table 11.4. Sample Actions to Understand Processes.

Action 4: Sample Manager/Team Actions	Sample Tools and Techniques

• Identify major activities/functions of department.
• Identify customers for all major activities/functions of department.
• Identify all activities/functions for each customer. (This is a cross-check that all activities/functions are identified.)
• Define for each function: objectives, priority, origin of work.
• List processes you manage or comanage.
• List other processes involving you and your staff.
• Flowchart processes you manage or comanage, to identify: actions, customers, interdependencies. Begin with the most important processes.
• Observe and listen carefully to people who perform jobs. They know the details of those current jobs best.
• Identify quality features of processes.
• Identify any major opportunities for improvement:
  —Within your department(s)/area(s).
  —Involving other departments (see Action Step 11).
	• Group discussion
	• Interviewing staff who perform work
	• Flowcharting
	• Brainstorming
	• Force field or barriers and aids analysis

Action Step 5: Identify internal and external customers and suppliers for processes.

External and internal customers and suppliers at each step of the process can easily be identified from the process flowchart. At each step, the person providing the service, product, or information is the supplier. The person receiving the service, product, or information is the customer. Typically the customer at one step in a process is the supplier in the next step of the process. For example, the admitting clerk is the customer of the patient providing information at the time of the admission. The admitting clerk then becomes the supplier to the inpatient unit clerk. Sample actions to identify customers and suppliers are illustrated in Table 11.5.

Table 11.5. Sample Actions to Identify Customers and Suppliers.

Action 5: Sample Manager/Team Actions	Sample Tools and Techniques

• For each activity of flowchart, identify:
  —Supplier (person providing service, product, or information; person at tail of arrow)
  —Customer (person receiving service, product, or information; person at point of arrow)
• Ask staff whom they provide services, products, or information to. What is provided to each customer?
• Identify relationships.
	• Flowcharting
	• Interviews

Action Step 6: Determine customer requirements.

Customer requirements are determined by frequently meeting and talking directly with customers. It is very hard to have too much communication with your customers. Most of us communicate far too infrequently and seldom about customers' current or future requirements. Mutual understanding is the key. The supplier should understand the customer's requirements, and the customer should understand the supplier's capabilities, potentials, and limitations. Suppliers can often provide new ideas and improvements, which improve the services, products, or information provided to the customer, if there is a mutual understanding of requirements and capabilities. Do not assume you know customer requirements. It is common for people to assume they know their customers' requirements without talking directly to them on a regular basis. Some sample actions to identify customer requirements are illustrated in Table 11.6.

Action Step 7: Choose key measures/indicators.

Once you have established the requirements of your customers, the question is how you or your customers will know whether you are meeting those requirements. You must establish measures or indicators to monitor progress. There is an old saying: "If it isn't measured, it isn't managed." There are virtually

Table 11.6. Sample Actions to Determine Customer Requirements.

Action 6: Sample Manager/Team Actions	Sample Tools and Techniques

• Interview customers about requirements. Ask questions and listen.
• Conduct focus groups of customers to determine customer requirements.
• Develop operational definitions.
• Ask key questions to define complete requirements:
  —What?
  —When?
  —Who?
  —For whom?
  —Where?
  —Why?
  —How? (systems, forms, tools)
• Suggest improvements.
• Define objectives.
• Determine priorities.
• Determine origin of work.
• Monitor customer opinion.
	• Interviews with customers
	• Questionnaires/ surveys
	• Focus groups
	• Quality function deployment
	• Pareto chart

an infinite number of possible things that could be measured. To keep everyone focused, however, it is important to select a few critical measures or indicators to monitor the degree to which you meet the customer requirements and process expectations. Key measures or indicators can be established externally or internally. These indicators do not provide all relevant information, but they should be used to determine when the process is out of control or a more detailed investigation is appropriate.

We are all familiar with the many requirements established by external organizations such as JCAHO, Health Care Financing Administration (HCFA) of the Department of Health and Human Services (HSS), state departments of public health, state departments of mental health, state and local fire marshals, professional associations, and third-party payers. An example may be the current JCAHO requirement that organizational policies be updated regularly. To some extent these requirements can be influenced, but for the most part they are simply requirements from a customer which must be met. Many of these requirements are reasonable; some should be viewed as minimum requirements. It is our responsibility to challenge requirements that do not make sense or that are counter to continuous quality improvement.

Internally established measures are equally important, especially those mutually established with your internal and external customers. If your customers work with you to establish the key measures or indicators, they will be satisfied that you have met or exceeded their requirements when those indicators exceed the desired levels. An example for referring physicians is that they will receive the following key information within forty-eight hours of discharge of any patient they refer to a physician or hospital: when the patient was seen, who saw the patient, the diagnosis, what procedures were done, the prognosis, and the required follow-up care. It has been our experience that referring physicians consider this type of information an integral part of the care we provide. You can then work to continuously improve the performance related to those measures. Sample actions to choose key measures or indicators are illustrated in Table 11.7.

Action Step 8: Measure and understand process capabilities.

Understanding process capabilities refers to measuring and understanding the results using key measures or indicators, over time. Through using graphs it is easier to perceive single points outside control limits, trends, or runs. No matter what your desired situation, it is important first to understand the capabilities of the current process, as measured by the key indicators. You can set goals and hope for anything, but the results are unlikely to change unless the process that produces those results is changed. Sample actions to understand process capabilities are outlined in Table 11.8. Descriptions and examples of run charts and control charts are provided in Chapters Twelve and Thirteen.

Operational definitions are very important. Virtually every Quality Improvement Team at UMMC, and other organi-

Table 11.7. Sample Actions to Choose Key Measures/Indicators.

Action 7: Sample Manager/Team Actions	Sample Tools and Techniques
• Identify measures/indicators of input from suppliers. • Identify measures/indicators of outputs to customers: — Quality measures. — Select few of most important indicators. — Begin with 1–2 most important measures. • Identify productivity measures. • Identify budget measures. • Develop operational definitions and methods of measurement for all measures. • Measure: features of customer requirements, other features (for example, JCAHO). • Verify appropriateness of measures: — Consistent with mission, goals, and objectives — Right level of detail and emphasis — Useful for decisions — Avoid excessive measurement — Minimize misuse to "beat" system — Meet RUMBA criteria: reasonable, understandable, measurable, believable, and achievable • Pilot test the measures.	• Interview customers • Checksheets • Pie/bar graphs • Run/control charts

zations with which we have communicated, discovered that different team members and people working in the process have varying operational definitions for the same terms. You should check operational definitions by asking each team member, and others working in the process, to give a definition of each key measure. For example, ask precisely what events are used to record the arrival and departure times in an outpatient clinic.

Once you have graphed the key indicators, and calculated upper and lower control limits, there are two key questions you should ask. If the process is not stable, which is indicated by single points outside the upper or lower control limits, trends of five or more points in sequence steadily increasing or decreasing, runs of five or more points in sequence above or below the

Table 11.8. Sample Actions to Understand Process Capabilities.

Action 8: Sample Manager/Team Actions	*Sample Tools and Techniques*
• Measure process.	• Checksheets
• Graph measurements:	• Pie/bar graphs
—If stable, use to predict. Ask about common causes.	• Histograms
—If not stable, ask about special causes.	• Run charts
• Require managers and staff to measure, submit, and discuss graphs of key measures.	• Control charts • Pareto charts
• Use graphs to ask questions, make decisions, and support changes.	• Stratification of measurements
• Identify:	• Stability assessment
—Problems	
—Constraints	
—Opportunities	
—Priorities	

average, or patterns, then you should ask what is causing the outlier, trend, or run. (Some use a sequence of seven points to indicate a run or trend. The number of points in a sequence to make this judgment is based on the probability number used.) If, on the other hand, the process appears to be stable, do not ask questions about assignable causes. You should ask how the whole process can be improved.

Another concern when establishing indicators is that they measure and reward the intended outcomes. You can verify the usefulness of the indicators by:

- Asking customers and suppliers for their questions about the indicators
- Asking how indicators might be misinterpreted or misused
- Asking which indicators have the highest priority
- Pilot testing the indicators

Action Step 9: Encourage ideas and "theories" of how to improve.

The key to substantial continuous improvement of quality, customer satisfaction, cost effectiveness, working environment, and other goals is to encourage ideas, or "theories" for improvement, from all employees, customers, and suppliers. Some sample actions to encourage ideas for improvement are illustrated in Table 11.9. All of us have more creative ideas together than any single person or group. Therefore, if your organization is to become a learning, continuously improving organization, you need to encourage ideas from everyone.

To prevent discouraging ideas, it is helpful to be aware of actions that discourage and encourage ideas. We inadvertently and unintentionally discourage ideas by some very subtle actions like:

- Telling people you do not have time to listen to their ideas
- Working on something else when an idea is being presented
- Frowning when you hear an idea

Table 11.9. Sample Actions to Encourage Ideas for Improvement.

Action 9: Sample Manager/Team Actions	Sample Tools and Techniques

• Ask for ideas at each meeting. Do not evaluate ideas as they are raised.
• Ask what those ideas or "theories" predict.
• Support people:
  — Offering ideas/"theories"
  — Testing ideas/"theories"
  — Making changes
• Share ideas and successful projects with managers and staff.
• Use questions like the following to make improvements:
  — Is output still required by customer(s)?
  — Can activity be eliminated?
  — Can activity be done less frequently?
  — Can activity be done a faster/easier way?
  — Can lower-skilled person perform part or all of activity? This represents work redesign or skill-mix change.
  — Can you use fewer/less-expensive supplies?
  — Are we billing appropriately for all services and information?
	• Brainstorming
	• Cause-effect, or fishbone, diagrams

- Prejudging ideas, or telling people their ideas have been considered before, and not providing specifics of why the idea was not used

Approaches that encourage ideas include:

- Ask for ideas regularly in meetings and privately.
- Give full attention to a person, and listen carefully when an idea is being presented.
- Smile and be encouraging.
- Schedule another time to listen to the idea if you do not have time now.
- Recognize people who propose ideas, even if some ideas do not work out.

Try to support a person proposing an idea, even if you think it is not a good idea—yes, even if you think it is a dumb idea. Do something like:

- Say "sounds interesting."
- Suggest sources of data or information related to the idea.
- Ask the person how he or she could do a small test of the idea, without significant risk to the department or organization.
  - If the idea does not work, as you suspected, the person will figure that out. However, he or she will see you as supportive of new ideas and will offer more ideas in the future.
  - If the idea does work, your organization will benefit, and you will learn through supporting others that more successes are accomplished.

Reduce steps that do not add value. When you flowchart processes in healthcare organizations, they are often very complex, with many steps. Efforts to reduce the number of steps in a process will normally result in improved reliability, improved quality, reduced rework and waste, reduced cost, and improved working relationships. Therefore, you should encourage ideas that reduce steps in a process. An example is illustrated in Figure 11.1. If a system has twenty-five steps, and the probability of each step being completed correctly the first time is 0.99, or 99 percent, the probability of the whole system working correctly the first time is 0.78, or 78 percent. The system will fail an average of 22 times out of every 100. If ten steps in the system are eliminated, with no improvement in the reliability of the remaining steps in the process, the probability of the whole system working correctly the first time is increased to 0.86, or 86 percent. The failures are reduced to an average of 14 out of every 100, for the simplified process. Many of the processes in healthcare organizations have far more than twenty-five steps. A system with a hundred steps and .99 probability of each step, for example, would have only a 0.37 probability, or 37 percent chance of working correctly the first time. Refer to Table 12.1 for guidelines on how to interpret a flowchart.

Action Step 10: Investigate methods to manage workload/demand.

A common problem leading to both poor quality for the customer and unnecessary costs is not matching your resources with the demand or workload. The greatest opportunity for improvement occurs by managing the workload/demand as early as possible. Understanding the demand or workload to meet your customers' requirements is key to providing timely, quality service, particularly in highly variable, people-dominated systems like healthcare. Sample actions to manage workload/demand are illustrated in Table 11.10. Additionally, a useful sequence of questions to analyze workload/demand requirements is illustrated in Figure 11.2. The approach is to first understand your customers' demands and, even earlier, what causes demands for your customers. If together you and each of your customers can understand that demand, you can better meet the requirements and minimize their costs and yours. The approach is to eliminate workload if not required by your customer, then to schedule the workload if possible, and if not possible to schedule, predict the workload as accurately as possible. This will allow you to schedule staff and other resources. For

Figure 11.1. Impact of Reducing Number of Steps in Process.

System with 25 Steps

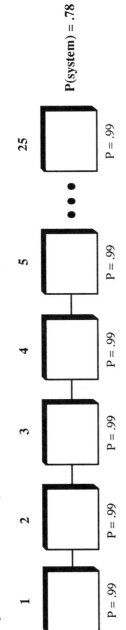

P(system) = .78

System with 15 Steps

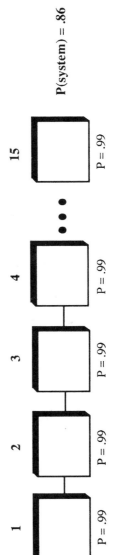

P(system) = .86

P = Probability of success first time. For example, P(1) = Probability step 1 correct first time.

Table 11.10. Sample Actions to Manage Workload/Demand.

Action 10: Sample Manager/Team Actions	Sample Tools and Techniques

• Eliminate activity by:
  − Determining what is unnecessary, with customer(s)
  − Transferring elsewhere, if appropriate and agreed to
• Schedule arrival or service time.
• Prioritize activity by time required (avoid "first come, first served" as only approach).
• Predict workload/demand:
  − Predict, whether or not you can manage, workload:
    – Timing
    – Magnitude of demand by hour of day, for example
• Match staffing to workload by:
  − Variable budgeting to match staff to workload, whether up or down
  − Methods to do variable staffing:
    – Request overtime (most cost-effective staffing to meet demand almost always involves small amount of overtime)
    – Call-in staff
    – Schedule vacation/time off
    – Ask staff to go home: partial paid or unpaid
	• Interviews with customers and suppliers
	• Interviews with staff
	• Scheduling with customers
	• Run chart
	• Control chart

example, in emergency services, you can statistically predict the approximate number of patient arrivals, and possibly the amount of room and staff time required, by hour of day, even though you do not know who the patients will be. Beyond scheduling for predicted workload, you can use different approaches to adjust the staffing on short notice, such as float staff, call-in staff, and sending staff home early (with or without partial pay).

Action Step 11: Evaluate and prioritize opportunities.

Priorities depend on the goals to be achieved and the criteria used to measure their achievement. That is the reason

Figure 11.2. Sequence of Questions to Analyze
Workload/Demand Requirements.

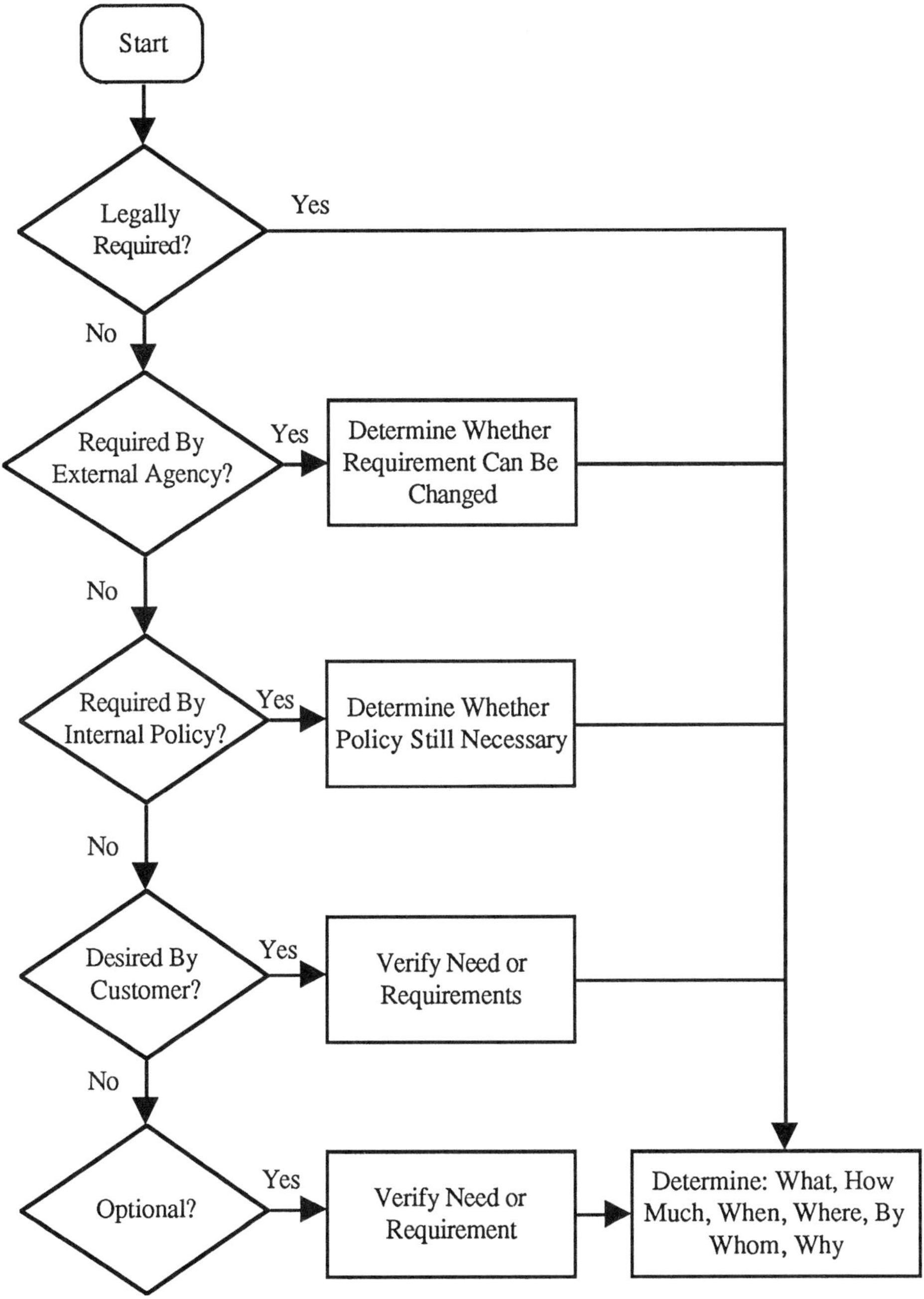

why it is important to develop alignment of organizational, departmental, and personal goals. Alignment of organizational, departmental, and personal goals is important to high quality.

Organizational goals are established by the organizational leaders, including the board, administrative, and physician leaders. To effectively meet customer requirements, input should be obtained from customers and employees when preparing or updating the goals. At UMMC the goals for the Total Quality Process were established by the Corporate and Divisional Lead Teams, which are composed of the administrative and physician leaders, with broad input from others.

Departmental goals are established by each department, based on the organizational goals. Input is required from internal and external customers and employees. Since these goals are closer to employees' daily work, the employees will have a greater personal commitment to the departmental goals than the organization's more general goals.

Personal goals are established by each person. The objective is to involve employees in developing the organizational and departmental goals, and to communicate those goals, so the employees' personal goals will be more consistent with the departmental goals. If organizational and departmental goals do not involve employees, and are not well communicated, each person will establish his or her own goals, which are unlikely to be aligned. Personal goals need not be identical with the departmental goals because everyone has goals in addition to those at work. However, employees' personal commitment is greatest to their personal goals. So it is beneficial if their goals are consistent with the organizational and departmental goals.

Once goals are established, criteria can be established to judge the relative priorities of different options or actions. Sample actions to evaluate and prioritize opportunities are illustrated in Table 11.11.

Action Step 12: Develop standard, approved method to perform each function.

For virtually any process, standardizing the methods and procedures within the process will reduce the variation of out-

Table 11.11. Sample Actions to Evaluate and Prioritize Opportunities.

Action 11: Sample Manager/Team Actions	Sample Tools and Techniques

• Measure and collect data.
• Evaluate usefulness of ideas/"theories."
• Define prioritization criteria, such as:
  — Within your control
  — Solvable within X months
  — Importance to patients or other customers
  — Dollar importance
• Listen to customers and employees concerning their prioritization criteria and why.
• Identify best similar processes in existence, through benchmarking.
• Involve people doing activities; they know the current processes best.
	• Pareto charts
	• Histograms
	• Nominal group technique
	• Benchmarking

puts and improve quality. Hence an important step for all daily operations is to standardize as many processes as practical. Sample actions to develop standard methods are illustrated in Table 11.12.

There is, however, an apparent paradox between standardizing processes and seeking continuous innovation and creativity. The relationship is best described using two interdependent processes called the Plan-Do-Check-Act (P-D-C-A)

Table 11.12. Sample Actions to Develop Standard Methods.

Action 12: Sample Manager/Team Actions	Sample Tools and Techniques
• Use most knowledgeable, skilled people to design improved process, preferably as a quality improvement team. • Test alternative methods, if alternatives exist. • Review potential impacts. Develop backup procedures, if required. • Develop/design standard methods. • Obtain approval, if required. • Document and communicate standard methods to all people involved.	• Brainstorming • Flowcharting

cycle and the Standardize-Do-Check-Act (S-D-C-A) cycle, as illustrated in Figure 11.3. The P-D-C-A process, most familiar for quality improvement efforts, is focused on improving a process through evaluating the current situation, planning counter-measures to make an improvement, implementing those countermeasures, checking whether the countermeasures were successful, and if so, acting to standardize the new process and methods. The S-D-C-A cycle begins with standardizing the process and methods, performing the work using those methods on a daily basis, checking to see that the process is following the standardized method and that the results are as expected, and acting to resolve any unusual or special events. The S-D-C-A cycle continues until another innovation or improvement is pilot tested, found to be better, and a new standard method is implemented. As will be discussed in Chapter Twelve, the "check" step of the S-D-C-A cycle can be thought of as the quality control or quality assurance process. Thus you switch back and forth between the P-D-C-A and S-D-C-A cycles every time an improvement or innovation is implemented.

Action Step 13: Check ideas for improvement.

This action represents the "check" step of the P-D-C-A cycle, although the same type of measurements are made regularly for the "check" or quality control step of the S-D-C-A cycle. It is best to test a new process option or method in a pilot area first. This will minimize any negative outcomes if the idea does not result in improvement, or if further refinement is required to improve the method before standardization to other areas. Sample actions to check ideas for improvement are illustrated in Table 11.13. One way to communicate the priority of continual improvement would be to include in managers' expectations that they test one or more improvement idea each year. Alignment could be improved by requesting that the improvements be related to key organizational and departmental goals.

Careful selection of pilot projects and test areas will develop important support and minimize risk. The following criteria are suggested to select pilot projects and test areas:

Figure 11.3. P-D-C-A and S-D-C-A Cycles.

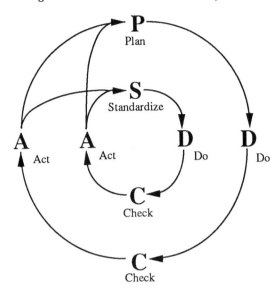

Source: Adapted from King, 1989b, p. 1-18.

- Address "pain" expressed by customers or employees working in a process. We have found that people are very willing to help, if the project has the potential to reduce or eliminate their personal pain.
- Select pilot projects and test areas to minimize the risk to the organization. This is particularly important if you or others feel the proposed change may not work.
- Allow the pilot process to return to the previous process, if the proposed countermeasures in the pilot test do not improve one or more of the following: customer satisfaction, quality, cost effectiveness, working environment, or other organizational or departmental goals. This means you try to avoid irreversible situations from an analytical or people perspective.
- Select projects that are consistent with the personal goals of the people and departments involved.
- Keep the financial commitment for the pilot test to a minimum.

Table 11.13. Sample Actions to Check Ideas for Improvement.

Action 13: Sample Manager/Team Actions	Sample Tools and Techniques
• Gain any necessary approvals and assistance to perform pilot test. • Pilot test, measure, and compare results to predictions from "theory." • Measure results. • Ask: What happened? — Did workloads increase or decrease? — Did quality measures increase or decrease? — Did productivity go up or down? — How did productivity compare to expectation? • Ask: Why it happened? — What were reasons for change? — Are changes: –Major or minor? –Broad or narrow impact? –Temporary or long-term trend? • Ask customers, suppliers, and employees how they feel about new process, in addition to the analytical measures. • Evaluate results and perceptions to see if benefits are greater than costs and disadvantages.	• Checksheets • Pie/bar graphs • Histograms • Run charts • Control charts • Pareto charts • Stratification of measurements • Stability assessment

Action Step 14: Take action, if within your control.

Each manager or supervisor has the authority to take actions, within limits, to implement improvements. Every manager and supervisor should be encouraged to test ideas and make changes as appropriate to improve quality and cost effectiveness. For many operational changes within a functional area, it may be unnecessary to form Quality Improvement Teams. The natural work team may be able to use quality improvement methods to test ideas and implement improvements without forming formal QITs. All employees should be encouraged to flowchart the processes in which they work, identify their customers, determine the requirements of their internal and external customers, and monitor key measures or indicators on a

Table 11.14. Sample Actions to Make Changes.

Action 14: Sample Manager/Team Actions	Sample Tools and Techniques
• Make changes, based on results. This is the "Act" of the Plan-Do-Check-Act cycle. • Continue to measure and monitor results of processes, to find and resolve special causes as necessary. This is the "Act" of the Standardize-Do-Check-Act cycle.	• Histograms • Run charts • Control charts • Pareto charts • Stability assessment

regular basis using charts. Sample actions to make changes are illustrated in Table 11.14.

Action Step 15: Ask for help to start a Quality Improvement Team.

If the problem or opportunity cannot be solved without more in-depth analysis, the manager or supervisor has a number of options. There is a continuum of quality improvement efforts, as illustrated in Figure 8.1. No matter which option is available or chosen, the existence of a process flowchart, defined customer requirements with measures/indicators, and data about the performance of the process will be much more useful than simply the perception that there is a problem. The options will depend on the level of implementation of TQM within your organization and the resources available. Some sample options are:

1. Establish a Quality Improvement Team. If your organization has a formally defined quality improvement process and teams, a QIT can be formed to address the problem or opportunity. Approval of a corporate or divisional lead team may be required to receive incremental staff or other resources.

2. Establish an Informal Team to Work on Problem or Opportunity. The approach is similar to a QIT and uses the same tools and techniques, but may not meet one or more of the criteria used to define a formal QIT. The team should still

include people who work directly in the process, a manager, and possibly a customer or supplier. The process flowchart will be helpful in identifying the people to be included.

In any situation, it will be helpful to attend any available training on TQM.

As stated earlier, a manager can initiate these actions in daily operations immediately to begin improving quality. However, you should recognize that completing and refining this process may take years of effort.

Actions for Staff

Medical staff and others focus their attention and actions toward their personal jobs and the processes in which they work. The actions available to staff are essentially a subset of the actions for managers, with a narrower focus. The objective is for employees to gain broader knowledge and skills to perform, evaluate, and improve their own jobs and the processes in which they work.

Action 1: Understand and live by values, vision, mission, goals, and expectations. As an employee or staff member, you should ask for and read the organizational and departmental statements related to the values, vision, mission, goals, and expectations of the managers and staff.

- Are the statements understandable to you? If not, ask for clearer statements or an explanation. If you cannot understand them, others will have difficulty also. Statements are often clear to the people who prepared them but unclear to others.
- Are the statements consistent with each other, in your view? If not, ask for clarification. It is typical that statements are written at different times by different people for different purposes, and they may not be consistent unless they have been carefully reviewed and edited.
- Are the statements consistent with your values and goals? If not, try to understand the organization's statements and your own values better. If your values remain inconsistent

with the organization's statements, you have two choices. First, try to get the organization's statements changed. Second, look for an organization with values similar to yours. This is not an immediate need, but over time such inconsistencies will lead to increasing frustration.

Refer to Table 11.1 for further actions and sample tools and techniques.

Action 2: Demonstrate commitment, sponsorship, participation, and common understanding for improvement of quality and cost effectiveness. The most effective way to develop knowledge that leads to commitment is to participate in education programs and meetings on Total Quality and other topics of importance to your organization. It is helpful to understand the general healthcare environment and issues facing your organization. Tell your friends about your positive experiences with teams, improved working environment, and supportive behaviors you observe with your manager and others. Similarly, you should raise negative experiences with your manager, with suggestions for improvement. Communication is critical for success of Total Quality. Refer to Table 11.2 for additional sample actions and tools and techniques.

Action 3: Develop mission and goals for your department. Although staff do not establish the departmental mission and goals by themselves, it is important that you participate in discussions about the mission and goals. Your ideas can be used only if they are heard. If you do not feel comfortable raising ideas directly, suggest that people write up ideas and submit them anonymously. Again, communication is key. Listen to the ideas of others and the role the organization expects of the department. Determine how your personal job contributes to the departmental mission. Once the mission is established, you should communicate and support the departmental mission on your daily job. Refer to Table 11.3 for additional sample actions and tools and techniques related to the mission.

Action 4: Identify and understand functions and processes within your department and involving other departments. What functions or processes do you personally participate in? Sample processes are admission, outpatient registration, outpatient surgery, in-patient care, medical record support, patient transportation, the billing process, food service, and facility environmental control. If you have trouble answering this question, ask your manager or others. There are many overlapping processes in a healthcare organization. Learn how to draw a flowchart of the processes in which you work. A flowchart is simply a diagram or picture of how things work. They do not have to be complex, do not have to use symbols, and do not require a computer. Refer to Chapter Twelve for a more detailed description of flowcharting. Make a simple flowchart of one process to begin. It is very helpful to understand how your job fits into the whole process, and it is both helpful and fun to communicate with others. Refer to Table 11.4 for additional sample actions and tools and techniques related to understanding processes.

Action 5: Identify internal and external customers and suppliers for processes. For each process, who are the people from which you directly receive a service, product, or information? They are your suppliers. In these cases, you are the customer. Who are the people to whom you directly provide a service, a product, or information? Those people are your customers. All people are customers of the people ahead of them in a process and a supplier to the people after them in the process. For example, if your manager explains how to do something, for that trans-action you are the customer and your requirements are to under-stand what is being explained. If your manager does not explain clearly so you understand, then he or she has not met your requirements. How many times have you been given incomplete instructions, only to have to do rework later? The purpose of this step is to identify all your customers for each process in which you work. Refer to Table 11.5 for additional sample actions and tools and techniques related to identifying customers and suppliers.

Action 6: Determine customer requirements. Talk directly to your customers, and ask each of them questions like:

• What are your requirements?
• What do I provide which you do not need? You can eliminate these, and save time and cost.

- What do you need that I do not provide? You may not be able to commit to provide everything desired, but at least you know the customer's perceived requirements and have established a dialogue.
- What do I do well?
- What do I need to improve, and what type of improvements are desired?
- What are your priorities among the things I provide for you?

By simply asking these questions of every person to whom you provide a service, product, or information, you will determine his or her requirements. If you cannot meet the initial requirements, please explain why, so at least your customers will understand the limitations under which you work. Refer to Table 11.6 for additional sample actions and tools and techniques related to determining customer requirements.

Action 7: Choose key measures/indicators. Determine the key measures or indicators that are being used by your department and the organization overall. Remember, you cannot measure everything. What is most important? Ask your customers what key measures or indicators are most important to them. This can be done at the same time as the requirements are determined by asking, "How will we judge whether your requirements are being met?" Discuss potential measures with your manager and customers. Refer to Table 11.7 for additional sample actions and tools and techniques related to measures/indicators.

Action 8: Measure and understand process capability. Measure key indicators on a regular basis. You should graph these indicators over time, so you can monitor the results of your efforts. If you are unfamiliar with graphs, you should ask for help with this as needed. Your manager, or a resource person in your organization, should be able to help. Again, graph only the key indicators; you could easily spend all of your time measuring and graphing data. Once you have the data graphed, watch for special events outside the control limits, trends of five or more points increasing or decreasing, or runs of five or more points in sequence above or below the average. These are indicators that an individual point or the process is unstable and requires special attention. If all points are within the control limits, it is not helpful to ask questions about individual points. Rather, ask how the whole process can be improved. Refer to Table 11.8 for additional sample actions and tools and techniques related to understanding process capability.

Action 9: Encourage ideas and "theories" of how to improve. Offer your ideas for improvement and encourage other employees to do the same. To communicate better the effectiveness of your ideas, try to provide:

- Purpose of proposed change
- How it relates to the organizational and departmental goals
- Description of the changes in functions, processes, organization, procedures, staffing, commodity usage, and other significant changes
- Estimated time and resource requirements for a pilot test
- Estimated time and resource requirements to standardize and implement broadly
- Estimated changes in outcomes toward goals, including customer satisfaction, quality, cost effectiveness, working environment, and competitive position

The organization will improve most quickly if everyone contributes ideas. Refer to Table 11.9 for additional actions and tools and techniques to encourage ideas.

Action 10: Investigate methods to manage workload/demand. Ask your customers and manager whether your workload can be managed to reduce variation in your demands. To the extent possible, you should try to schedule your workload, and if that fails you can use the demand data to predict when workload will occur. Possibly, you could consider variable work hours as a way to meet varying workload. Refer to Table 11.10 for actions and tools and techniques to manage workload/demand.

Action 11: Evaluate and prioritize opportunities. Measure and collect data on ideas for improvement generated by you, those you work with in your department, and other departments. Discuss with your manager the criteria to prioritize potential changes in processes. Read and talk to others to identify similar processes, in your organization or elsewhere, with the best-known results. This is known as benchmarking and is further discussed in Chapter Fourteen. For example, you may read about a good example in a magazine. Then you could gather ideas about how to improve your job. Note that many of the supportive processes in hospitals are also found in other industries, such as hotels. Refer to Table 11.11 for additional actions and tools and techniques to prioritize opportunities.

Action 12: Develop standard, approved method to perform each function. Almost all processes will generate more consistent results if a standardized approach is used. So you should develop the most effective approach, methods, and operational definitions to accomplish your proposed changes, verify that these are consistent with departmental requirements, then document them as the standard approach. Involve the most knowledgeable and skilled people to develop the standard method, then have others review the proposed standard method for questions and improvements. Once the function is finalized, everyone who performs it should be trained in the standard method. Refer to Table 11.12 for additional actions and tools and techniques related to standard methods.

Action 13: Check ideas for improvement. You may need to obtain approval to test your ideas either from your manager or managers in other departments. You will need to document carefully the results from the current system, what happened when your proposed changes were tested, and the results, both from factual basis and from the perceptions of the people involved. Remember, improving the working environment for staff is itself a meaningful goal. Refer to Table 11.13 for additional actions and tools and techniques to check ideas for improvement.

Action 14: Take action, if within your control. Based on the results of the pilot study, make any changes that are within your control. Often you will need to coordinate the changes with your customers, suppliers, other staff, and manager(s). As part of the implementation, you should develop a process to measure the results. If you need help to implement changes, ask for it.

It will take time to improve communications and trust among managers and staff, and for staff to become knowledgeable and empowered to improve quality on their daily jobs. However, this is both important to your customers and rewarding to staff.

Conclusion

The actions described in this chapter can be undertaken before managers and staff are broadly trained in the philosophy, analytical knowledge and skills, and people knowledge and skills associated with TQM. The methods are simple, improve communication, and improve data for when more formalized quality improvement efforts are undertaken. It is not expected that all of these actions will be undertaken simultaneously for all the processes within an area; actions must be prioritized. You will find that communications among suppliers and customers about operational definitions and their mutual requirements and capacities will improve quality, cost effectiveness, and working environment even before more formal efforts are undertaken. Although not as visible or obvious as formal QI projects, these daily efforts by managers and staff to improve quality can accomplish substantial improvements over time. Again, remember that this is an ongoing effort that will take years to refine fully.

Chapter Twelve

Quality Improvement Methods

This chapter presents selected principles and methods for quality improvement efforts. We will provide practical guidance for managers and staff within healthcare organizations. However, this is not intended to be a detailed presentation of the methods. Additional education and practice will be required to become proficient with the methods. References are provided for more complete coverage of each topic.

This chapter includes concepts related to quality improvement methods and selected tools and techniques used during a QI project. The methods are presented in the sequence they are often used. In Chapter Thirteen we will present a sample case study for an admission process to demonstrate use of the methods, tools, and techniques.

Several places throughout this book we have emphasized that TQM represents the balance of a customer-focused, continual-improvement philosophy, analytical skills, and people skills with a structure and organization to support TQM (see Figure 2.1 in Chapter Two). While the analytical tools presented are powerful, the addition of appropriate concern for the people involved is required to address QI projects effectively.

Principles for Improvement

There are several principles that underlie quality improvement efforts. These principles, which are theoretically based, provide an overall focus and specific actions for managers, staff, and quality improvement teams. The principles evolved through our training programs jointly developed with Edward D. Rothman, University of Michigan professor of statistics, and through the experiences of our QITs.

Purpose. A process must have a purpose or aim. Yet many organizations within the healthcare industry have no well-communicated purpose. The purpose of any process should be consistent with and supportive of the organizational and departmental vision, values, and mission to meet customer requirements.

Customers judge quality and value. The customers of our processes, products, services, and information are the ones whose judgment about quality and value are most important. Your external customers will make decisions about whether to return and what to tell their friends and acquaintances based on their judgments. Your organization should monitor measurements of your processes to assure quality, but you must get direct input from both internal and external customers to determine whether their perceptions match yours.

Measurement. Measurement is necessary to make judgments about a process, event, or object. It is very difficult to manage a process without measurement of that process. Measurement is meaningful only if there are consistent operational definitions and a specific method of measurement. Measurement is further discussed in the next section.

Reduce process variation. One approach to improve quality is to reduce variation. The average of any quality measure alone is an inadequate statistical measure. Increased variation reduces the ability to plan, reliability, and quality of the process. An example of waiting time to see your physician will be used to demonstrate this principle. Assume your objective is to wait ten minutes or less. Consider two alternatives, each with an average waiting time of ten minutes. For one alternative the waiting time is precisely ten minutes each time, with no measurable variation. Your requirements are met every time, and you can plan your schedule accurately. The second alternative has an average wait time of ten minutes, but with a high variation. You might not have to wait at all, or you might wait as long as sixty minutes. In this case, your requirements are met only part of the time, you cannot accurately plan your schedule, and the measured quality has decreased, even though the average wait time is the same. The quality of a product or service exists when it does what it claims to do every time, with minimal variation. Hence the principle is to take actions that reduce variation.

Consistent operational definitions. Consistent operational definitions are important to quality improvement. Any term can have many definitions. An operational definition is the precise definition used within your organization for any given term. Unless an effort is made to establish and communicate common definitions, operational definitions may vary substantially among people within your organization. We will use the operating room scenario to illustrate this point. The authors have firsthand knowledge of several operating room projects. At the beginning of each of these projects, different events were used as the basis for recording the operation start time by different circulating nurses. Thus the variation of the recorded operation start times was greater than the actual operation start times due to variation in the operational definitions used by staff as a basis for recording the start times. Virtually every quality improvement team at UMMC has found inconsistencies in one or more operational definitions of terms and measurements related to the process being studied.

Eliminate process steps that do not add value. All steps in a process add variation and resource cost to that process. If a step in a process does not add value, that step should be eliminated to decrease variation and improve quality. As an important byproduct, removal of process steps that do not add value reduces the cost of the process.

Reduce number of suppliers. Reducing the number of suppliers for a particular transaction or process reduces variation in a process. Each supplier uses somewhat different methods, equipment, materials, and staff, which causes more variation among suppliers than within any supplier's product or service. A single supplier is best but not always possible or practical. This is an extension of Deming's fourth point of ending the practice of awarding business on the basis of price tag alone (Deming, 1986, p. 23).

Work on root cause rather than symptom. When a customer's expectations are not met, you have multiple options to resolve the situation. Often actions are directed toward the symptom, such as dealing with customer complaints. This approach may be necessary in some cases and may ultimately satisfy the customer, but causes costly rework. It is far more effective to ask "why" questions about the process that produced the result. Ask, "why is there large variation in the accuracy of the information?" rather than "what can we do about the large variation?" An admitting example may illustrate this point. The patients, physicians, and other customers are dissatisfied with the large average waiting times in the admitting lounge; their requirements are seldom being met. One approach is to assign or hire staff to attend to the needs of the patients and their families while waiting, provide meals for patients and their families, and provide an apology in the form of a flower, card, and possibly a visit after the patient is admitted. These actions may satisfy that patient and family but are costly and do nothing to prevent such delays in the future. It is far more effective to determine the steps, or root causes, in the admitting system that cause delays. Then eliminate the root causes of delays, which will reduce waiting times for all patients.

Make improvements upstream where actions are more effective. Improvements made earlier in a process, or upstream, are more effective at improving quality and reducing costs. This is a corollary of the principle of working on the root cause rather than the symptoms. The output of each step of a process becomes the input of the next step in the process. Therefore, working upstream is equivalent to working on the causal system of a step in the process. A billing example may be helpful. The quality problem in the billing office may be long delays in collecting payments from insurance companies, which in turn causes delays in sending patients bills for balances due on services provided months earlier. This problem can be approached at several steps in the billing process. The last, and least effective, is to approach patients very apologetically and possibly write off charges of some upset patients. This approach is time-consuming, costly, and results in lost revenue. An approach earlier in the process is to assign billing and medical records staff to expedite billing. This is a more effective approach but still represents extra process steps and cost. The best approach is to provide admitting, outpatient registration, and medical records staff with up-to-date lists of requirements for all insurance policies so they can initiate early inquiries and facilitate billing. This "upstream" approach is the most effective at improving quality or services and reducing rework and waste.

Look at entire process for opportunities. When looking for opportunities for improvement, it is important first to look broadly at an entire process, to avoid sub-optimization. This will allow identification and prioritization of those steps in the process that cause the greatest quality problems or offer the greatest opportunity for improvement. Then individual teams can work on improvements based on established priorities. An analogy to the weakest link in a chain may help explain this principle. You can strengthen any link of the chain, except the weakest link, with no impact on the overall strength of the chain. You must strengthen the weakest link to strengthen the chain. Making improvements in the best portions of a process may produce little or no improvement in the overall reliability and quality of the process outputs. Thus it will be more effective for a team to work to improve a step in the process that is most critical to the overall value of meeting the external customer's requirements.

People in the process have the greatest knowledge. The people working directly in a process have the most specific knowledge and information about the portion of the process they currently perform. We have found that when a quality improvement project includes the people who perform the activities, we gain a much better understanding of the process. The knowledge of these employees is particularly valuable when flowcharting the process and generating ideas for improvement. For example, the people with the most accurate definition of the start time for a surgical procedure in the operating room are the circulating nurses who record the time on the operating room record.

Others may have an idea about the time, but the only people who know for sure are those that record the time.

Work on lowest cost changes first. There will be many specific problems or opportunities to be addressed, and several different options or proposed solutions for each problem. By asking staff to work on low-cost changes first, you may provide incentives to seek root causes of problems. Based on our experiences at UMMC and several other healthcare and non-healthcare organizations, there is an initial tendency to jump to a quick solution and throw resources at the symptoms of a problem rather than determining the real root causes. It is common for a person or team to say, "just give me more staff and we can improve our quality measure," which addresses the results or symptoms of a problem. As a person or team searches for lower-cost alternatives, they look further upstream for the root causes, and better proposed solutions are normally discovered. At UMMC we have implemented a few QIT recommendations that require incremental funding, but the large majority had negligible implementation costs, yet resulted in financial benefits in addition to improved quality.

Ask for questions, not answers. One useful principle is to ask customers, suppliers, and others about their questions relating to any change in process or new process. This principle was introduced to us by Edward D. Rothman, and has proven to be useful. At UMMC the task team developing a plan to use attrition as a means for staff reduction used this principle when collecting information. Managers and staff were asked about their questions and concerns related to a potential attrition plan. The plan was then developed to address their questions and concerns. If you ask someone for questions about a process change, you will receive many of the questions that person feels are relevant. If, on the other hand, you ask that person for a solution to a problem, you will receive a single solution. This causes two difficulties. First, you will not identify as many relevant questions, concerns, and issues to be addressed by the new process. Second, each person will be vested in the solution he or she provided. Selection of any other solution will result in everyone who did not suggest that "solution" being disenfranchised. There is an analogy to this principle, called "Getting to Yes," or mutual gains bargaining, which has been used in our nursing union negotiations at UMMC (Fisher and Ury, 1983). Instead of asking for answers or positions, each side is asked to provide a list of interests and concerns. Both sides then work together to develop a list of possible solutions that will address the interests and concerns. This approach allows discussion of the issues without win-lose conflicts.

Rework time is indicator of system performance. Within healthcare organizations, the use of staff time for rework is an indicator of process effectiveness. If staff spend much of their time doing rework, it is likely that the process requires change. The organization should survey employees about types of rework they see and how this might be reduced or eliminated. An accounts receivable example will be used to illustrate this point. All employees could be asked to keep a log of their activities for one week. The frequency of calls, record requests, and other activities related to incorrect patient or insurance information is a measure of rework related to inaccurate admission or registration processes. The frequency of different types of rework can then be used to prioritize the portions of the process to improve first.

Cycle time is a good overall indicator. An operational definition of cycle time for a healthcare organization may be the complete time from initiation of a service, product, or information until it is delivered to the customer's satisfaction. For example, the cycle time for an outpatient visit might be measured from the time the patient arrives at the outpatient clinic until the patient leaves the last point of service, such as the outpatient pharmacy. Cycle time is a good overall indicator of the performance of a process. Keki Bhote (1991, p. 42) states that "cycle time is an excellent 'integrator' of quality, cost, delivery, and effectiveness. . . . If quality is poor, cycle time is lengthened because of checks, rework, etc. If cost is high — generally, because of poor quality, poor efficiency, long set-up and change-over times, and long equipment down times — cycle time is also lengthened. If there is poor delivery, cycle time is again lengthened because of waiting or queue time. Finally, if the effectiveness of a process is poor, it takes longer to perform the task, further lengthening the cycle time."

Stratification of data helpful to identify opportunities. Stratification is a method of breaking down data into meaningful categories for analysis (GOAL/QPC, 1988, p. 76). Clinic waiting time data in Exhibit 12.1 will be used as an example. Stratifying the same data by one categorization method may provide little insight into the causes, as illustrated by the day-of-the-week stratification in Figure 12.1. Stratifying the same data by different categories may provide information about causes and potential improvement, as illustrated by the clinical service stratification in Figure 12.2. The approach is to stratify the same data by several categorizations, to see which reveals the most information. It may be helpful to solicit ideas from people working in the process, through brainstorming, for example, about potential factors that will affect the quality measure, such as waiting time.

Prediction. Management requires prediction, and prediction is improved with a statistically stable system. Run charts, control charts, and other measurements reflect historical or current performance. These are helpful for planning to the extent that they help us predict. One of the shortcomings of many management information systems is that they report only historical data and do not include mechanisms for predicting future demand and performance necessary for management to plan. Your information systems should be modified to provide predictions of the key planning criteria for each department or function.

Supportive environment is important. A supportive environment is necessary to encourage ideas for improvement. Although ideas for improvement are often available within your employee population, a facilitating environment to enhance creativity and innovation often does not exist. Based on our experience and the experience of other organizations and consultants, this is the key barrier to implementing Total Quality in many organizations. The culture must be supportive for quality improvement efforts to be effective. This was addressed further in Chapter Six.

Exhibit 12.1. Sample Clinic Waiting Time Data.

Patient	Day of Week	Clinical Department	Wait Time in Clinic
1	Mon	General Medicine	10
2	Mon	Cardiology	18
3	Mon	General Surgery	30
4	Mon	Orthopedic Surgery	60
5	Mon	Pediatrics	8
6	Mon	Obstetrics/Gynecology	15
7	Tue	General Medicine	15
8	Tue	Cardiology	21
9	Tue	General Surgery	25
10	Tue	Orthopedic Surgery	55
11	Tue	Pediatrics	10
12	Tue	Obstetrics/Gynecology	17
13	Wed	General Medicine	12
14	Wed	Cardiology	23
15	Wed	General Surgery	28
16	Wed	Orthopedic Surgery	45
17	Wed	Pediatrics	15
18	Wed	Obstetrics/Gynecology	12
19	Thu	General Medicine	13
20	Thu	Cardiology	20
21	Thu	General Surgery	22
22	Thu	Orthopedic Surgery	57
23	Thu	Pediatrics	14
24	Thu	Obstetrics/Gynecology	16
25	Fri	General Medicine	11
26	Fri	Cardiology	17
27	Fri	General Surgery	27
28	Fri	Orthopedic Surgery	52
29	Fri	Pediatrics	13
30	Fri	Obstetrics/Gynecology	15

Average Clinic Wait Times

Mon	23.5	General Medicine	12.2
Tue	23.8	Cardiology	19.8
Wed	22.5	General Surgery	26.4
Thu	23.7	Orthopedic Surgery	53.8
Fri	24.0	Pediatrics	12.0
		Obstetrics/Gynecology	15.0

Figure 12.1. Sample Waiting Time by Day of Week.

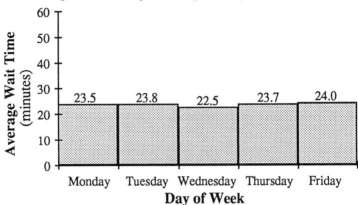

Measurement Considerations

Measurement values are meaningless unless there are consistent operational definitions and measurement methods. For any measurement, you should address the questions of "what," "how," and "why." There are an infinite number of things that can be measured, and you could easily spend all of your time measuring different characteristics. For example, clinic waiting time could be measured using several criteria. The beginning of wait time could be measured as the time the patient arrives at the parking lot, patient arrives at the clinic door, clerk completes

Figure 12.2. Sample Waiting Time by Clinical Department.

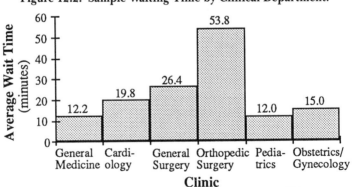

the check-in process, or the scheduled patient arrival time, if the patient arrives early. The end of the same wait time could be measured as the time the patient is called from the waiting room, the time the intake process is completed, the time the patient is put in an exam room, or the time the physician first sees the patient. These times could be measured using single or multiple measuring methods and devices. If multiple devices are used, there is almost certainly a significant variation in the measurement based on the differences among the watches, clocks, or other measuring devices. An example is the time measurement of events as a patient moves through an outpatient visit. If each employee who records the time on the data collection form uses his or her own watch, there will be a substantial variation, unless the watches are synchronized at the beginning of each data collection period. Another approach we have used in multiple studies is to attach a digital clock to the clipboard containing the data collection form, so each employee uses the same watch. The point is that measurements should be carefully selected, defined, and implemented. Even then there must be an awareness that these limited measures cannot fully measure all situations. Many of the most important things are unknowable and ummeasurable.

The following considerations are offered to limit and prioritize the things that are measured. You should focus on key quality and performance indicators important to your customers.

Measure customer requirements. The requirements of external and internal customers are vitally important to the long-term success of your organization. Therefore, the most important customer requirements, from the perspective of the customer, should be the basis for key quality and value indicators. Try to focus on the vital few rather than attempt to measure every possible characteristic. The only way to understand fully the customer requirements is to communicate directly with the customer—ask him or her! Then discuss what and how you can jointly measure whether those requirements are being met, and what will be done with the information. Unless the information can be used to take action, the information is of little value.

Measure health status. Given the high cost of medical care, the large numbers of uninsured people, and the relatively unimpressive measures of U.S. health status, many are calling for healthcare organizations to take a more active role in the health of their communities. There is a need for new coalitions of healthcare providers to address the total health of their communities, including hospitals, nursing homes, home health agencies, public health agencies, school health departments, industrial health departments, physicians, and others. Does the vision and mission of your organization formally address the health status of your community, or are they limited to the provision of selected medical services and products? An increasing portion of most healthcare organizations' business involves care provided outside of an inpatient setting, such as ambulatory care, industrial health, and home care. We suggest that measures of health status of the population within your service area or region are relevant measures of the collective success of all healthcare providers in your area. Examples of health status include infant mortality rate, prevalence of substance abuse like alcohol and drugs (including inappropriately used prescription drugs), number of school days missed, and percentage of working-age population physically unable to work. Integration of health status measures into the evaluation of healthcare organizations is in its infancy and will require much development.

Begin with few measures. Rather than attempt to measure everything, prioritize and start with very few measures. Starting with one to four measures judged most important by the key customers within the respective processes can address your attention to the most important issues first. Focus first on those characteristics of your service, product, or information about which your customers have "pain" and complaints. From a top-down organizational perspective, it is best to begin with key customers and processes critical to your organization, then to expand to other customers and processes.

Measurement and monitoring should be cost effective. You could easily spend all of your time measuring, monitoring, and analyzing data. However, measurement is seldom the product, service, or information desired by your customers. From their perspective, measurement per se is not a major contributor of value. Hence you should select the vital few key measures for each process. Measurement and monitoring costs must be judged in relation to the expected benefits. Bhote states: "A cardinal rule in measurement is that the cost of the measurement should be at least one order of magnitude lower than the expected tangible benefits" (1991, p. 60). Thus the measurement costs should never exceed 10 percent of the expected tangible benefits. It is best if automated data collection can be accomplished as a byproduct of providing patient care or other service.

Descriptions of Selected Quality Improvement Methods

The purpose of this section is to summarize some of the most useful quality improvement methods. The following selected quality improvement methods typically used by QITs are described:

- Process flowchart
- Run chart and control chart
- Brainstorming
- Affinity diagram
- Multivoting
- Prioritization matrix
- Checksheets
- Histogram and Pareto chart
- Cause-effect, fishbone, or Ishikawa diagram
- Proposed options matrix
- Force field analysis
- Cost-benefit analysis

Chapter Thirteen presents a quality improvement case study that illustrates and gives examples of most of these methods.

Process Flowchart

A process flowchart is one of the most useful tools to improve the quality and cost effectiveness of any process. A flowchart is a graphical representation of all the steps in a process. The purpose of a flowchart is to establish a representation of what actually happens. This process helps identify productive and nonproductive activities. When the chart is assembled, the team can then ask questions like: What is the purpose of this activity? Does it add value? Can it be done better? Who can do it best?

A flowchart can be used to represent the flow or movement of people, products, equipment, information, and other things. A flowchart can represent a past process, current process, alternative processes for consideration, a desired process, or a standardized process.

We have found that developing a flowchart of a process causes several improvements, including the following:

- Every person learns that he or she does not understand the complete process in detail. Every team member has said something like, "I didn't know it happened that way." Only the people who perform that activity understand the current process in detail.
- Every person learns that other team members know some aspect of the process better than he or she does. This leads to greatly improved mutual respect and communication, which extends far beyond the team's project.
- Every person learns more about the whole process, and how his or her job fits into the whole.
- Steps in the process that do not add value are normally discovered. Steps in the process that are unnecessary or redundant, or cause errors, rework, and waste are also identified. These can often be eliminated immediately with little additional effort and produce quick improvements. Several opportunities for improvement are often identified as the flowchart is being prepared.
- Ideas for improvement outside the scope of the team's project are often identified, and individual team members will pursue those improvements outside the team.

Symbols for Flowcharting. It is useful, but not necessary, to use symbols within a flowchart. We found that some new team members were intimidated by the use of flowcharting symbols. In these cases, the flowchart was created with short word phrases connected by arrows to show the direction. As those team members became more comfortable with the process of flowcharting, a few simple standard symbols were introduced. The UMMC quality improvement teams in general use only the four simple symbols included in Figure 12.3.

Approach to Flowcharting. The specific approach will depend on the subject and objectives of the analysis, but the following general approach is often useful. This approach is

Figure 12.3. Commonly Used Symbols for Process Flowcharts.

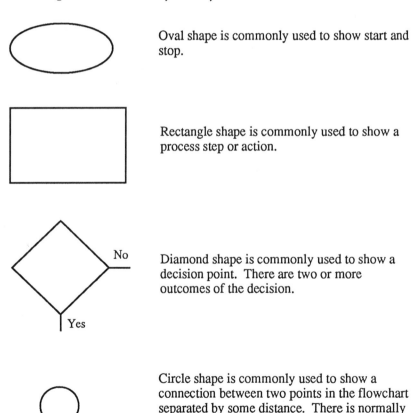

Oval shape is commonly used to show start and stop.

Rectangle shape is commonly used to show a process step or action.

Diamond shape is commonly used to show a decision point. There are two or more outcomes of the decision.

Circle shape is commonly used to show a connection between two points in the flowchart separated by some distance. There is normally a number or letter in the connector to show which things relate to each other.

oriented toward flowcharting a current process, but the same approach can also be used for future alternatives and recommended processes.

- Develop a very general flowchart first, then expand to the level of detail appropriate for the situation. Different levels of detail are appropriate, depending on the requirements and planned use of the flowchart. This step will help identify the people involved with the process. If a flowchart is too general, you will miss the opportunities for improvement. If the flowchart is too detailed, you will expend unnecessary resources. Given the potential benefits of process improvement, it is better to err toward more detail. Illustrations of a very simple flowchart and a more detailed version of the same process are illustrated in Figures 12.4 and 12.5.
- Involve the people who perform the activities, either as part of a team or to provide information. They know their part of the process best.
- Act out the process. Pretend to be a patient, piece of paper, or product, and go through the whole process from beginning to end. Ask questions like, "what happens to me now?"; "what happens if I don't meet the requirements?"; "where do I go next?"; "who helps/sees/processes me?" (note that this is the next customer in the process); "what am I used for?" If there is no meaningful use for the final output, it may be possible to eliminate all preceding steps in the process.
- Collect all forms or documentation used in the process, and identify the sources of the data for the forms and who enters the information. The resulting data and statistics can be no more accurate than the information entered when collected. Also, determine whether there are other sources of similar information.

Separate flowcharts may be required for the flow of patients, employees, equipment, suppliers, information, and other characteristics.

One helpful approach is to use a standard format to state

Figure 12.4. Sample Simple Flowchart.

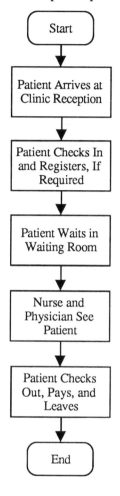

process steps, using a subject, verb, and object. A sample format would be:

- Form: (person) (action verb) (object) (for whom)
- Example: (clerk)   (prepares)   (form)   (for patient)

This format is helpful for understanding the supplier-customer relationship and for analyzing the flowchart for improvement

Figure 12.5. Sample More Detailed Flowchart.

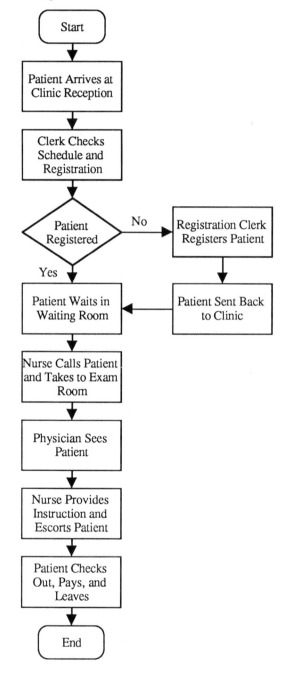

opportunities. Using this format, the person who performs the action is the supplier of that process step, and the person for whom it is done is the customer.

A specialized form of flowchart known as a critical path is discussed in Chapter Fourteen. In this case, each step is assigned a time and/or resource use, and the path from the beginning to the end of the process that takes the most time is known as the critical path.

Guidelines to Interpret Flowchart. Creating a flowchart will improve communication and understanding, but the real benefit comes from the review of the process for potential improvements. Sample guidelines to review and interpret a flowchart are given in Table 12.1.

Benefits of Flowcharting. Some sample benefits of flowcharting processes are:

- Documents process
- Allows differing levels of detail
- Provides logical summary of process
- Improves communication
- Enhances respect and teamwork, as everyone recognizes he or she does not fully understand process
- Allows everyone to see how he or she contributes to providing the final service, product, or information
- Increases mutual respect among individuals working in the process
- Provides excellent approach and format to review purpose, value, and outputs of every step in the process, by highlighting feedback or rework paths, decisions lacking clear actions, duplicate activities, and multiple approvals
- Can represent and/or compare current process, alternative processes, or planned process
- Identifies suppliers and customers at each step of process

Selected references for more information on process flowcharting are *The Memory Jogger* (GOAL/QPC, 1988), *The Team Handbook* (Scholtes, 1988), *Juran's Quality Control Handbook* (Juran

Table 12.1. Guidelines to Interpret Process Flowchart.

Topic	Method/Approach	Interpretation/Action
Final Use of Service/ Product/ Information	Review whether final service, product, or information useful to customer.	If not useful: • Evaluate customer requirements, or • Eliminate whole process If useful, what would enhance value?
No/Limited Value	Review each step to determine if value added, in the view of: • Next customer in process • External customer	If no value: • Eliminate step • Document changes and benefits
Feedback or Rework Paths	Review for return paths, especially those with large frequencies of activity.	Return paths normally involve some type of rework. Revise process to reduce requirement for rework.
	Check how far back in process a feedback/rework path goes.	The further back in a process it goes, the greater the impact.
Path That Goes Nowhere	Look for paths that go nowhere.	If required, complete path. If not required, eliminate.
Decisions Lacking Clear Actions	Review all decisions (diamond-shaped boxes). Are there clear actions or outcomes for each?	Common problem of infrequent outcomes being undefined or poorly defined.
Duplicate or Repeated Activities	Look for duplicate, repeated, or similar activities in flowchart.	Consolidate, if possible. Coordinate. Use fewer suppliers.
Multiple Reviews/ Approvals	Look for multiple review or approval steps.	Normally these do not add value.
	Look for forms handled several times.	Reduce review/approval steps. Empower people to make approvals lower in the organization.
Few Parallel Activities/ Many Serial Activities	Review precedent requirements of all serial activities (one following another)	If serial activities do not have precedent requirements, do them in parallel, to reduce time.

Table 12.1. Guidelines to Interpret Process Flowchart, Cont'd.

Topic	Method/Approach	Interpretation/Action
Verify Connections	Check with both supplier and customer to verify mutual understanding of connections on flowchart.	If understanding is different, correct.
Number of Decisions	Count number of decisions (diamonds).	Larger number of decisions means more complex process. Determine whether complexity is required.
Review Verbs Used	Review verbs in boxes: • Manual actions • Automated actions • Transportation • Search/look • Other	Verbs provide insight about types of changes. Complex or multiple verbs may indicate more detail required.
Focus Upstream First	Look at upstream (early) decisions and activities first.	The earlier a decision/assumption occurs, the greater its impact. Earlier correction lowers effort and cost.
Elapsed/Cycle Time	Review elapsed/cycle time of activities and groups of activities. Review total elapsed/cycle time of process.	Longer elapsed times offer greater opportunity for improvement.
Delays/Waits	Review all delays/waits in flowchart.	Determine impacts of delays/waits. Reduce delays/waits. Focus on those in critical path, or in critical processes, first.
Outside Review of Flowchart	Have people other than those performing process or preparing the flowchart: • Review the flowchart • Use flowchart to perform process	People unfamiliar with process will often ask questions that improve flowchart. If flowchart cannot be used to perform process, improve flowchart.

and Gryna, 1988), and the *Handbook of Industrial Engineering* (Salvendy, 1982).

Run Chart and Control Chart

A run chart is a graph of measurements made over time, which is normally shown as a line graph. The purpose of the run chart is to look at the performance of a process over time. A process is defined as statistically stable if there has been no change in the underlying process that generated the measurements. We normally do not know whether there has been a change in the underlying process, so we use the measurements plotted on a run chart or control chart to make a judgment of whether there has been a change.

A control chart is simply a run chart with the addition of statistically determined upper and lower control limits used to make a judgment of whether the individual measurements deviate sufficiently from the average that there has been a likely change in the process. A sample control chart is illustrated in Figure 12.6. The primary purpose of a control chart is to determine which of two different questions is appropriate:

1. *Is there a special or assignable cause for the observed value?* There are a number of measurement results that indicate a process is not stable, as illustrated in Figure 12.6.

- Single point outside control limits. The fourth point is greater than the upper control limit. Therefore the process is judged to be unstable, and the cause for that point should be investigated.
- Run. More than five points in a sequence, points 11–16, are below the mean. Based on this run below the mean, the process is judged to be unstable, and the cause for these points should be investigated. The number of points in a run or trend required to judge a process as unstable is based on the probability used.
- Trend. Five points in a sequence, points 16–20, are constantly increasing. Based on this increasing trend, the pro-

Figure 12.6. Sample Control Chart.

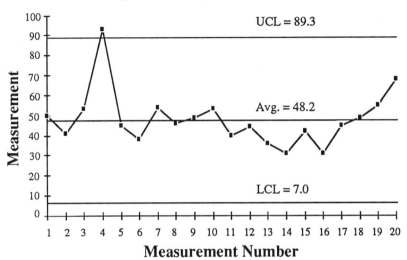

cess is judged to be unstable, and the cause for this increasing trend should be investigated.

• Pattern of measurements. A repeating or other pattern is also an indication that the process has nonrandom variation and is unstable. For example, a series of points one above the mean, one below the mean, one above, and so on, is a nonrandom pattern.

2. *Is there a common cause?* If individual points are not outside of the control limits and runs are not occurring, the process is likely to be stable, and you should ask questions about how the overall process can be improved. It is inappropriate and unhelpful to ask questions about why specific points are above or below the average. Asking such questions about individual points when the process appears to be stable is called management tampering, and leads to increased variation and decreased quality. Continuing with the example, excluding point 4, the first ten points appear to be from a stable process. In this case, attention should be directed to improving the process overall, not to investigating individual points.

Control charts help you look in the right place and ask the right question, but are not useful to solve problems or improve performance. Bhote points out that "control charts are seldom used in Japan. They are not a problem-solving tool" (1991, p. 67).

A good rule of thumb for calculating upper and lower control limits for single measurements of continuous variables is to use:

—Upper control limit (UCL) = the mean + 3 times the standard deviation. If the process is stable, there is only a 0.1 percent probability that a measurement will exceed this UCL.

—Lower control limit (LCL) = the mean – 3 times the standard deviation, but should not be less than zero. If the process is stable, there is only a 0.1 percent probability that a measurement will be less than this LCL.

Therefore, if a point is outside the control limits, the judgment is made that the process has changed, is no longer stable, and we should look for a special or assignable cause for the point.

There are several rules to be more precise about the upper and lower control limits, which can be determined from a number of statistical references including those listed at the end of this section. For example, if a variable is the average of samples of size N, then the standard deviation for the average is divided by the square root of N.

Selected references for more information on run charts and control charts are *The Memory Jogger* (GOAL/QPC, 1988), *The Team Handbook* (Scholtes, 1988), *Juran's Quality Control Handbook* (Juran and Gryna, 1988), the *Handbook of Industrial Engineering* (Salvendy, 1982), the *Team Leader Training Course* and *Facilitator Skills Training Course* (Qualtec, Inc., 1989a, 1989b), and *Total Quality Leadership Program* (University of Michigan Medical Center, 1992b).

Brainstorming

The purpose of brainstorming is to generate ideas, concerns, problems, or options. Brainstorming is referred to as a form of divergent thinking because the purpose is to expand the number of ideas being considered. Some basic ground rules can make the exercise more effective. Brainstorming is normally divided into four phases:

1. *Preparation Phase.* Explain the purpose of the brainstorming exercise, and give the team a minute or two to think silently about the question being posed. It is a good idea to put the purpose of the brainstorming exercise on a flipchart, so it is visible to all participants.
2. *Generation Phase.* Go around the table, in order, giving each team member a chance to contribute one idea. These should be recorded on a flipchart, overhead, or other medium that is visible to all and that can be used later to document the ideas. Remember to ask the person recording ideas to take a turn also. During the generation phase, ideas should be generated and recorded without explanation, judgment, or discussion. Participants are allowed to "pass," if they do not have an idea at the moment of their turn. Continue to go around until you hear several passes. Then ask if anyone else has any final ideas to contribute.
3. *Clarification Phase.* During this phase, the team goes over the list to make sure everyone understands the ideas on the list. The purpose is to understand, not criticize or comment on, the ideas.
4. *Evaluation Phase.* During the final phase, the team reviews the complete list to eliminate any that are irrelevant, duplicative, or outside the scope of the issue being considered. Duplicative ideas may be consolidated. The final list should represent all of the independent ideas the team could generate.

The power of brainstorming is that you can generate ideas from several people who have very different roles and perspectives, which develops a sense of participation and ownership. The final list should be transcribed and distributed to all participants.

More information on brainstorming can be found in the works recommended for further reading on run charts and control charts listed above.

Affinity Diagram

An affinity diagram is an approach to combine ideas into similar groups. You normally begin with a list of many topics, generated by brainstorming or another approach, to identify as many ideas as possible. Affinity diagramming is a form of convergent thinking because the purpose of an affinity diagram is to group the ideas logically into a smaller set of categories. The approach works best with a small group of people. Participants silently rearrange the items, which are written on cards on a table or posted on movable cards or Post-It notes on a wall chart, into groups of similar ideas. Each person participates, and the movement continues until each person feels comfortable with the groups of ideas. Then the team discusses appropriate header titles for the groups of similar topics. The process is like the opposite of outlining, where you start with the most general heading and build increasing levels of detail.

Selected references for more information on affinity diagramming are *The Memory Jogger Plus +* (Brassard, 1989), the *Team Leader Training Course* and *Facilitator Skills Training Course* (Qualtec, Inc., 1989a, 1989b), and *Total Quality Leadership Program* (University of Michigan Medical Center, 1992b).

Multivoting

Multivoting is used to reduce a large number of ideas or options to a manageable few judged important by the participants. Usually the number of ideas is reduced to three to five. Multivoting is also a form of convergent thinking because the purpose is to reduce the number of ideas being considered. The rules may vary somewhat but generally use the following approach:

> *Round One.* Each team member of participant may vote for as many items as he or she considers to have merit. The

votes are added, and those with relatively larger numbers of votes are circled for further consideration. The
other items are dropped from further consideration.
Subsequent Rounds. For the second and subsequent rounds,
the number of items remaining is totaled, and each
team member is given a number of votes totaling half of
the total. For example, if eleven items were circled in
phase one as having the greatest merit, then for round
two each person would be given five or six votes (usually the team will round up, giving each person six
votes). Each member then votes for half the items on
the list he or she considers most important. The votes
are added, and those with relatively larger numbers of
votes are circled for further consideration. This process is repeated with decreasing numbers of items on
the list until the list is reduced to three to five items.

One of the real powers of multivoting is that you end up
with a short list of items to pursue further rather than being
forced to vote down to a single item. This builds more consensus
than a formal voting process where there are winners and losers.
Never continue the multivoting process until only one item
remains. This forces participants to give up items they consider
important, which may reduce their support of the team effort.
Also, additional data will be collected on the short list of items to
determine which one represents the largest problem or opportunity. We would offer one caution based on experiences with
many teams. During the consolidation phase of brainstorming
and during the rounds of multivoting, team members may
consolidate the ideas too much. The result is broad topics rather
than a specific issue to address. The categories should be sufficiently specific that they can be addressed by a team.

Selected references for more information on multivoting
are *The Team Handbook* (Scholtes and others, 1988), the *Team
Leader Training Course* and *Facilitator Skills Training Course*
(Qualtec, Inc., 1989a, 1989b), and *Total Quality Leadership Program* (University of Michigan Medical Center, 1992b).

Prioritization Matrix

The basic approach of quality improvement is first to identify and prioritize the general topics for improvement, then to refine the priority topics into more and more specific topics.

A prioritization matrix is a general tool used to prioritize among issues, problems, opportunities for improvement, or proposed solutions. The purpose is to use a structured approach to evaluate which issue requires the greatest attention. The same general approach has many uses, with modification of the criteria and issues being considered. This tool is a form of convergent thinking, to reduce the number of options being considered. A sample prioritization selection matrix is illustrated in Exhibit 12.2. Different components of the matrix will be explained.

Issues. The various issues or topics being considered, and

Exhibit 12.2. Prioritization Matrix.

	Prioritization Criteria				
Issue	*Criterion A*	*Criterion B*	· · ·	*Criterion N*	*Overall Score*
	A	B		N	A*B*···*N

Scale: 1–5: 1 = None, 2 = Somewhat, 3 = Moderate, 4 = High, 5 = Very High.

which need to be prioritized. Sample uses of this type of matrix are to prioritize:

- General issues or themes
- Specific quality gaps, problems, or opportunities for improvement
- Options or proposed solutions for improvement

Prioritization Criteria. The criteria to be used to prioritize the issues are listed across the matrix as column headings. Sample prioritization criteria are:

- Customer impact, or interest by key customers
- Need to improve, or urgency of issue
- Frequency of occurrence
- Probability of success
- Financial impact

At times the relative values of the different criteria are substantially different. In these cases, different weights can be assigned to each of the criteria at the top of each column. For each issue (row) the score for each criterion is then multiplied by the relative weight for the respective criteria (column).

Scores. Each issue is scored based on its relative merit as judged by each criterion, based on consensus of the team. Samples of different types of scales are:

- Score from 1 to 3, with 3 being the most important. For example, 1 = low, 2 = medium, and 3 = high.
- Score from 1 to 5, with 5 being the most important. For example, 1 = none, 2 = somewhat, 3 = moderate, 4 = high, and 5 = very high.

At times you may want to enter actual financial estimates or other measures of the criterion. Be cautious, however, that the scores for the different criteria have similar scales to avoid the values of one criterion from overpowering the others. One useful approach to do this is to convert them proportionately to a percentage or scale relative to the other criteria.

Overall Score. The overall score can be calculated in different ways. Some of the more common approaches are to:

- Multiply the scores for each of the prioritization criteria, and enter the product in the overall score column for each of the issues.
- Sum the scores of the prioritization criteria for each of the issues.
- Use a weighted sum of the criteria. In this case, the score for each issue and criterion is multiplied by the relative weight of the criterion, and that number is entered into the matrix adjacent to the score. The weighted scores are then summed across the columns for each issue to get an overall score.

Approach. The following is a suggested approach to using a prioritization matrix to establish relative priorities.

1. List the issues, quality gaps, or options to be considered in the left column. A sample blank prioritization matrix for prioritizing opportunities for improvement is illustrated in Exhibit 12.3.
2. Brainstorm the list of criteria to evaluate the issues. After brainstorming the list, the criteria should be evaluated to make sure there is no overlap and whether different weights will be required. List the criteria along the top row of the matrix. The sample criteria in Exhibit 12.3 are impact on the customer, need to improve, and probability of success, which are defined at the bottom of the exhibit.
3. Select a scoring approach and scale. In the sample matrix, the criteria are treated relatively equal, so no relative weights were established. A scale of 1–5 is illustrated.
4. Score each issue with its relative value for each of the criteria. In the sample matrix, scores of 1–5 are assigned as each issue, quality gap, or opportunity for improvement is evaluated relative to each criterion.
5. Calculate an overall score. In the sample matrix, the overall

Exhibit 12.3. Sample Blank Prioritization Matrix.

Quality Gap or Improvement Opportunity	Prioritization Criteria			Overall Score
	Impact on Customer A	*Need to Improve* B	*Probability of Success* C	A*B*C
Issues: After multivoting, there are 3–6 issues, problems, or improvement opportunities that remain.	*Impact on Customer:* A rating based on the team's present knowledge and judgment of the direct effect of this issue on customer satisfaction.	*Need to Improve:* A rating based on the team's present knowledge and judgment of the difference between the present performance and that needed to meet the customer's valid requirements.	*Probability of Success:* A rating based on the team's judgment of the probability of successful implementation of this improvement opportunity.	*Comparative Score:* The product of the Impact on Customer*Need to Improve*Probability of Success
Teams should consider only those issues they can affect.	Higher ratings are given to issues that have a more direct effect on customers.	Higher ratings are given to opportunities with greater need to improve.	Higher ratings are given to improvement opportunities that have the highest probability of success.	The improvement opportunity receiving the highest ranking should be selected for further investigation, unless there is a strong reason otherwise. Establish an indicator and measure actual value versus valid requirements. If there is a difference, proceed. If not, select the next highest ranked improvement opportunity.

Scale: 1–5: 1 = None, 2 = Somewhat, 3 = Moderate, 4 = High, 5 = Very High.

score is the product of the three criterion scores for each quality gap.

A sample completed prioritization matrix for an admission process is illustrated in Table 13.1.

Selected references for more information on the prioritization matrix are the *Team Leader Training Course* and *Facilitator Skills Training Course* (Qualtec, Inc., 1989a, 1989b), and *Total Quality Leadership Program* (University of Michigan Medical Center, 1992b).

Checksheets

Checksheets are used primarily to collect data on the frequency of occurrence of selected events. A checksheet, for example, could be used to determine the frequency of occurrence of the three to five problems or opportunities identified during multivoting. Checksheets are normally used in a quality improvement process to collect frequency data later displayed in a Pareto chart. The team should define all the terms and methods of measurement to assure uniform data collection. Two examples of completed checksheets are included in Figures 13.2 and 13.7.

Selected references for more information on checksheets are *The Memory Jogger* (GOAL/QPC, 1988), *The Team Handbook* (Scholtes and others, 1988), *Juran's Quality Control Handbook* (Juran and Gryna, 1988), the *Handbook of Industrial Engineering* (Salvendy, 1982), the *Team Leader Training Course* and *Facilitator Skills Training Course* (Qualtec, Inc., 1989a, 1989b), and *Total Quality Leadership Program* (University of Michigan Medical Center, 1992b).

Histogram and Pareto Chart

A histogram displays the frequencies or numbers of different events or measurements as a bar chart. The bars of a histogram are often arranged by some logical characteristic of the data, like day of week or hour of day. A Pareto chart does the same thing with two additional features. First, the frequencies are displayed decreasing from left to right, so the most frequent events, or tallest bars, are at the left. Second, the cumulative frequency is also plotted on the graph as a line. A Pareto chart is used to display visually the significance of different factors, to separate the many from the vital few. This is similar to the "80–20 rule," which ascribes 80 percent of the potential improvement to 20 percent of the issues. A sample Pareto chart is illustrated in Figure 12.7.

A Pareto chart is commonly used to display the frequency of problems or opportunities to select a theme or problem to work on, and to display the frequency of root causes once a problem has been selected. More information on Pareto charts and histograms can be found in the works recommended for further reading on checksheets listed above.

Cause-Effect, Fishbone, or Ishikawa Diagram

A cause-effect diagram is a graphic tool used to organize possible causes of the observed effect or problem. This tool is also called a fishbone or Ishikawa diagram. A sample completed cause-effect diagram, including the problem statement and major bones or branches, is illustrated in Figure 13.6. The effect is written at the right side of the main backbone. Then major types of reasons or causes are drawn as spines along the backbone, resembling fishbones. You can use typical major types of reasons, or develop others appropriate to your needs. It will be easier to work with the cause-effect diagram if the major categories are independent and uniquely different. Examples of major categories of causes are:

Four M's:	*Four P's:*	*Another Alternative*
• Method	• Policies	• People
• Manpower	• Procedures	• Methods
• Material	• People	• Information
• Machinery	• Plant	• Materials
		• Facilities

The purpose of the major categories is to stimulate ideas about potential causes of the effect that you plan to change.

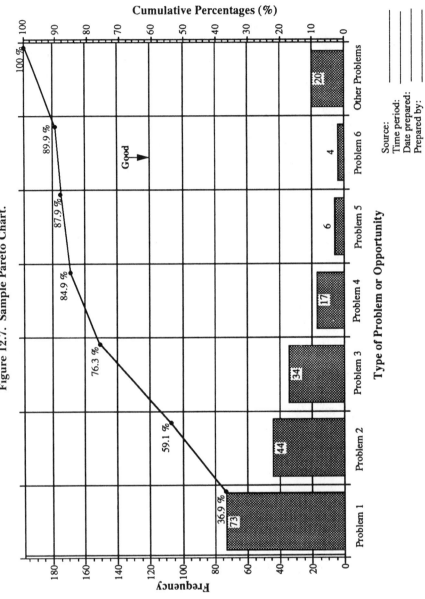

Figure 12.7. Sample Pareto Chart.

Brainstorming is a useful approach to generate ideas. Then, as each idea is listed, ask the question "why" and write those reasons down on smaller bones or branches of the diagram. The question "why" is repeated until there is no additional logical answer to the question. The most important of these end points, as determined by data on frequency, impact, or opinion, are called the "root causes." The root causes should be circled for easy identification. As a rule of thumb, the question "why" should be asked five times. During this process, the team may decide to add or delete bones or branches to identify fully causes of the stated problem.

An alternative graphic approach is to use a hierarchy outline of the causes leading to the effect. The fishbone diagram is very helpful for illustrating the concepts to the team, but can become very busy as many possible causes are added to the figure. Also, the fishbone diagram is more difficult to update and change. An outline approach can also be used. An example of this type of outline is illustrated in Exhibit 13.5. Each successive indent answers the next subsequent question of "why."

Before completing the cause-effect diagram, each branch should be checked for logic in two directions:

1. As you proceed downward from more general to more specific, each subsequent branch should answer the question "why."
2. As you proceed upward from more specific to more general, it should make sense that each subsequent branch is a "cause" of the one above it.

Selected references for more information on cause-effect diagrams are *The Memory Jogger* (GOAL/QPC, 1988), *The Team Handbook* (Scholtes and others, 1988), *Juran's Quality Control Handbook* (Juran and Gryna, 1988), the *Handbook of Industrial Engineering* (Salvendy, 1982), the *Team Leader Training Course* and *Facilitator Skills Training Course* (Qualtec, Inc., 1989a, 1989b), and *Total Quality Leadership Program* (University of Michigan Medical Center, 1992b).

Proposed Options Matrix

Options or proposed solutions are the changes planned to reduce or eliminate the root causes of the problem, or opportunity for improvement. There are normally many potential options, and your objective is to identify them and select those that offer the greatest opportunity for improvement.

    Options List. The first step is to develop a list of potential options or proposed solutions that remedy verified root causes, meet customers' valid requirements, and are cost-beneficial. The following approaches are helpful to generate the list of proposed solutions:

1. Review the flowchart of the process in detail to identify options or potential solutions. This may require a more detailed flowchart be developed related to the identified root cause(s). Review each step in the flowchart for whether that step adds value from the perspective of the customer(s). If not, eliminating those steps, and possibly reorganizing the remaining work, is an excellent option.
2. Brainstorm possible options and potential solutions with your team. It may be helpful to solicit input from a wide variety of people knowledgeable about the portions of the process related to the identified root cause.
3. Use the best practices of similar processes as benchmarks to identify potential changes. Benchmarking is explained further in Chapter Fourteen.

    Options Matrix. The options matrix is a useful tool that summarizes and scores practical methods of implementing changes, the effectiveness of the changes, and the feasibility of the changes to prioritize the options or proposed solutions. The options matrix is a form of a prioritization matrix described earlier. A sample blank options matrix is illustrated in Exhibit 12.4. A sample completed options matrix is illustrated in Table 13.3.

    More information on the options matrix is included in

Exhibit 12.4. Sample Blank Options Matrix.

Description				Relative Score (e.g., 1–5)				Action
Quality Gap	Root Cause	Option or Proposed Solution	Methods (How)	Financial Impact A	Effectiveness B	Feasibility C	Overall A*B*C	
The quality gap or opportunity selected for improvement.	Root causes from cause-effect diagram.	Options or proposed solutions aimed at root causes. To extent possible within team's ability to implement.	Specific task(s) to implement. Addresses "how."	Relative net financial impact of costs and revenues.	Rating of effectiveness to reduce root cause.	Rating of time, cost, acceptance, and probability of success.	Product of effectiveness and feasibility.	Indicate Yes or No whether action will be taken.

Scale: 1–5: 1 = None, 2 = Somewhat, 3 = Moderate, 4 = High, 5 = Very High.

Total Quality Leadership Program (University of Michigan Medical Center, 1992b).

Force Field Analysis

For the selected option(s) or proposed solution(s), it is useful to identify forces that support or oppose implementing the option(s). This approach is also called barriers and aids analysis. Forces opposing implementation are those processes, people, environmental factors, and other things that inhibit or slow implementation of the option(s). Forces supporting implementation are the same types of things that facilitate or speed the implementation. The purpose of this analysis is to identify all of the things affecting implementation of the option(s), so you can address them in your action plan. The steps in a force field analysis are to:

1. Identify the option.
2. Use brainstorming to list potential driving or supporting forces, and opposing or restraining forces.
3. Rank the strength of each supporting or opposing force as high, medium, or low.
4. Match similar supporting and opposing forces in the force field matrix.
5. Evaluate the relative strengths of the various forces, to identify items that require the team's attention.
6. Develop an action plan.

A sample blank force field analysis matrix is illustrated in Exhibit 12.5, and a sample completed force field analysis matrix for the admission case study is illustrated in Table 13.4.

Selected references for more information on barriers and aids and force field analysis are *The Memory Jogger* (GOAL/QPC, 1988), *Juran's Quality Control Handbook* (Juran and Gryna, 1988), the *Team Leader Training Course* and *Facilitator Skills Training Course* (Qualtec, Inc., 1989a, 1989b), and *Total Quality Leadership Program* (University of Michigan Medical Center, 1992b).

Exhibit 12.5. Sample Blank Force Field Analysis Matrix.

Option or Proposed Solution	Negative Forces (Oppose Option Implementation)	Positive Forces (Support Option Implementation)

Cost-Benefit Analysis

The cost-benefit of options should be understood before beginning implementation. Although most managers fear quality improvement teams will identify very expensive and infeasible options, most organizations, including UMMC, have not experienced this. The purpose of the cost-benefit analysis is that the team members consider the full impact of their recommended actions. One-time and annual costs and benefits should be considered. Financial services, management engineering, and other analytical staff can provide valuable additional assistance for this analysis, if required by the team.

Selected references for more information on cost-benefit

analysis are *Juran's Quality Control Handbook* (Juran and Gryna, 1988), the *Handbook of Industrial Engineering* (Salvendy, 1982), the *Team Leader Training Course* and *Facilitator Skills Training Course* (Qualtec, Inc., 1989a, 1989b), and *Total Quality Leadership Program* (University of Michigan Medical Center, 1992b).

Fault Analysis

A fault analysis investigates all of the possible ways the proposed option could fail. It can be simply represented as a matrix, with the options or actions to implement the options in the left column, the potential fault or failure in the middle column, and possible actions to address the fault in the right column. Brainstorming is a good approach to generate potential faults and possible actions to address those faults. If, for example, a computerized patient registration is being planned for a satellite clinic, faults might include delayed implementation, hardware failure, software errors, or staff not understanding how to use the system. Possible actions should be developed to address each of these. Some failures can have catastrophic consequences if not considered in a fault analysis.

Chapter Thirteen

A Case Study of Quality Improvement

The purpose of this admitting case study is to provide an example of a quality improvement project that demonstrates selected analytical tools and techniques and people-management methods. Admitting is used as an example because many healthcare organizations have difficulty managing the admission/discharge process because of the complexity of the process and the number of different people involved in it. Therefore, the case study has direct relevance to most healthcare organizations. Also, many people within these organizations have some knowledge of the admission process.

The case study is presented as a story, describing team dynamics as well as the analytical tools and techniques. The QI story is presented in the format of the UMMC Quality Roadmap illustrated in Figure 8.2 in Chapter Eight. At each step of the case study, typical tools, techniques, and outputs are demonstrated with sample data. The same types of tools and techniques are used in virtually all QI processes and are often used multiple times during a project. Throughout the case study we have also included some helpful hints and guidelines.

Case Study Background Information

Brief background information is provided to give you a sense of the environment in which the case study is conducted. However, the approach used for this case study is relevant in vastly different situations.

Hospital. The organization is a 350-bed community hospital in an urban area, with several medical training programs for resident physicians and nurses. Based on its excellent clinical reputation, the hospital has an overall inpatient occupancy of 82 percent. The adult medical/surgical acute care units have an average occupancy of over 88 percent and are frequently full Monday through Thursday.

Admitting. The admitting department receives and admits two types of patients:

1. Patients scheduled for admission, whose arrival time is known and scheduled. This case study will focus on these scheduled admissions.
2. Patients not scheduled for admission. These are patients whose need for immediate admission is identified by a physician in emergency services, an outpatient clinic, or a physician's office on or shortly before the day of admission. This group also includes patients transferred via helicopter or ambulance. This case study will not address these unscheduled admissions.

The admitting department has received a large number of complaints from patients and families, attending and resident physicians, and many others about several problems, including long delays and wait times, inadequate seating space, transportation of patients, and the patient scheduling system. As a consequence of the patient complaints, staff in the several departments relating to admission, discharge, and transfer of patients have been blaming each other for the delays. Most complaints are unspecific about the several different problems.

A Quality Improvement Team was formed to investigate the problems related to patients scheduled for admission and to develop a plan for improvement.

Team Formation

The director of admissions was selected by the Corporate Lead Team to be the team leader since he or she was the co-owner of the process for scheduled admissions. Given the widespread criticism and the volume of complaints, this QI effort was viewed as important to the organizational goals. Thus this team was formed from a top-down direction. Other members of the QIT were selected by the team leader, based on a rough flowchart of the scheduled admission process, because their jobs were part of the process. The members included:

- Housekeeper, who cleans patient rooms
- Housekeeping manager, who determines the policies and priorities for cleaning patient rooms
- Admission clerk, who processes the patients in admitting and who attends to the patients and families while they are waiting
- Nursing inpatient unit clerk, who serves as an important communication link
- Resident, or house officer, who initiates discharge orders for patients being discharged
- Nurse from inpatient nursing unit, who interacts with the physicians, patients, and families to obtain and communicate orders for the discharge, supplies, drugs, and other things required before the patient can leave
- Transporter, who transports patients being discharged and admitted

Since team members were from different departments, the team was referred to as a cross-functional team. Sample criteria for the size and membership of QITs are illustrated in Exhibit 13.1. A number of other people who were not team members were consulted about processes in their areas that impacted the admission process. Examples included the director of radiology, the pathology manager, a pharmacist, and a materiel services supervisor.

The team leader had attended multiple education programs on TQM, including a Total Quality leadership program specifically designed to provide skills for leading a formal team or other QI effort. In addition, the Corporate Lead Team assigned a trained facilitator to assist the team leader and team. The team leader and team facilitator met three times before the

**Exhibit 13.1. Sample Criteria for Size and Membership
of Quality Improvement Teams.**

- Size of team is five to nine members, with six to seven being best. Team dynamics work best at this size. Larger groups seldom work effectively as a team. Other people may serve as consultants to the team.
- Team leader is an owner or co-owner of process being studied.
- Members should be key customers and suppliers of steps in the process, the people who actually do steps of the process.
- Avoid teams of managers only. They do not have the detailed knowledge of the process. Also, employees will support the team's findings more if employees are team members.
- Steps of flowchart used to define all customers and suppliers of process.
- Good idea to begin with smaller team to define problem statement or statement of improvement opportunity, because it may be beneficial to add additional key customers or suppliers as the problem is refined. Also, the selected team members should have the option of adding people who they think are critical to the team's success.
- Input from other customers and suppliers should be sought by team.

first team meeting to select the team members, to review the QI process, to plan the meeting agendas, and to discuss how to resolve potential conflicts among the team members. One-hour team meetings were scheduled weekly at a time acceptable to all team members.

At the first meeting, the team leader had all team members introduce themselves and discuss their role in the scheduled admission process, although only one of them was not familiar with the others. The team leader also asked if there was anyone else who should be part of the QIT. Although the team leader then used an icebreaker to relax the team members, all of them remained relatively quiet. Everyone was polite, but there was a feeling of tension in the room. During this initial meeting, the team was in the form stage of development (Tuckman, 1965).

During the next three to five meetings, there were intermittent implications and occasional open accusations of who was at fault for the problem of long waiting times. It seemed that everyone knew who was the problem, and it was someone else. There was a clear lack of trust among the team members. During these meetings the team was in the storm stage of its development (Tuckman, 1965). The team leader, with the help of the team facilitator, used the following approaches to reduce the tension and to focus the team on process improvement:

- Provided sixteen hours of education on the QI process, which included information on the following:
  - Seven-step quality improvement process.
  - Examples to demonstrate that at least 85 percent of quality improvement opportunities are due to process improvement, not people. This was done in an effort to reduce the implications that people in the different departments were at fault.
  - Introduction of new terminology, including *quality gap* and *opportunity for improvement*, to reduce the "search for the guilty."
  - Team dynamics topics.
- Helped the team establish a set of rules of conduct. Each team can amend the rules of conduct if it wishes, but a sample set of rules of conduct are illustrated in Exhibit 13.2 (Qualtec, 1988, pp. 2–6; University of Michigan Medical Center, 1992b).
- Asked all team members to explain the functions they perform and the process, quality gaps, problems, opportunities for improvement, barriers to change, and personal frustrations from their own perspectives. Other team members were asked to listen, but not to comment or rebut the state-

Exhibit 13.2. Sample Rules of Conduct.

- Show respect for all team members.
- Seek first to understand, then to be understood.
- Share responsibility.
- Criticize ideas, not people.
- Keep an open mind.
- Question and participate.
- Come on time and be prepared to contribute.
- Complete your teamwork assignments.
- Listen actively.
- Be constructive.

Sources: University of Michigan, 1992; Qualtec, 1989b; Covey, 1990.

ments while each person was speaking. Although these discussions were somewhat tense, they did open every team member's eyes. All members began to realize that they did not understand the whole process.

- Asked team members what people not represented on the team would be good sources of input and information during the quality improvement project.

After the initial discussions and education, the team leader and team facilitator agreed it was best to focus the attention of the team members on the QI process. This would provide the team members with a meaningful approach and draw the attention away from the long-standing arguments over who was to blame for the problems.

Step 1: Recognize the Process

The objective of Step 1 of the UMMC quality improvement process is to identify and analyze major work processes and customers. The team leader and team facilitator encouraged the team to first flowchart the admission process in order to understand it.

Flowchart Admission Process

As the team discussed flowcharting, some things became evident. First, a key influencing factor on admission problems was the discharge process. Therefore, the team decided to flowchart both the discharge and admission processes. Actually, there were several subprocesses involved in both, such as performing radiology exams on patients as they are admitted. Second, some team members did not feel comfortable with the technique of flowcharting. One or two team members were uneasy with the flowchart symbols (see Figure 12.3 in Chapter Twelve), so the initial charts were prepared simply describing the process with words. As the team members became more comfortable, the symbols were used. The primary effort of flowcharting the process was assumed by two of the team members who had previous experience with flowcharting. The team struggled with what level of detail was required in the flowchart, because it seemed that ever increasing detail was possible. The decision was made to err on the side of too much detail and to describe the process carefully.

The discharge process flowchart was initiated with the notice of discharge of the previous patient in the respective bed. A flowchart is simply a picture of the flow of activities, materials, patients, or information within a process. The process can be drawn on paper, drawn on a flipchart, entered into a computer flowchart program, or created using Post-It notes on a wall or large piece of paper. The latter approach makes it easier if the team as a whole wishes to create a flowchart. In this case, however, two team members who created the flowchart took notes on legal pads, created the flowcharts in a computer, then passed out copies for the team members and others to review. A simple flowchart for the admission/discharge process is illustrated in Figure 13.1. The actual flowcharts were very detailed and covered many pages.

After the flowcharts were completed, the team spent time reviewing them for opportunities for improvement. The analyses of the flowcharts included topics like those described in Figure 12.1 in Chapter Twelve. Some of the possible improvements were raised during the brainstorming session and are discussed later in this chapter.

Identify and Select Improvement Opportunities

The team decided to use brainstorming to create a list of potential problems or improvement opportunities related to the scheduled admission process. As described in Chapter Twelve, the brainstorming included three different phases:

- Preparation Phase. The team agreed on and posted the purpose of the brainstorming session on a flipchart.
- Generation Phase. All team members contributed to generating a list of problems or improvement opportunities re-

Figure 13.1. Simple Flowchart of Admission/Discharge Process.

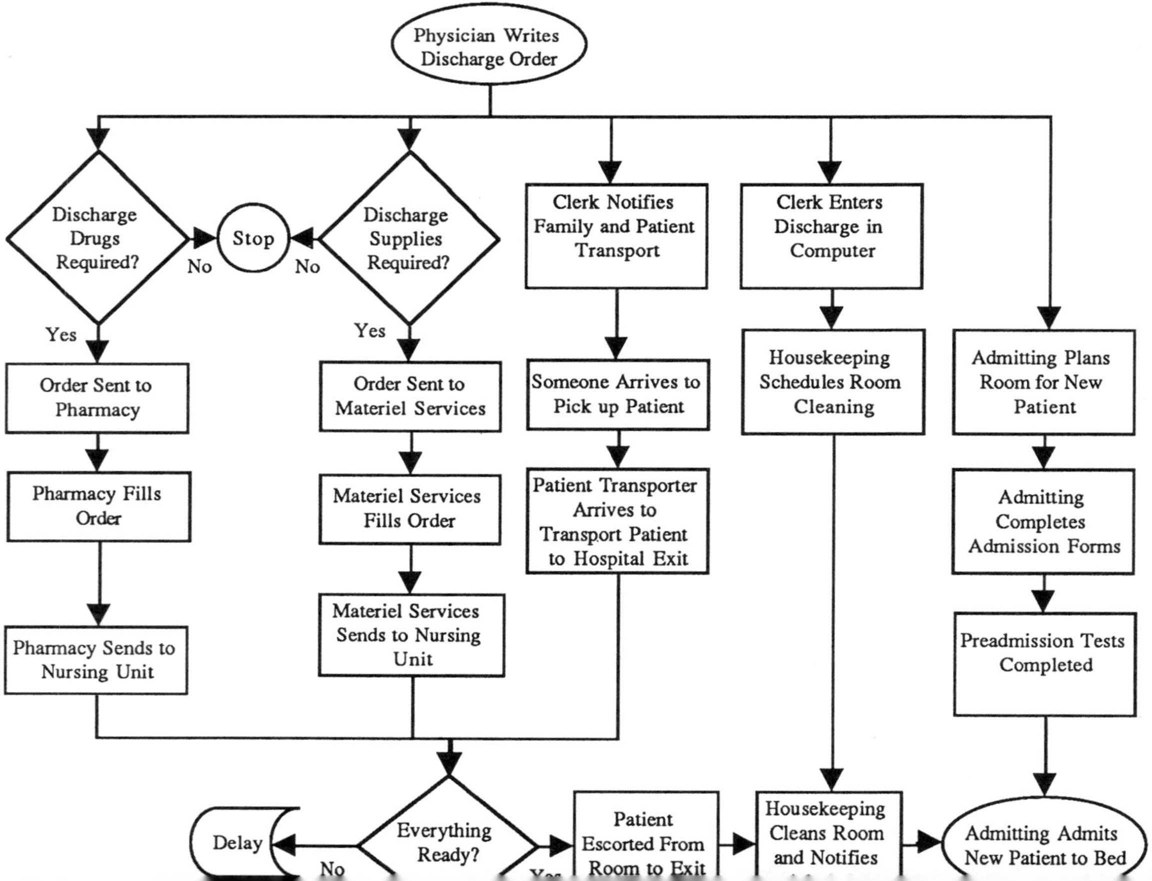

lated to scheduled admissions. One of the team members recorded these ideas.

- Clarification Phase. The team went over the list to make sure everyone understood each of the ideas on it.
- Evaluation Phase. The team reviewed the list and eliminated duplications and irrelevant ideas.

The team then used multivoting to reduce the list to five improvement opportunities for further analysis: excess waiting time for patients, inadequate space, patient scheduling system, transportation of patients, and physician relations.

A prioritization matrix was then developed to prioritize among the remaining improvement opportunities, as illustrated in Table 13.1. Each of the improvement opportunities was scored on a scale of 1–5, with 5 being the most important, for each of the three criteria used by the team: impact on customer, need to improve, and probability of success. The scores were based on the collective knowledge of the team members, along with the information from the flowchart and other data.

Step 1 Questions

During each step of the QI process, the team leader encouraged the team members and others, especially managers of affected areas, to ask questions in order to understand better the progress and results. In addition, after Steps 2, 4, and 7 of the process, the Corporate Lead Team reviewed the team's progress and asked similar questions. In addition to actively leading the TQM process, one of the most important things leaders and managers can do is ask good questions. If, for example, you ask teams and staff about trends of data over time, they will maintain run charts or control charts of important quality measures. If, on the other hand, you never ask about trends of data, they will conclude that such data are unimportant or of low priority.

Such questions are important for understanding the issues involved. Sample questions during the "Recognize the Process" step and some sample answers are:

Table 13.1. Prioritization Matrix of Admitting Problems.

Quality Gap or Improvement Opportunity	Impact on Customer	Need to Improve	Probability of Success	Overall Score
	A	B	C	A*B*C
Excess waiting time for patients	5	5	3	75
Inadequate space	4	4	2	32
Patient scheduling system	3	4	3	36
Transportation of patients	3	3	3	27
Physician relations	2	4	3	24
Improvement Opportunity: Teams should consider only those improvement opportunities that they can affect.	*Impact on Customer:* A rating based on the team's present knowledge and judgment of the direct effect of this improvement opportunity on customer satisfaction. Higher ratings are given to improvement opportunities that have a more direct effect on customers.	*Need to Improve:* A rating based on the team's present knowledge and judgment of the difference between the present performance and that needed to meet the customer's valid requirements. Higher ratings are given to improvement opportunities with greater need to improve.	*Probability of Success:* A rating based on the team's judgment of the probability of successful implementation of this improvement opportunity. Higher ratings are given to improvement opportunities that have the highest probability of success.	*Comparative Score:* The product of the Impact on Customer*Need to Improve*Probability of Success The improvement opportunity receiving the highest ranking should be selected for further investigation, unless there is a strong reason otherwise. Establish an indicator and measure actual values versus valid requirements. If there is a difference, proceed. If not, select the next highest ranked improvement opportunity.

Scale: 1–5: 1 = None, 2 = Somewhat, 3 = Moderate, 4 = High, 5 = Very High.

1. Who was involved in creating the flowchart? Has direct input been received from every customer and supplier group represented on the flowchart? Not every person needs to be a member of the QIT but should have input, even if not on the team. Also, by posting the QI storyboard in a visible location, input can be obtained from all employees and managers who wish to contribute to the effort.

2. Are there any steps in the flowchart that do not add value? Eliminating steps that do not add value is the quickest and easiest way to both improve quality and reduce costs. The team found several steps in the process that did not add value.

3. What criteria were used to prioritize among the improvement opportunities, and why were those criteria used?

4. What additional information is required?

5. What type of support does your team need?

Step 1 Lessons Learned

As the team completed Step 1, a number of observations and lessons emerged. Some examples are:

- Discussion. There was a lot of discussion among team members, which created many ideas.
- Avoid jumping to conclusions. There were a lot of ideas and data, with team members expressing different operational definitions, understandings, and processes. Jumping to conclusions was a major problem. There was also a tendency at this stage to jump to conclusions about the options or potential solutions before there had been a good definition of the problem, any analysis of data, or any investigation of root causes. The lesson was to avoid jumping to conclusions or options.
- Begin with the big picture. It was important to begin by considering the major issues related to the overall vision and

goals of the organization and the admission process. It was also clear that the discharge process was an integral part of the admission problems. It was easy to focus too quickly on the little things and end up "rearranging the deck chairs on the Titanic."

- Need to prioritize. Many different problems and opportunities are identified, but which one should be worked on first? In fact, the team jumped back and forth among several different problems until the prioritization matrix was used to structure the discussion and to prioritize among the many issues.
- The structure of the standardized seven-step QI process helped guide and prioritize the discussion and analyses.

Step 2: Organize the Data

The objective of Step 2 is to stratify and describe the current processes, customers, and gaps in quality, then to develop a statement of improvement opportunity. The team now focused on collecting more data to verify the findings in the prioritization matrix, to understand the current process, and to determine the quality gap.

Frequency of Problems or Opportunities

The team designed checksheets to collect data on the frequency of different problems or improvement opportunities. A checksheet is a simple tool used to collect data on the frequency of events or problems. The team listed the improvement opportunities selected in Step 1 on a form, leaving space for staff to count the frequency of occurrence for each problem. Each of the terms was defined, with a method of measurement. For example, the wait time for a patient scheduled for admission was measured by staff in the admitting lounge beginning when all admission forms and testing were complete and ending when the patient left the admission lounge for his/her inpatient bed. When someone complained, it was recorded as a problem. The team then solicited help to collect the data. Baseline data were

Figure 13.2. Checksheet of Admitting Problems.

Type of Problem	Count of Occurrences	Total
Inadequate Space	𝍸 𝍸 𝍸 𝍸 𝍸 𝍸 IIII	34
Long Wait Times for Scheduled Patients	𝍸 𝍸 𝍸 𝍸 𝍸 𝍸 𝍸 𝍸 𝍸 𝍸 𝍸 𝍸 𝍸 𝍸 III	73
Long Wait Times for Unscheduled Patients	𝍸 𝍸 𝍸 𝍸 𝍸 𝍸 𝍸 𝍸 IIII	44
Not Enough Admitting Clerks	𝍸 I	6
Transporter Not Available	𝍸 𝍸 𝍸 II	17
Admission Tests Not Ordered	IIII	4
Other	𝍸 𝍸 𝍸 𝍸	20

collected for one month. A sample checksheet of admitting problems is illustrated in Figure 13.2.

One of the team members volunteered to prepare a Pareto chart to display the data from the checksheet graphically. A Pareto chart is similar to a histogram in which the reasons are plotted from highest to lowest frequency, from left to right. The cumulative frequency is plotted as a line above the frequency bars. The Pareto chart of the number of admitting problems is illustrated in Figure 13.3.

Control Charts Related to Admission Wait Times

Since the problem of long wait times for scheduled admissions occurred most frequently, the director of admitting asked his/her staff to collect and graph data on actual wait times for scheduled patients. The wait time data for scheduled patients are given in Exhibit 13.3, and a control chart of these wait times illustrated in Figure 13.4. The graph of the control chart was created to:

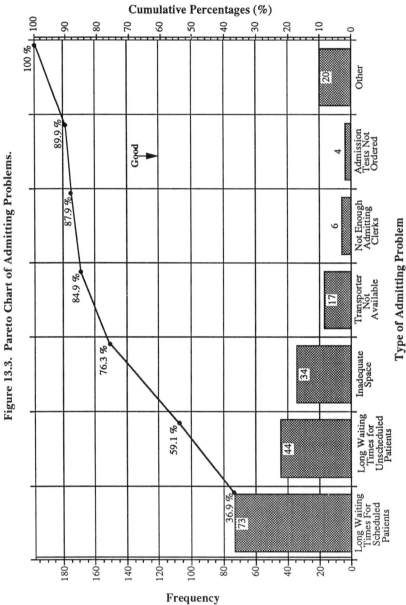

Figure 13.3. Pareto Chart of Admitting Problems.

Cumulative Percentages (%)

Frequency

Type of Admitting Problem

100 %

89.9 %

87.9 %

84.9 %

76.3 %

59.1 %

36.9 %

Good

73

44

34

17

6

4

20

Long Waiting Times For Scheduled Patients

Long Waiting Times for Unscheduled Patients

Inadequate Space

Transporter Not Available

Not Enough Admitting Clerks

Admission Tests Not Ordered

Other

Source: Admitting department; *Time period:* July 1990–July 1991; *Date prepared:* July 1991; *Prepared by:* EJG[R]C.

Exhibit 13.3. Admission Lounge Wait Times: July 1990–July 1991.

Month	Average Lounge Wait Time (minutes)	
	1990	1991
January		133
February		123
March		112
April		116
May		130
June		125
July	138	130
August	174	
September	104	
October	117	
November	109	
December	122	

Average or mean (July 1990 to July 1991) = 125.6 minutes
Standard deviation (July 1990 to July 1991) = 17.6 minutes
  (17.57/sq. root 30 = 3.2)

Source: Admitting department
Time period: July 1990–July 1991
Date prepared: July 1991
Prepared by: EJG/RJC

- Cover a wide range of possible wait times (0–180 minutes)
- Leave space to plot data after options or proposed solutions have been tested
- Indicate direction of "good" performance on graph with an arrow pointing in the "good" direction
- Include on each graph a small block that identifies data collection period, who prepared graph, date prepared, and source of information

The primary purpose of a control chart, with upper and lower control limits, is to help you ask the correct questions about the process. Control limits for the wait time data are also illustrated in Figure 13.4. A good rule of thumb for calculating upper and lower control limits is to use:

Figure 13.4. Control Chart of Average Admission Lounge Wait Time: July 1990–July 1991.

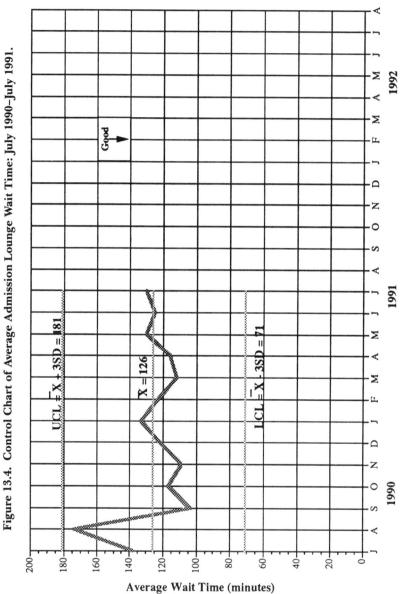

Source: Admitting department; *Time period:* July 1990–July 1991; *Date prepared:* July 1991; *Prepared by:* EJG/RJC.

— Upper control limit (UCL) = the mean + 3 times the standard deviation.

— Lower control limit (LCL) = the mean − 3 times the standard deviation, but should not be less than zero.

There are several rules to be more precise about the upper and lower control limits, which can be determined from a number of statistical references. For example, if a variable is the average of samples of size N, then the standard deviation for the average is divided by the square root of N. A person knowledgeable in statistics may be helpful with this.

For this, or any other, control chart, two questions are appropriate:

1. *Is there a special or assignable cause for the observed value?* If an individual point lies outside the upper or lower control limits, a run of 5 points in a row lies above or below the overall average, a trend of 5 points in a row is steadily increasing or decreasing, or there is a repeating pattern (such as alternating high and low points), it is appropriate to ask questions about the special cause for these values.

2. *Is there a common cause?* If individual points are not outside the control limits, and runs, trends, or patterns are not occurring, you should ask questions about how the overall process can be improved. It is inappropriate and unhelpful to ask questions about why *specific* points are above or below the average. Asking such questions about individual points when the process appears to be stable leads to what is called management tampering.

The waiting time was considered by the team to be a key quality measure for service to scheduled patients. However, if internal measures are used, it is important to verify that they are consistent with the direct customer perceptions. Therefore the team also collected data on patient complaints about the admitting process.

The team collected and summarized the patient complaints for the same time period as the wait time data, as shown in Exhibit 13.4. Then a control chart of the patient complaint data was prepared, as illustrated in Figure 13.5.

From the data it was clear to the team that there was a major problem with excessive wait times for patients scheduled for admission. The average wait time of over two hours indicated a major quality gap. The patient complaint data confirmed that the patients were unhappy with the delays. The team prepared a written statement of the problem: average wait time of over 120 minutes in the admission lounge is unacceptable and must be reduced. The team set an initial target to cut the wait times in half, although they did not consider an hour wait time acceptable either. Continued improvement would be necessary.

At the conclusion of Step 2, Organize the Data, the team was invited to discuss its findings and proposed plan with the

**Exhibit 13.4. Number of Complaints About Admissions:
July 1990–July 1991.**

	Number of Complaints	
Month	1990	1991
January		59
February		75
March		37
April		35
May		26
June		3
July	33	52
August	41	
September	12	
October	26	
November	25	
December	51	

Average or mean (July 1990 to July 1991) = 36.5 minutes
Standard deviation (July 1990 to July 1991) = 19.5 minutes
  (19.47/sq. root 30 = 3.55)

Source: Admitting department
Time period: July 1990–July 1991
Date prepared: July 1991
Prepared by: EJG/RJC

Figure 13.5. Control Chart for Number of Patient Complaints: July 1990–July 1991.

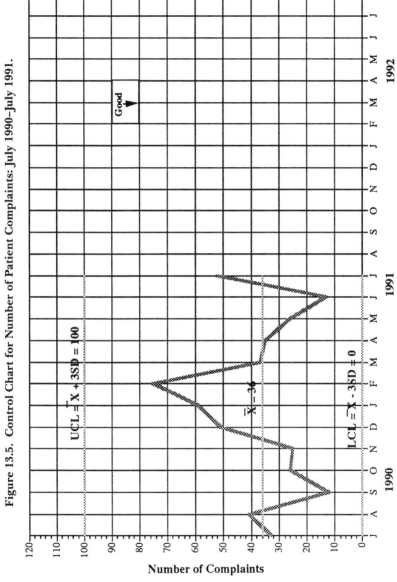

Source: Admitting department; *Time period:* July 1990–July 1991; *Date prepared:* July 1991; *Prepared by:* EJGRJC.

Corporate Lead Team. Some of the team members were very nervous because they had never made a presentation to the organization's administrative and clinical leaders before. The Corporate Lead Team gave the team several compliments and asked how they could provide support to the team. After presentation to the Corporate Lead Team, the team leader celebrated the team's progress by having a pizza party, which the team members thought would be fun.

Step 2 Questions

The following are questions that may be addressed by managers during the Organize the Data step:

1. What did your team select as the operational definitions of the quality measures? Remember, a measurement is meaningful only with an operational definition and a method of measurement. The definition of waiting time selected by the team was the amount of time, in minutes, from the completion of all processing and testing, when the patient is ready to go to his or her bed, until the patient leaves the admission lounge. Many different definitions are possible. One of the deciding factors is whether a practical method can be used to measure the waiting time. For example, one team member suggested starting from the time the patient arrived at the hospital until he or she was in bed, but there is no practical method of measuring this. The more places and people involved in collecting data, the more difficult it is to maintain control of the measurement process.

2. What are the indicators or measures related to the process: quality indicators? cost-effectiveness indicators? The quality indicators used by this team included waiting time of patients; complaints of patients, families, physicians, and staff; poor working environment; and error rate during the admission process.

3. Do the control charts of the measures indicate that the process is stable? Indications of an unstable process are special events outside the control limits, runs of five or more points in a row above or below the mean, trends of five or more points in a row increasing or decreasing, or repeated patterns. The team felt the waiting time and patient complaint processes were stable. It should be noted that stability is not inherently good or bad; it simply means that the underlying process remains unchanged. In this case the wait times were stable at an unacceptably high level.

4. What are the appropriate questions to ask if the control chart indicates that the process is stable or unstable? If unstable, what is the special cause of the observed data? If stable, what are the common causes of the process causing the observed data?

5. Are the potential problem/opportunity statements interdependent? If so, which ones cause the others?

6. How does the control chart for patient complaints (perceived poor quality) compare with your control chart of waiting times? At this stage the relationship was unclear to the team members, because the team was looking for relationships among small, random variations of the two processes. Later in Step 5, Measure the Change, the relationship will be clearer.

7. What additional relevant facts should be collected and considered?

8. What type of support does your team need?

Step 2 Lessons Learned

Some of the lessons learned by the team during Step 2, Organize the Data, were:

- Prioritize problems. There were many different problems, and it was important to select the one that would be addressed first. If this is not done, the team will go into a state analogous to "cardiac fibrillation," in which different team members repeatedly raise different problems and issues, and the team becomes ineffective.
- Compare internal and external quality measures. When possible it is useful to compare your internal quality measures, such as waiting time, with the customers' perceptions of your service. They may be different.

Step 3: Analyze Root Causes

The objective of Step 3 is to identify the underlying factors, or root causes, that contribute to the identified quality gap. The team spent two meetings generating a cause-effect diagram of the potential causes of long wait times. This tool is also called a fishbone or Ishikawa diagram. A cause-effect diagram is normally initiated with major types of reasons, such as people, methods, information, materials, and facilities, which were used by this team. The aim is to select major headings that will include all possible causes. The major headings should be as independent as possible to avoid confusion.

The team then brainstormed the potential factors that would cause long waiting times. These were written along the major bones or branches of the diagram. For each cause listed, the team asked "why," then wrote those reasons down as smaller bones or branches on the diagram. A rule of thumb is to ask "why" five times in a row. When you reach a point where there is no additional logical answer to the question "why," you have reached what is called a "root cause." The root causes should be circled for easy identification. Brainstorming should include each of the major headings or bones. During this process, the team may decide to add or delete bones or branches to fully identify causes of the stated problem, in this case long waiting time. The cause-effect diagram generated by the team, including the problem statement and major bones or branches, is illustrated in Figure 13.6.

Figure 13.6. Cause-Effect Diagram for Long Wait Times.

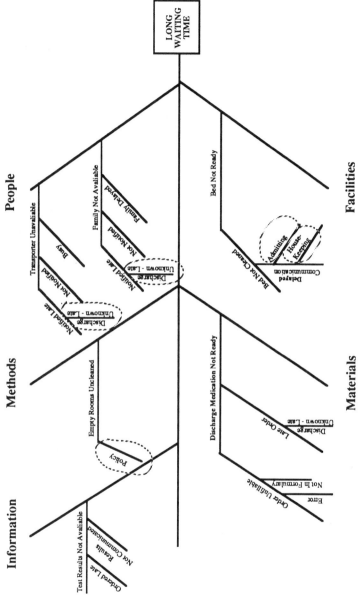

Source: Admitting department; *Time period:* July 1990–July 1991; *Date prepared:* July 1991; *Prepared by:* EJG/RJC.

An alternative graphic approach is to use a hierarchical outline of the causes leading to the effect. The fishbone diagram is very helpful for illustrating the concepts to the team, but can become very messy as many possible causes are added to the figure. Also, the fishbone diagram is more difficult to update and change. The sample outline format illustrated in Exhibit 13.5 is another useful way of illustrating the causes. Each successive indent answers the next subsequent question of "why."

Once different root causes were identified, the team again faced a priority question. Normally the best approach is to collect data on the frequency of the different root causes. It is not uncommon that the measured frequency of the different root causes is different from that suspected by the team members. A checksheet was created to collect data on the frequency

Exhibit 13.5. Sample Hierarchical Outline Format of Cause-Effect for Long Wait Times.

Effect: Excess waiting time for scheduled patients
Cause: The following are possible causes of the effect.
People
    Transporter unavailable
        Not notified
            Discharge unknown
        Notified late
            Discharge known late*
        Busy
            Other duties are higher priority
            Inadequate number of transporters
    Family not available
        Not notified
            Discharge unknown
        Notified late
            Discharge known late*
        Family delayed
    No staff to attend discharged patients before they leave
    Multiple supervisors in admitting slow communication
Methods
    Empty rooms left uncleaned
        Policy that afternoon and midnight shift housekeepers not clean
        rooms*

    * Indicates root cause.

of root causes of long wait times, as shown in Figure 13.7. The frequencies of each problem were summed and used to create a Pareto chart.

From the checksheet, a team member prepared a Pareto chart of the individual and cumulative frequencies of the root causes of long wait times, illustrated in Figure 13.8.

Step 3 Questions

Sample questions and issues that may be asked by the team or managers during the Analysis step are:

1. What defines a "root cause"? When you ask the question "why" repeatedly and you reach a point where there is no further reasonable answer to that question, you have reached what is called the root cause. The root cause is often significantly deeper than the apparent symptom of the problem.

2. What data should be collected relating to root causes? As illustrated above, it is helpful to collect data on the frequency and consequences of their occurrence. Above we addressed only the frequency of the root causes. The impact or

Figure 13.7. Checksheet of Frequency of Root Causes of Long Wait Times.

Root Cause	Count Of Occurrences	Total
Methods Room Cleaning Policy	ЩҐ ЩҐ ЩҐ ЩҐ ЩҐ ЩҐ lll	33
People and Materials Discharge Unknown	ЩҐ ЩҐ ЩҐ ЩҐ ЩҐ ЩҐ ЩҐ ЩҐ ЩҐ llll	49
Facilities Housekeeping Communication	ЩҐ ЩҐ ЩҐ ЩҐ ЩҐ ЩҐ ЩҐ ЩҐ ЩҐ ЩҐ ЩҐ ЩҐ ЩҐ ll	67
Admitting Communication	ЩҐ ЩҐ ЩҐ ll	17

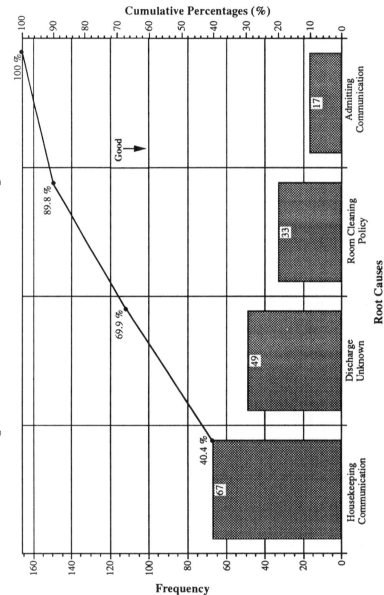

Figure 13.8. Pareto Chart of Root Causes of Long Wait Times.

Source: Admitting department; *Time period:* July 1990–July 1991; *Date prepared:* July 1991; *Prepared by:* EJGRJC.

consequences of the problems caused by each root cause should also be considered.

3. Which root cause(s) should be addressed first? The root cause that has the greatest negative consequences should be addressed first, unless there are reasons for doing otherwise. For example, long or very costly countermeasures may indicate that another root cause should be addressed first.

4. What type of support does your team need?

Step 3 Lessons Learned

The team learned a number of lessons during the Analyze Root Causes step. Some examples are:

- Do not jump to solutions. There is a tendency for teams to look at the major symptoms and immediately start working on solutions or countermeasures for them rather than continuing to ask the question "why." Options to address symptoms are usually obvious but are often expensive solutions. It is tedious and takes a lot of time to continue to ask the question "why."
- Consider consequences of root causes. The consequences of root causes should be considered in addition to just the frequency of their occurrence.

Step 4: Determine Options

The objective of Step 4 is to select and test proposed options or solutions that will reduce the quality gap associated with the root cause(s). After the team had ranked the root causes, its attention was turned to this objective.

Select Options to Remedy Root Causes

The team first developed a list of options or potential solutions that might remedy the verified root causes, meet customers' valid requirements, and be cost beneficial. The team did the following to develop the list of options:

— Reviewed the flowchart of admission and discharge processes in detail to identify potential improvements. Each step in the flowchart was reviewed to determine whether that step added value from the perspective of the customer(s).
— Brainstormed possible options.
— Did a survey of admission practices in similar organizations and used the best identified practices of similar processes as benchmarks to identify potential changes. Benchmarking is explained further in Chapter Fourteen.

A selected list of the options is illustrated in Table 13.2. The countermeasures included on the list were then used as a basis for an options matrix.

An options matrix is a form of a prioritization matrix that summarizes and scores options and methods of implementing changes, the effectiveness of the changes, and their feasibility. This was done to prioritize the options. An options matrix for some of the countermeasures the team selected is illustrated in Table 13.3.

Flowchart of Revised Procedures

Once the options for initial improvement were identified, the process flowcharts were revised to reflect the planned changes. The revised flowchart served as a basis for explaining process changes to implement the options and later served as a basis for standardization in Step 6, Apply to Workplace. The team would reconsider additional options during Step 7, Plan for the Future.

Table 13.2. List of Options to Reduce Wait Times.

Options or potential solutions were listed under the topic headings from the cause-effect diagram.

People
  Promote earlier discharge information: tentative discharge, actual discharge.
  Reorganize to consolidate management.
  Establish mechanism to assure earlier communication to families.
Methods
  Change room cleaning policy so afternoon and midnight shift housekeepers clean rooms vacated after 4:30 P.M.
Information
  Develop and implement a mechanism to notify ancillary departments that patient is being discharged, so they can expedite results reporting.
Materials
  Develop and implement a mechanism to notify pharmacy that patient is being discharged, so pharmacy can expedite discharge medications.
Facilities
  Initiate discharge suite for patients whose transportation is delayed.
  Reduce people in communication chain for cleaning room:
    Issue pagers to housekeepers.
    Train housekeepers to use computer system.
  Reduce communications delays in admitting:
    Change process to direct calls about clean rooms to bed assignor.
    Change priorities of people who receive telephone calls to expedite information on clean rooms.

Force Field Analysis

For the selected countermeasure(s), the team decided to identify the different forces that support and oppose implementation of the selected options. The team displayed these graphically as a matrix with the negative forces on one side and the positive forces on the other. This is known as a force field analysis; the resulting matrix is displayed in Table 13.4. (GOAL/QPC, 1988, pp. 72–73). This technique is also referred to as a barriers and aids analysis (Qualtec, 1989b, Unit 4, p. 18). The purpose of this analysis is to identify all the forces that support and oppose implementing the countermeasure, so the team can address

Table 13.3 Matrix of Options to Reduce Wait Times.

Description				Relative Score (eg, 1–5)				Action
Quality Gap	Root Cause	Option or Proposed Solution	Methods (How)	Financial Impact A	Effectiveness B	Feasibility C	Overall A*B*C	
Reduce admission wait time for scheduled patients	Delayed housekeeping communication about cleaning beds	Reduce numbers of communications	Assign pagers to housekeepers	4	5	5	100	Yes
Same as above	Same as above	Eliminate housekeeping supervisors from communication chain	Page housekeepers directly	3	5	4	60	Yes
Same as above	Policy to clean empty rooms only on day shift	Clean rooms whenever they become vacant	Reprioritize work on evening and night shifts	3	5	4	60	Yes
Same as above	Discharge unknown by patient family	Notify families of pending and actual discharge	Assign responsibility to notify family	3	4	4	48	Yes
Same as above	Same as above	Same as above	Assign responsibility to notify patient	3	3	4	36	Yes
The problem or opportunity selected for improvement.	Root causes from cause-effect diagram.	Countermeasures aimed at root causes. To extent possible within team's ability to implement.	Specific task(s) to implement. Addresses "how."	Relative net financial impact of costs and revenues.	Rating of effectiveness to reduce root cause.	Rating of time, cost, acceptance, and probability of success.	Product of effectiveness and feasibility.	Indicate Yes or No whether action will be taken.

Scale: 1–5; 1 = None, 2 = Somewhat, 3 = Moderate, 4 = High, 5 = Very High.

Table 13.4 Force Field Analysis Matrix.

Option or Proposed Solution	Negative Forces (Oppose Option Implementation)	Positive Forces (Support Option Implementation)
Reduce numbers of communications	Requires more pagers and pager volume	Housekeepers may prefer more autonomy
	Requires regular training of housekeepers	Admitting will support reduction of delays
		Administration will support reduced time and costs
Reduce housekeeping supervisors from communication chain	Housekeeping supervisors feel lack of control, and oppose change	Administration will support reduced time and costs
	Must use another method to monitor housekeeping quality	
Clean rooms whenever they become vacant	Additional workload on afternoon and evening shifts	Admitting and nursing will support earlier bed cleaning
	Requires housekeeping policy change	Operating rooms and post-anesthesia care unit will support reduced delays
Notify families earlier of pending and actual discharge	People who receive full responsibility for notifying families may feel overworked	Stress will decrease for all if families notified earlier
	Requires more coordination among UMMC staff	Admitting will support earlier discharges
		Patients and families will appreciate earlier notification

them in the action plan. These may involve facilities, people, dollars, external environment, and other factors.

Cost-Benefit Analysis

Before proceeding with the implementation plan, the team performed a rough cost-benefit analysis of implementing the proposed option. The purpose of this analysis was to consider the full financial impact of the recommended actions. Financial services, management engineering, and other analytical staff can provide valuable assistance for this type of analysis, if it is needed by the team. Most team members felt uncomfortable doing the complete cost-benefit analysis, so they obtained some help from financial services. The team members identified the various costs and benefits associated with the implementation, then worked with financial analysis to estimate the net impact of those costs and benefits. Sample categories of costs and benefits considered were:

- One-time operational costs and benefits of implementation.
- Annual operating costs and benefits.
- Capital costs and benefits related to implementation. It is common to consider the depreciation as annual costs or to figure a return on the capital investment.
- Financial costs and benefits to other departments or processes. For example, improving service to outpatient clinic patients may generate more clinic visits, which in turn may generate more outpatient pharmacy revenue.

In today's environment of prospective payment systems, it may be necessary to work with financial services to determine the net financial impact of implemented changes.

Action Plan

The team then prepared a detailed action plan to test the proposed options. Some sample topics included in their action plan were:

- Actions to implement change(s) and people responsible for those actions
- Implementation procedures
- Time schedule for testing the options or proposed solutions
- Measures and methods of measurement to be used to evaluate the proposed options
- Study period for the pilot test of the options
- Data analysis methods
- Education and training required
- Resource requirements, including people, facilities, equipment, dollars, and any other internal and external resources required for successful testing of the options
- Approvals required, internally and externally
- External coordination and support required

The completed action plan was then reviewed with all the people involved with the pilot test of the options.

Reviewing the Action Plan

Before proceeding with implementation, the team presented its findings, conclusions, and action plan to the affected line managers and the Corporate Lead Team for their approval and support. Before this presentation, some of the team members were concerned that the line managers or Corporate Lead Team would not support their proposed quality improvement options and plan. If the teams are not supported, the members will view their effort as wasted and management as not listening to what they believe to be a good plan, which breaks down trust. The purpose of the presentation to the Corporate Lead Team should be to enable it to understand the potential implications and to determine how to support the implementation, not to decide whether to support the pilot study.

Implementing the Countermeasures

After presentation to the Corporate Lead Team, the admission team implemented each of the options in the options matrix, following the proposed action plan. One person was assigned overall responsibility to coordinate the pilot test of the options and the data collection. However, many people were involved in the actual implementation.

Step 4 Questions

Sample questions that may be answered by the team and managers during the Determine Options step are:

1. What additional factors, if any, should be included in the options matrix? In addition to the practical methods, effectiveness, and feasibility, the team might also look at factors like the impact or consequences of the change and the availability of resources to implement the changes.

2. Is it possible that the best long-term solution would be to scrap the entire current process and implement an entirely new one? If so, how can you determine when to do this? The question of the best long-term solution is an important one. Although the quality improvement process we are using can improve virtually any situation, the improvement may not be worth the effort. For example, if your organization has an old payroll system custom written for your organization twenty years ago, and patched several times since, it may be best to select or develop an entirely new payroll system than to make small improvements to the current one. This decision involves evolutionary versus revolutionary change. The best approach is to make sure the current process addresses the vision, goals, and requirements of your customers and your organization.

3. What types of changes were made to the process flowchart? Sample changes could include elimination of steps that do not add value and reducing the amount of activity on rework loops.

4. What types of financial and nonfinancial costs and benefits were identified as relating to the selected countermeasures?

Step 4 Lessons Learned

The team learned a number of lessons related to the Determine Options step. Some examples are:

- Low-cost countermeasures. Although there was a fear that the team would recommend very costly options, this did not occur. The team tried less costly options first, then considered more expensive options later.
- Option cost of addressing symptoms versus root causes. Options or proposed solutions to remedy root causes are almost always less costly than options that address the symptoms directly. Using this admitting case study as an example, it is less costly to improve communications to speed room cleaning than to employ patient relations staff to address patient complaints, take flowers to patients, and other activities addressing the symptom of unhappy patients. Another way of stating this is to work on problems "upstream," or earlier in the process.

Step 5: Measure the Change

The objective of Step 5 is to measure results and the success of the proposed option(s) and determine whether to standardize the process. Alternatively, the measurement may show no or minimal improvement, in which case the team will want to look at other countermeasures. The key is that results must be measured. In order to judge whether there has been any improvement, the same measures should be available for the period before the countermeasures were implemented.

The team measured several aspects of the revised admission/discharge process during testing of the options, including times required for different activities. However, the two major measures were the average waiting time and the patient complaints, for which the team had data before the options were implemented.

Results of Improvements

The team collected data on two key measures: the waiting time in the admission lounge and the patient complaints related to the admission process. They collected data on other relevant measures related to the admission/discharge process, such as quality of products and services, external and internal customer satisfaction, cost effectiveness, working environment, and comparative position with other healthcare organizations, but they are not summarized here. In order to illustrate the long-term impact, the results summarized here cover not only the pilot test period but more than a year after the process changes were standardized.

Exhibit 13.6 illustrates admission lounge wait times from July 1990 through August 1992. The complete graph of admission lounge wait times from July 1990 through August 1992 is illustrated in Figure 13.9. One question the team faced was when to recalculate the control limits for the control chart. Control limits are meaningful only when a process is stable. A process is judged stable when there is no evidence of single point outliers, upward or downward trends, runs above or below the mean, or patterns of data. Therefore, the control limits have little meaning during a period of instability, such as the rapid reduction of wait times shown in Figure 13.9. Control limits cannot be meaningfully recalculated until the process stabilizes at a new level. Therefore, the team was monitoring rapid improvement without any control limits during the transition period.

The team also measured the patient complaints for the same time period. Exhibit 13.7 illustrates sample patient complaints from July 1990 through August 1992. The complete graph of patient complaints from July 1990 through August 1992 is illustrated in Figure 13.10.

It was clear from the results during the test period, and subsequently, that the proposed solutions were effective at reducing both the wait times and the patient complaints. From this the team concluded that their internal measure of waiting time, which was measured for every patient, is a good measure of

Exhibit 13.6. Admission Lounge Wait Times: July 1990–August 1992.

Month	Average Lounge Wait Time (minutes)		
	1990	*1991*	*1992*
January		133	27
February		123	11
March		112	20
April		116	17
May		130	18
June		125	12
July	138	130	16
August	174	62	12
September	104	38	
October	117	22	
November	109	22	
December	122	30	

Average or mean: July 1990 to July 1991 = 125.6 minutes
August 1991 to August 1992 = 23.6 minutes
Standard deviation: July 1990 to July 1991 = 17.6 minutes
(17.57/sq. root 30 = 3.2)
August 1991 to August 1992 = 13.9 minutes

Source: Admitting department
Time period: July 1990–August 1992
Date prepared: August 1992
Prepared by: EJG/RJC

quality as perceived by the patients. The team members were very enthusiastic because the options they proposed were reducing wait times. Several previous efforts to reduce wait times had been unsuccessful.

Step 5 Questions

The team and managers may want to ask questions like the following related to the Measure the Change step:

1. What other measured changes should be considered?
2. Should the tested options be standardized?

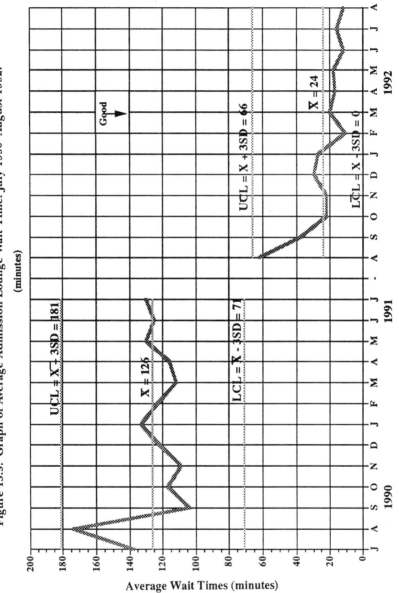

Figure 13.9. Graph of Average Admission Lounge Wait Time: July 1990–August 1992.

(minutes)

Average Wait Times (minutes)

UCL = X̄ - 3SD = 181

X̄ = 126

LCL = X̄ - 3SD = 71

Good →

UCL = X̄ + 3SD = 66

X̄ = 24

LCL = X̄ - 3SD = 0

1990   1991   1992

Source: Admitting department; *Time period:* July 1990–August 1992; *Date prepared:* August 1992; *Prepared by:* EJG/RJC.

Exhibit 13.7. **Number of Complaints About Admissions:**
July 1990–August 1992.

	Number of Complaints		
Month	1990	1991	1992
January		59	2
February		75	0
March		37	4
April		35	0
May		26	1
June		13	0
July	33	52	2
August	41	4	0
September	12	1	
October	26	2	
November	25	0	
December	51	3	

Average or mean: July 1990 to July 1991 = 37.3 complaints
                      August 1991 to August 1992 = 1.5 complaints
Standard deviation: July 1990 to July 1991 = 18.2 complaints
                      (18.2/sq. root 30 = 3.3)
                      August 1991 to August 1992 = 1.5 complaints

Source: Admitting department
Time period: July 1990–August 1992
Date prepared: August 1992
Prepared by: EJG/RJC

Step 5 Lessons Learned

The team learned a number of lessons related to this step, such
as:

- Use the same measures. To the extent possible, it is important to use the same measures of quality before and after the
  countermeasures are implemented. This may not be possible for all of the measures, if major systems changes are
  made.
- Improve multiple measures simultaneously. The team found
  that implementing the options simultaneously improved

Figure 13.10. Graph for Number of Patient Complaints: July 1990–August 1992.

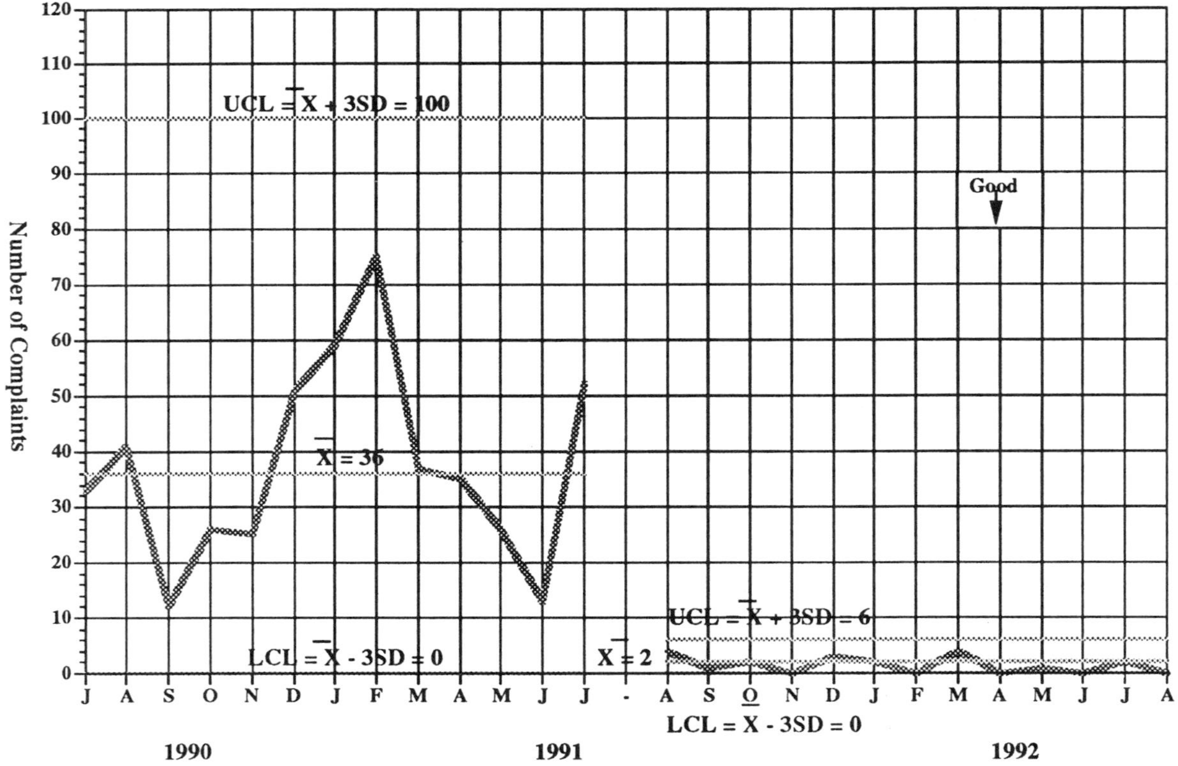

Source: Admitting department; *Time period:* July 1990–August 1992; *Date prepared:* August 1992; *Prepared by:* EJG|RJC.

measures of quality, customer satisfaction, cost effectiveness, and working environment.

- Results speak loudly. As the changes began to cause reduced wait times, there was a gradual recognition by physicians and staff that the improvements were working. Physicians and admitting department staff were receiving fewer complaints from patients, their families, and other staff. As a consequence, the working environment improved and there was improved trust among staff.

Step 6: Apply to Workplace

The objective of Step 6 is to standardize and maintain successful aspects of piloted quality improvements to prevent the recurrence of root causes.

With enthusiasm running high, the team members and other people working in the admission/discharge process were tempted to move on to something else without standardizing the changes to maintain the gain. The team then did the following:

- Identified and selected "successful" aspects of the options that had been pilot tested. Some minor aspects of the options did not work well, and those were discarded.
- Developed and tested the standard process and procedures. The flowcharts were revised, and the required written policies and procedures were prepared.
- Evaluated the quality indicators to determine which one would be used routinely. It was decided that the wait time data would be the key indicator and that the other service time indicators would not be routinely collected.
- Investigated whether the wait time data collection could be automated. Given the information processing priorities, this had to be delayed.
- Developed a full-scale implementation plan. Given that there were few changes, this plan was very similar to the action plan for the pilot test.
- Secured approval to implement the standardized options.

This was done when the team presented to the Corporate Lead Team after Steps 6 and 7.
- Managed implementation of the standardized process. This involved training, new forms, and a new monitoring process. The changes were widely communicated.

Step 6 Lessons Learned

The team learned a number of lessons in the Apply to Workplace step, including:

- Different perceptions. Different people have differing perceptions of the success of the options.
- Standardization requires substantial effort. There is a substantial amount of work required to standardize the process. It is common for the team to celebrate the successful results but not invest the additional effort needed to assure that the countermeasures have been standardized.

Step 7: Plan for the Future

The objective of Step 7 is to generalize improvements to other areas, investigate additional improvements, communicate findings, and celebrate achievements. Step 7 involves four distinctly different types of activities.

Generalize to Other Areas

After developing the plan to standardize the tested options, the team worked to identify improvements that could be generalized to other areas. First the team identified potential departments, groups, or processes that might potentially benefit from the tested options. Then a summary of the options and results were communicated specifically to those groups and more generally to others. It was somewhat frustrating to the team that they could only identify the opportunities in other areas, since they could not implement changes in them. However, during their final presentation to the Corporate Lead Team, they highlighted potential benefits to other areas. As an example, the team considered who else could benefit from the method of issuing pagers to housekeeping staff to reduce the number of people involved in the communication chain. The team identified that maintenance staff could also benefit from this approach, reducing the need for nurses to call the maintenance office and leave a message for the maintenance staff.

Investigate Additional Improvements

At this stage the team went back through the Quality Roadmap they had followed and reviewed each of the tables and figures they had generated. The options matrix was reviewed to determine whether another option should not be tested. Upstream, the cause-effect diagram was reviewed for other root causes. And further upstream, the prioritization matrix of problems was reviewed. This review is conducted using the same tools and techniques, and most of the analyses have already been performed. The team now looked for what to work on next. The team decided to work on the admission scheduling system next. The QI process then began again. The team membership was reviewed, and three members were changed. A systems analyst from information processing and a scheduling clerk from the operating room were added to the team.

Present Findings and Recommendations

The team was invited to present the complete Quality Roadmap to the Corporate Lead Team. In addition, line managers from affected departments were invited.

Celebrate Achievements

Celebration after Steps 6 and 7 was more formalized for the team. However, the team leader, facilitator, and members all agreed that small celebrations at the conclusion of each step of the QI process had been important. The process had taken a long time, and the positive reinforcement was necessary to maintain their enthusiasm.

Concerning celebration, it is important that the team members decide what they would like for a celebration. Different people have far different interests. In the end, however, we found that the greatest enthusiasm and recognition came from implementing the changes recommended by the team.

Conclusion

This case study about the admission/discharge process demonstrates the approach to a QI project and the use of many QI tools and techniques. It also highlights some of the human dimension issues the team faced.

The following are several overall lessons from this case study:

- The QI process takes time. Completion of the total process may take from four to twelve months. Teams that tackle large, ill-defined projects may take even longer.
- Enthusiasm may fade. Given the large amount of time and effort involved before options are tested, it is common for team members to lose enthusiasm.
- Stay in process. It is important to continue to follow the seven-step QI process and use the applicable tools and techniques. Given the many issues and opportunities that face most teams, it is easy to lose focus and take even longer to get through the process.
- The QI process is useful in daily work. Given the knowledge and practical applications described in the last two chapters, we hope you see the usefulness of the QI tools and techniques in your daily jobs, in addition to their usefulness for quality improvement teams. TQM is not restricted to team efforts; it includes quality planning and use of quality improvement methods in daily operations.
- Endless opportunities exist for improvement. You can continually improve any of the many processes in which you work.

Chapter Fourteen

Advanced Applications of TQM

This chapter addresses some of the more advanced applications of TQM and some alternatives for applying these useful approaches. These strategies include full implementation of TQM looking outside your organization for expectations, targets, and improvements; integrating many different quality improvement efforts; and coordinating expectations and deployment. To gain from the opportunities of advanced TQM methods, your organization must look outside itself to expectations and capabilities of external customers and suppliers, and learn from other organizations with exemplary processes and results. In Chapter Two we described TQM as the integration of a customer-focused, continual improvement philosophy, analytical thinking and skills, people orientation and skills, and a structure and organization (see Figure 2.1 in Chapter Two).

The concepts discussed in this chapter are at the leading edge of TQM implementation among all industries in the world. Consequently there are few implemented examples of these methods within the healthcare industry. However, we will present some examples and specific actions to expand your TQM thinking. We have neither the space nor expertise to address all of these advanced applications in detail in this book. References are provided as sources for additional, more detailed descriptions of the methods presented.

Cooperation Versus Competition

TQM requires cooperation among your suppliers, your organization, your customers, and even your competitors. Cooperation within your organization is necessary for a successful TQM process. There are many potential opportunities for improvement, if your organization is willing to cooperate and share information and practices with others.

Before undertaking relationships with other organizations through partnerships, benchmarking, or other efforts, your organization should address its philosophy concerning cooperation versus competition. In today's times of constrained resources and decreasing use of acute inpatient facilities, there is strong competition among healthcare organizations. Inpatient occupancy rates are falling, causing economic hardships, downsizing, and even hospital closures. While many believe that a competitive approach is good, it can be shown that competition on every aspect of your business reduces communication, slows learning, and leads to wasteful duplication and underutilization of resources. Cooperation, on the other hand, can increase learning and enhance your organizational performance. To collaborate effectively, you should decide what things you are willing to share with whom.

For meaningful participation in networks and other partnerships, and for benchmarking and other efforts, your organization must be willing to communicate and share. No organization is willing to continue participating in a network or other relationship if it does not gain from it. Some examples of a cooperative approach are:

- Networks. These are arrangements in which participants share methods, QIT successes and failures, leadership challenges, cultural barriers and aids, and ideas for improvement. Typically, member organizations pay a fee to join, and each organization bears its own expenses and takes turns at hosting meetings.
- Benchmarking. Participants develop a partnership and share detailed information about their results and the pro-

cesses and methods that created them. Both the strengths and weaknesses are shared openly.

- Just-in-time integrated systems developed with supplier and customer participation. Participants must share detailed information and plans for new products and processes, which requires a high level of trust. There are shared risks and opportunities among the parties.

Factors to consider that may affect the selection of organizations with whom you will cooperate are:

- Financial Position. The stronger your financial position, the easier it is to focus on the best long-term solutions.
- Scope of Services and Uniqueness. The greater the scope and uniqueness of services, the more difficult it is for other organizations to duplicate those services.
- Relative Prices. Those organizations with a distinct price or cost advantage may want to guard how that is accomplished from competing organizations.
- Service Area. The geographic area served by your current and planned services will define the region in which other healthcare organizations could draw patients that could potentially come to yours. For highly specialized services, the service areas can be very broad. There is regional and even some national competition now to provide specialized services like coronary artery bypass surgery. Some organizations are comfortable sharing only with organizations outside their service area.
- Other Healthcare Providers. The number of healthcare providers within your service area and the services offered by them may affect cooperative efforts.
- Degree and Type of Innovation. The more innovative your organization, the less concerned you should be about sharing information with others. Even if another organization copies a process, by the time the changes are implemented, you will have developed something better. The type of innovation may also affect your decisions. An organization may innovate to develop new services and products or to mini-

mize costs of well-established ones (Marszalek-Gaucher and Coffey, 1990, pp. 38–39).

- Degree of Mutual Interests. Organizations that benefit simultaneously clearly benefit most by cooperation.
- Trust. Cooperative efforts require trust, and your willingness to enter cooperative efforts will be based on your trust of the organizations involved.

Action Step: Discuss in detail the degree of external cooperation your leadership will support, including the types of processes, information, strengths, and weaknesses you are willing to share with whom.

Partnerships to Improve Quality

One of the first steps to extend TQM beyond quality improvement teams and other QI efforts within your organization is to participate in partnerships to improve quality. A partnership can take many forms. Some of the more common forms include involving suppliers and customers in your quality improvement efforts, developing networks of organizations working on Total Quality, developing just-in-time (JIT) integrated systems with suppliers and customers, and formal joint ventures.

Developing Partnerships with Suppliers and Customers

A ready source of quality improvement ideas is available from suppliers and customers. Cross-functional QITs involve internal suppliers and customers of the processes being improved. However, you should also consider external suppliers and customers to improve your processes. Healthcare organizations have conducted patient and physician opinion surveys for many years. But these represent relatively inactive participation and often focus on perceptions of what happened rather than opinions about desired services or what could happen. These external suppliers and customers can contribute much more through participation in focus groups and serving on QITs. When customers and suppliers are involved, loyalty is enhanced. Baxter International, for example, has representatives serve on materials management Quality Improvement Teams at the University of Massachusetts Medical Center, Worcester, Massachusetts, and many other healthcare organizations to improve the quality and cost effectiveness of service.

Networks

An effective approach to accelerate your learning and develop partnerships is to join or form networks focusing on quality improvement. There are many regional and national networks to choose from. Several of the healthcare systems are developing Total Quality resources and networks. Some examples of networks and organizations are listed in Exhibit 14.1. Certainly the networks of healthcare organizations will provide the most directly applicable experience. However, you should look at networks of other types of organizations as well. Our experience indicates that the more you learn about TQM, the more you realize that you can learn from organizations in any industry. In fact, some of the best benchmarking candidates are from non-healthcare industries. When considering advanced TQM methods, non-healthcare organizations have more experience to share.

Action Step: Join a network of organizations implementing TQM. Joining a regional network provides substantial benefits at low cost.

Winners of Quality Awards

Former Malcolm Baldrige and Healthcare Forum/Witt quality award winners are excellent organizations to get information from and to benchmark with. Many of these organizations sponsor one-day seminars each month to share award-winning strategies.

JIT Integrated Systems with Suppliers and Customers

An extension of involving suppliers and customers on QITs is to develop just-in-time integrated systems with suppliers and cus-

Exhibit 14.1. Selected List of Total Quality Networks and Organizations.

Network/Organization	Description
American Productivity & Quality Center 123 N. Post Oak Lane Houston, TX 77024-7797 713-681-4020	Network of 50 + organizations working on benchmarking and other TQM topics.
American Society for Quality Control 611 E. Wisconsin Avenue P.O. Box 3005, Milwaukee, WI 53201-3005 414-272-8575	Professional organization
Association for Quality and Participation 801-B West 8th Street Cincinnati, OH 45203 513-381-1959	Professional organization
GOAL/QPC Healthcare Application Research Committee GOAL/QPC 13 Branch Street, Methuen, MA 01844 508-685-3900	Committee of healthcare and consulting organizations working to develop advanced TQM applications
Hospital Corporation of America One Park Plaza, Nashville, TN 37202-0550 615-320-2759	Network of HCA and other hospitals
Humana CQI Network Humana Building 500 W. Main St., Louisville, KY 40202 502-580-1000	Network of Humana hospitals and other organizations
Industrial Management Council 930 East Avenue, The Hutchinson House Rochester, NY 14607-2296 716-244-8834	Network of industrial and healthcare organizations

Institute for Healthcare Improvement and
   Quality Management Network (formerly
   National Demonstration Project on Quality
   Improvement in Health Care)
P.O. Box 550, Brookline, MA 02146
617-730-4770
	Network of healthcare and other organizations to improve quality

Intermountain Health Care 36 South State, #2200 Salt Lake City, UT 84111 801-533-3730	Network of Intermountain Health Care hospitals and selected non-IHC organizations
Maryland Hospital Association 1301 York Road, Suite 800 Lutherville, MD 21093-6087 410-321-6200	Sample hospital association

Exhibit 14.1. Selected List of Total Quality Networks and Organizations, Cont'd.

Network/Organization	Description
Midwest Business Group in Health 8303 W. Higgins Road, Suite 200 Chicago, IL 60631 312-380-9090	Sample business coalition
National Association for Healthcare Quality (formerly National Association of Quality Assurance Professionals, Inc., NAQAP) 5700 Old Orchard Road, 1st fl. Skokie, IL 60077 708-966-9392	Professional association that promotes quality through conferences, certification, etc.
National Institute of Standards and Technology Administration Building, Room A537 Route 270 & Quince Orchard Road Gaithersburg, MD 20899	Agency of the Commerce Department's Technology Administration
Philadelphia Area Council for Excellence (PACE) 1234 Market Street, Suite 1800 Philadelphia, PA 19107-3718 215-972-3977	Network for TQM exchange, education, and communication
Quality & Productivity Management Association 550 Frontage Road, Suite 395 Northfield, IL 60093 708-501-2650	Provides regional meetings and networking
Quality Improvement Network I, II, & III (QIN) The Healthcare Forum 830 Market Street, San Francisco, CA 94102 415-421-8810	Three networks of healthcare organizations focusing on quality improvement
Quorum Networks P.O. Box 24347, Nashville, TN 37202 615-340-5836	Network of Quorum and other healthcare organizations
Southern California Health Care Coalition Contact: Total Quality Management Naval Hospital, San Diego, CA 92134 619-532-8219	Network of military and community hospitals in southern California to share education on quality
SunHealth Alliance SunHealth Corporation 4501 Charlotte Park Drive Charlotte, NC 28217 704-529-3300	Network of SunHealth healthcare organizations

Exhibit 14.1. Selected List of Total Quality Networks
and Organizations, Cont'd.

Network/Organization	Description
University of Wisconsin Center for Health Systems Computer Network 1300 University Avenue, Madison, WI 53706 608-262-3768	Maintains computerized data base of shared quality improvement projects
U.S. Quality Council I & II Conference Board Contact: R. M. Parent & Associates 109 Driscoll Way, Gaithersburg, MD 20878 301-926-4147	Network of twenty-one organizations, each dedicated to sharing quality learning

tomers. An extension of Deming's fourth point, "end the practice of awarding business on the basis of price tag alone" (Deming, 1986, p. 31), is to develop long-term relationships with a single supplier of a product or service. These partnerships can lead to improved quality and cost effectiveness for both parties. The principle is to develop relationships with suppliers so that required products, services, and information arrive just in time for use to reduce costs associated with the inspection, storage, handling, and expense of inventory waiting for use.

As an example of this technique, the University of Michigan Hospitals (UMH) developed a preferred vendor relationship with UARCO to produce forms. That relationship provides on-site UARCO representatives to help managers with forms design and ordering. It also allowed UMH to substantially reduce inventories of forms, reduce storage space, close a print shop, and save $280,000 per year. The same has been done with sutures and other operating room supplies. A number of suppliers to healthcare organizations have developed Total Quality processes and may be able to integrate with your TQM process. Examples we have knowledge of include Abbott, Baxter International, Johnson & Johnson, and 3M Corporation.

Action Step: Contact your suppliers and ask whether they have experience with TQM and are willing to work together to help improve quality and cost effectiveness.

Benchmarking

Benchmarking is the process of measuring a characteristic of your organization against the same characteristic of another organization known for its quality. David T. Kerns, chief executive officer, Xerox Corporation, states that "benchmarking is the continuous process of measuring products, services, and practices against the toughest competitors or those companies recognized as industry leaders" (Camp, 1989, p. 10)

The purpose of benchmarking is to improve processes and outcomes. Benchmarking helps you see the need to change, determine the priorities for change, and develop a model for change. It helps an organization become more externally focused. Benchmarking can also stimulate innovation and creativity as people see effective ideas in other organizations.

Why participate in benchmarking? There are two parts to this question: why benchmark with others, and why become a benchmark? If you identify an organization doing something substantially better than yours, your reason to participate is to learn and improve your processes and results. But why participate as the organizational benchmark? First, the detailed external review and critique of your processes will stimulate improvements of your already excellent processes. Another point is that no organization is best at everything. Your organization can certainly learn something from the organization wishing to benchmark some of your processes.

Many healthcare organizations have traditionally contacted similar organizations to gather information about what they are doing. This is a simple type of competitive benchmarking. As used here, however, benchmarking is more detailed and resource intensive than a telephone survey or questionnaire sent to a group of organizations. The best results are achieved when an organization acts as a partner and explores processes in depth, learning and improving over time.

Robert Camp defines four types of benchmarking (1989, pp. 61–65):

- Internal benchmarking to replicate best practices within your organization.
- Competitive benchmarking to identify and benchmark the best practices among competitors.
- Functional benchmarking to identify and benchmark comparable functions, even if in other industries.
- Generic process benchmarking to identify most important business practices to achieve greatest gains. With limited resources, look at where other companies are directing their activities. Xerox, for example, has identified sixty-seven basic business practices to be improved and is directing most of their improvement efforts toward those business practices.

Concepts of Benchmarking

Before discussing a process for benchmarking, some of its key concepts will be briefly described.

- Understand your own organization and its processes before benchmarking to others.
- Search widely for benchmark processes and organizations. Look beyond your geographic area, your competitors, and the healthcare industry. However, do not overlook small organizations; they are often very skilled in specific processes. For example, studying the way processes are accomplished in a small, high-volume physician's office may provide substantial insight into work redesign and simplification processes. Also, it is helpful initially to benchmark similar processes within your organization.
- Expand thinking of managers — get out of the mind-set that the way we do something is "the only way" to do it.
- Benchmarking involves two types of comparisons:
  - Comparison of outcomes or results. Which organizations have the best outcome, and what are those outcomes? For example, which healthcare organizations have the lowest cost per outpatient visit, by type of visit, and what are those costs?

—"How" is that performance achieved? What are the detailed processes that accomplish the results? This information is far more important than benchmarking to outcomes alone.

- Benchmarking is like reverse engineering. You must dissect the processes you are benchmarking to understand them sufficiently to apply what you have learned. It is inadequate to benchmark on outcomes or general processes only.
- Benchmarking is a two-way partnership. You must be willing to share detailed information about your processes and results—you must have approval and information to share.
- Benchmarking is an evolving process, not a one-time process or cookbook recipe.
- Establish long-term benchmarking relationships, sometimes called strategic benchmarking.
- Benchmarking is to learn, not just copy. If you just copy a process from somewhere else it may not be totally appropriate in your organization. Your organization can make substantial improvements by just achieving the best-in-class performance of the processes you benchmark. However, by the time you have implemented the copy, there will be a new "best-in-class." The objective is to learn, and to adapt and improve the best practices found elsewhere, if possible.
- Employee involvement is key for benchmarking, as for other aspects of TQM. Employees who do the work know those processes best.

Process for Benchmarking

We have listed below some of the key steps in a benchmarking process. As you can see, there is a lot of work to be done before conducting a benchmark visit. There is a tendency for people to want to make a "field trip" to an excellent organization. If acceptable to that organization to begin the relationship, such a trip is a good place to start. But the trip will fail to provide good benchmarking information because you have not done sufficient homework to know the correct questions or to share any information with your benchmark partner. Based on successful industrial experience, and limited experience in the healthcare industry, a successful benchmarking process should include the following steps.

Secure leadership commitment. Leadership commitment to benchmarking is the first step, as with any other portion of TQM or other corporate undertaking. Leadership should define how it sees benchmarking contributing to the organization's goals. As with other aspects of TQM, benchmarking needs one or more champions.

Identify what will be benchmarked. Identify what will be benchmarked, the information required, and who in your organization will use the information. This selection should be tied to your strategic or hoshin planning process for prioritization, since no organization has the resources, capabilities, or time to excel at everything. Sample criteria to select what will be benchmarked are importance to key customers; critical processes or critical success factors to meet customer requirements; consistency with values, mission, and goals; areas of known problems, weaknesses, or inferior performance; information that could influence key plans or actions; and ease of study and change. What is most important to improve? A process must be sufficiently specific to be successfully benchmarked. Benchmarking on too broad a topic will be very difficult to focus and time-consuming. Sample sources for locating best-in-class are professional associations, trade organizations, government agencies, Total Quality publications, consultants, and network participants.

Form and train a team. Form a team familiar with the process to be benchmarked. The characteristics of a benchmarking team are similar to those of a Quality Improvement Team: five to six members, including people who are most familiar with the process; team leader trained and as experienced as possible with benchmarking; positive, "can-do" attitude; attentive to detail; good listeners; and ability to implement or influence change. For a team to be successful, it must have sufficient time, support, and resources to complete the benchmarking assignment. You may want to use an external consultant or a potential benchmarking partner to work with the first teams on the best approach. Train the team members in a process to do internal evaluation, to search for the best-in-class organization to benchmark, and to do the benchmarking process. The team should then write a statement of purpose relating to the customers, scope of the study, and planned outputs.

Identify measures. Identify the measures of results and processes to be used. These will be refined as the team does its literature research, studies processes internally, and studies the benchmark organizations.

Document current process and results. Document the processes in your organization in detail: goals, priorities, processes, operational definitions, customers, customer requirements or expectations, quality and other performance indicators, and trends of results measured for each of your major organizational goals, such as customer satisfaction, issues, strengths, and weaknesses.

Benchmark internally. Benchmark to similar processes within your organization first, which Robert Camp calls *internal benchmarking*. There is often large variation among similar processes within an organization. Starting within your own organization improves communication, provides more questions for the benchmark team, leads to quick improvements, and reduces variation within your organization.

Identify organizations to be benchmarked. Do research to identify potential organization(s) to be benchmarked. Sample criteria in selecting benchmark partners are best-in-class performance on processes key to your organization, degree of competition with your organization, availability of information, and of course willingness to participate. The research should include information about processes, past performance, planned changes, and projections. Sample sources include the library, professional associations, healthcare and other industry publications, academic journals, seminars or conferences, materials about potential benchmark organizations, and industrial experts. The American Productivity & Quality Center, in Houston, Texas, for example, has established an international benchmarking clearinghouse.

The team should look for best practices in any industry

with processes similar to yours. For example, virtually all industries have billing services, so it may be beneficial to look outside the healthcare field. "While some companies have had good experiences benchmarking within their own industry, it is usually in staff, not line, functions" (Biesada, 1991, p. 30). Even if some topics will not be shared, there may be substantial benefit to benchmarking with leading healthcare organizations.

Top leadership, such as the chief executive officer or chief operating officer, should contact organizations with which you would like to benchmark. Later, the detailed study can be conducted by people most familiar with the processes being benchmarked, but the executives should still participate. Leaders and team members should also attend, invite others to your organization, and visit award-winning quality organizations.

Research benchmark organizations. Before making a benchmark visit, the benchmark team should conduct research on the organization, its processes, its customers, and its results. This will help identify which organizations to visit and which characteristics to study within those organizations.

Perform external benchmarking. Benchmark to one or more external organizations, including phone conversations to discuss process and data elements, personal meetings and interviews, and surveys. The objective is to understand in detail the results and characteristics of the processes that produce those results.

As soon as possible after the benchmark visit, possibly beginning on the way home, debrief everyone on the team about what they observed. Sometimes seemingly minor observations are keys to understanding a successful process.

Analyze gaps. Focusing on the key processes benchmarked, your team should compare your baseline process with the process benchmarked. It is more important to compare "how" the results were obtained than to compare the results only. A detailed list of characteristics should be developed, comparing your organization's performance with that of the benchmark organization's for each characteristic. Given the historical changes in measures, the team should also project the gap for future years. An example of a benchmark gap analysis is illustrated in Figure 14.1 (Camp, 1989, p. 151). Your team is likely to find some characteristics of the process for which your organization is considered better. Remember, the objective is to learn how to improve, not to copy. The findings should be summarized and discussed with leadership. The team may have to overcome substantial denial. "Denial is not an unusual reaction for a company stunned by the gap between its operational performance and that of a best-practice company. In fact, it is the typical first step in the rehabilitation process" (Biesada, 1991, p. 29).

Develop action plan. Based on the analysis of gaps and on the strategic plan for your organization, the team should develop an action plan for change, including objectives, priorities, actions, responsibilities, schedule, and expected results.

Implement action plan. Those people with authority and responsibility should implement the changes and monitor the progress of process changes and results. The benchmarking team may serve some ongoing role as part of the implementation process.

Repeat benchmarking process. The benchmarking process should be refined and repeated periodically, so that both benchmark partners will continue to learn.

Figure 14.1. Sample Benchmark Gap.

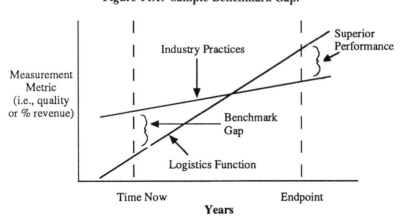

Source: Reprinted from *Benchmarking* by Robert Camp, copyright 1989, with permission of the publishers Quality Resources, White Plains, New York, and ASQC Quality Press, Milwaukee, Wisconsin.

Reasons for Failure or Poor Results from Benchmarking

Given the complexity of the benchmarking process, the relationships with external organizations, and the difficulty of making major organizational changes, there are many opportunities for failure. Some of the most common reasons for failure or poor results from benchmarking are the following.

- Leadership's not considering benchmarking important to achieve the organization's goals, or not supporting the benchmarking team or the required changes.
- Unwillingness of all benchmarking partners to share detailed information.
- Focus on outcome or result measures rather than the process characteristics that produced those results.
- Too broad a benchmarking topic used, for example, ambulatory care rather than the registration process for ambulatory care patients.
- Using too narrow a scope of companies for potential benchmarking. This limits learning; for example, a hospital benchmarks only to competing hospitals in its geographic region.
- Not involving employees with the greatest knowledge of the processes being benchmarked. This is similar to not involving people who do work on quality improvement teams.
- Approaching benchmarking as a one-time effort rather than an ongoing, long-term effort. Xerox is said to have over eight hundred benchmarking projects under way at any given time. To some extent, every Quality Improvement Team should consider some level of benchmarking when developing countermeasures.
- Denial of the need to change, the need to benchmark, or the benchmark results.
- No action or changes after all of the effort to do benchmarking.

Commonly Cited Benchmarks

Some of the commonly cited benchmark organizations for different types of products, services, and processes are listed below (Whiting, 1991, p. 130; Biesada, 1991, pp. 36–47).

- Accounting: Motorola
- Advertising: Benetton Group
- Asset management: Emerson Electric
- Billing: American Express
- Compensation and benefits; Herman Miller
- Customer service and retention: American Express, Federal Express, MBNA America, Nordstrom
- Distribution: Federal Express, L.L. Bean, Super Valu Stores, Wal-Mart
- Employee training: Merck Sharp & Dohme
- Facilities, most advanced: Yamazaki Mazak (Japan)
- Healthcare cost management and promotion: Coors, Johnson & Johnson, Kodak, Travelers
- Information systems management: American Airlines/Sabre
- Manufacturing: Hewlett-Packard, IBM, Motorola, Toyota
- Product development: Hewlett-Packard, Honda, Intel
- Quality management: Motorola, Xerox
- Sales/marketing: IBM, Marion Merrell Dow, Xerox
- Technology transfer: 3M

Action Step: Identify a key process needing improvement and a potential benchmarking partner. If you join a network, one or more of those organizations may be willing to participate.

The potential to initiate meaningful clinical benchmarking is increasing. Several research projects focused on clinical quality initiatives and outcomes management are beginning to show results (Ellwood, 1988; InterStudy, 1990a, 1990b; Hudson, 1992).

Selected References on Benchmarking

Some useful references on benchmarking are *Benchmarking: The Search for Industry Best Practices That Lead to Superior Performance*, by Robert Camp (1989); "Benchmarking: As Competition Is Heating Up, So Is the Search for World-Class Performers," by Alexandra Biesada (1991); and "Benchmarking: Lessons from the Best-in-Class," by Rick Whiting (1991).

The American Productivity & Quality Center in Houston, Texas, is working with over fifty organizations establishing a clearinghouse of benchmarking case studies and information, and is an excellent source. The SunHealth Alliance in Charlotte, North Carolina, has established a formal benchmarking process among several of its hospitals.

TQM Evaluation

Regular measurement and evaluation of your services, products, information, and processes are key to continuous improvement. Although internal measurement is a basic element of TQM, this section has been included in the advanced applications chapter because of the external comparisons discussed here. A process that is not measured is not likely to be well managed or improved. Evaluation criteria may be established internally, or externally developed criteria may be used. A TQM audit instrument and process are helpful approaches to evaluate your organization's status and progress related to Total Quality Management. Benchmarking, discussed in the previous section, is a specialized form of evaluation compared to those organizations with best-in-class performance.

Internally Developed Evaluation Criteria or Indicators

Internal evaluation criteria or indicators basically come from three sources: internal customer requirements, professional groups, and management. The professional groups could also be considered important internal and external customers of your processes.

By developing and reviewing flowcharts of processes within your organization, you can identify external and internal customers and suppliers involved in each of those processes. Discussions, measurement, and analysis of the key requirements for each internal customer will yield internal quality and performance indicators, which serve as key criteria for evaluation.

Professional groups establish criteria for credentialing, performance, and evaluation within your organization, in addition to external evaluation criteria established by similar professional groups external to it. Examples include the professional credentials required for a professional to practice within your organization.

Management also establishes criteria for your organization. These tend to focus more on operations than on professional practice. Key management criteria also serve as internal evaluation criteria.

Externally Developed Evaluation Criteria or Indicators

In the long run, the most important criteria or indicators for your organization are those of your external customers, including patients, patients' families, admitting physicians, referring physicians, third-party payers, professional associations and organizations, accreditation organizations, and regulatory agencies. These customers collectively determine whether your organization will continue to serve those external customers.

Action Step: Establish regular communication opportunities and forums with each of your key customer groups. Use focus groups, surveys, personal interviews, and other feedback methods to listen and dialogue.

Mandated external criteria or indicators, such as those of the JCAHO, are familiar to all healthcare organizations. Similar criteria are used by professional review organizations (PROs), state departments of health, state mental health departments, third-party payers, and other organizations to assess quality and value of care. These external requirements must be met, even if you consider them unreasonable, until your organization and others convince those organizations to change their requirements. To our knowledge, only the JCAHO has begun to emphasize quality improvement. JCAHO is beginning to address the transition from quality assurance (QA) to quality improvement and is introducing accreditation standards in 1992 and 1994 reflecting that change (Joint Commission on Accreditation of Healthcare Organizations, 1991b).

Of greater assistance to evaluate your progress on TQM are the guidelines introduced for quality awards and used by industrial organizations emphasizing quality improvement. The following are examples.

Healthcare Forum/Witt Award: Commitment to Quality. The Healthcare Forum and Witt Associates Inc. first granted this award in 1988 to recognize healthcare organizations that have demonstrated commitment and progress toward continual quality improvement. The application form, available from The Healthcare Forum, San Francisco, California, identifies several judging criteria under the following six major categories, with the indicated distribution of 100 total points (The Healthcare Forum, 1991, p. 3):

A.   Executive summary
B.   Leadership and strategic planning (20 points):
     1.   Leadership
     2.   Strategic planning
C.   Quality assurance of products and services (30 points):
     1.   Medical quality assurance
     2.   Patient service quality
D.   Human resource utilization (15 points)
E.   Quality results (15 points)
F.   Patient and community needs assessment (20 points)

These evaluation criteria emphasize identifying and meeting community healthcare needs in addition to providing quality services and products. Former Healthcare Forum/Witt Award winners were listed in Chapter Five. For copies of the award application, contact the Healthcare Forum (listed under the Quality Improvement Network in Exhibit 14.1).

Malcolm Baldrige National Quality Award. This national quality award was first awarded in 1988 to emphasize and recognize quality improvement among U.S. organizations. Awards are offered in three categories—manufacturing, service, and small business—but not-for-profit organizations, including most healthcare organizations, are ineligible. However, the application guidelines provide excellent guidance for any organization to do a self-evaluation of its Total Quality efforts. The following core values and concepts underlie all requirements (National Institute of Standards and Technology, 1992, pp. 2–4):

- Customer-Driven Quality. Quality is judged by the customer.
- Leadership. A company's senior leaders must create a customer orientation, clear and visible quality values, and high expectations.
- Continuous Improvement. Achieving the highest levels of quality and competitiveness requires a well-defined and well-executed approach to continuous improvement.
- Employee Participation and Development. A company's success in meeting its quality and performance objectives depends increasingly on work force quality and involvement.
- Fast Response. Success in competitive markets increasingly demands ever-shorter cycles for new or improved product and service introduction.
- Design Quality and Prevention. Quality systems should place strong emphasis on design quality—problem and waste prevention achieved through building quality into products and services and into the processes through which they are produced.
- Long-Range Outlook. Achieving quality and market leadership requires a company to have a

strong future orientation and a willingness to make long-term commitments to customers, employees, suppliers, stockholders, and the community.

- Management by Fact. Pursuit of quality and operational performance goals of the company requires that process management be based upon reliable information, data, and analysis.
- Partnership Development. Companies should seek to build internal and external partnerships to better accomplish their overall goals.
- Corporate Responsibility and Citizenship. A company's quality system objectives should address corporate responsibility and citizenship.

The application guidelines provide very useful evaluation criteria in the following seven categories, with the indicated distribution of 1,000 total points (National Institute of Standards and Technology, 1992, pp. 16–32):

1. Leadership (90 points)
2. Information and analysis (80 points)
3. Strategic quality planning (60 points)
4. Human resource development and planning (150 points)
5. Management of process quality (140 points)
6. Quality and operational results (180 points)
7. Customer focus and satisfaction (300 points)

The Malcolm Baldrige criteria and those for the Healthcare Forum/Witt Award application are detailed and useful when evaluating your organization. Copies of the Malcolm Baldrige National Quality Award Application Guidelines are available from the National Institute of Standards and Technology (see Exhibit 14.1). The Anchor Health Care HMO at Rush-Presbyterian-St. Luke's Medical Center, for example, is using external reviewers to assess their organizational progress compared to the Malcolm Baldrige National Quality Award criteria.

Please refer to Appendix A, which gives an evaluation form tailored to healthcare organizations, based on the Baldrige criteria.

Industrial Quality Guidelines. Many industrial organizations have established quality guidelines and criteria for their suppliers. To date the primary focus has been on internal and external suppliers of products, but attention in several organizations is now extending to service suppliers. We believe that in three to five years healthcare organizations will be expected to meet similar quality guidelines as other suppliers. In Michigan, for example, the automobile manufacturers are the major industry, so their guidelines are relevant to Michigan healthcare organizations. Both Ford Motor Company (1990) and General Motors Corporation (1990) have large notebooks of detailed guidelines and criteria. Certainly, former Malcolm Baldrige award winners like Milliken & Company, Xerox, Globe Metallurgical, Motorola, Westinghouse Electric Corporation, Wallace Company, Federal Express Corporation, IBM Rochester, and Cadillac Motor Car Company have similar quality guidelines and criteria. Such guidelines and criteria are also useful for evaluating quality improvement in healthcare organizations.

Action Step: Meet with representatives of key business, industrial, and service organizations within your area to obtain and understand all applicable quality guidelines used for their suppliers.

TQM Audit

One approach to formalize an evaluation of your organization's status and progress implementing Total Quality Management is to perform a TQM audit. This approach gives the entire organization a snapshot of its strengths and weaknesses related to TQM evaluation criteria. You could develop your own audit tool based on the Healthcare Forum/Witt, Baldrige, and industrial quality criteria. Alternatively, you could use a tool developed by others. Periodic use of the audit tool would highlight areas progressing and needing further attention.

Many healthcare organizations may want to include quality audit criteria not emphasized in the industrial quality evaluations. These include professional practice, regulatory requirements, physicians as customers/suppliers, continuity of care, customer expectations, social expectations, education requirements, and research and development requirements.

Regular Evaluation Process

More important than the source of the evaluation criteria is following the concepts and regular use of those criteria to evaluate progress. The evaluation can be done for different purposes and at several different levels of detail.

An important step to reduce confusion is to assemble and communicate a complete list of all internal and external evaluation criteria. All applicable criteria for each process, professional entity, and/or department should be listed. Then these criteria should be clarified and reviewed to eliminate duplication, categorize, and prioritize which criteria are the most important. Some criteria, for example, may be minimum requirements for licensing or accreditation, and therefore must be met, but may not be particularly relevant to continuous quality improvement. A decision must be made as to which of the multitude of criteria will be used as a basis for regular evaluation of your organization.

One purpose of routine quality audits is to gain a general understanding of how your organization measures up against internal and external quality guidelines and criteria. This can be accomplished with relatively little effort. Another purpose is to do a more detailed analysis to identify specific opportunities for improvement during the next year. This type of evaluation requires substantially more effort but will yield specific plans for improvement.

For the quality evaluation to be taken seriously, it must be treated as important by senior leadership. Thus the results of the evaluation should have significant impact through leadership attention, recognition and reward systems, and resource allocation.

Action Step: Evaluate your progress on quality improvement annually using a combination of internally and externally developed criteria.

Integrated TQM Model

The term Total Quality Management is used in many different ways. Some have a broad definition, others a very narrow one. One risk is that an organization uses one or two TQM elements, and is misled to think that it has a complete TQM process. Having an integrated TQM model helps in understanding the complete scope of TQM and planning your process, even if only parts are currently being used.

TQC Wheel

One model developed by GOAL/QPC is called the Total Quality Control (TQC) Wheel (King, 1989a, p. pref. 7; King, 1989b, p. 1-8). This TQC Wheel is illustrated in Figure 14.2. Some highlights of this model are:

- The customer is the focus of the whole model.
- Cross-functional management includes methods that focus on coordination across the organization, such as quality function deployment (QFD), which is described later in this chapter. This is referred to as horizontal integration.
- Hoshin planning addresses the vertical integration to focus your whole organization on a few strategic breakthroughs. Hoshin planning is addressed later in this chapter.
- The daily control methods address measurement, standardization, and work groups involved in daily work.

The advantage of the GOAL/QPC TQC Wheel is the integration of many quality improvement methods.

This model has one significant weakness in that it addresses very few of the critically important people-management methods, which must be integrated with the analytical methods. The seven management tools do address methods to organize ideas, like affinity diagrams and tree diagrams, but important

Figure 14.2. TQC Wheel.

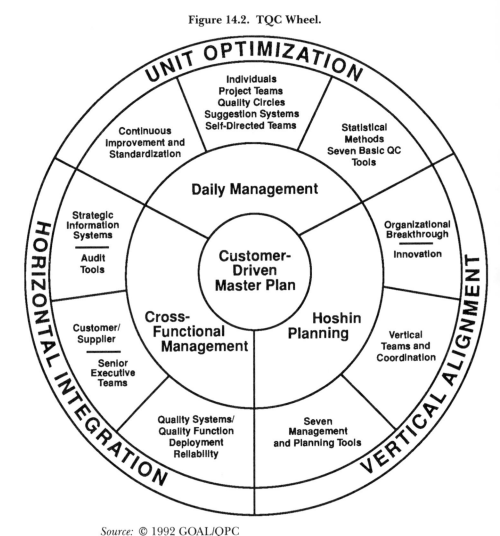

Source: © 1992 GOAL/QPC

team-management skills are not addressed. The GOAL/QPC
Healthcare Application Research Committee, which includes
UMMC, is investigating approaches to show the integration of
people methods with the TQC Wheel.

Evolutionary Versus Revolutionary Change

To be successful over the long run, your organization should integrate quality improvement methods to achieve incremental evolutionary improvement with methods to address major breakthroughs or revolutionary change. The seven-step quality improvement process described in Chapters Twelve and Thirteen, the Plan-Do-Check-Act (P-D-C-A) cycle, and the Standardize-Do-Check-Act (S-D-C-A) cycle are very effective at steadily improving your services and products. Over time these approaches will accomplish major improvements. Although these methods may yield occasional major breakthroughs, they are not designed for that purpose.

One useful approach to expand the horizon of thinking to seek real breakthroughs, or revolutionary change, is called Breakthrough Thinking, developed by Gerald Nadler and Shozo Hibino. They identify seven principles of breakthrough thinking (Nadler and Hibino, 1990, p. 88):

1. The Uniqueness Principle: Each problem is unique and requires a unique solution.
2. The Purposes Principle: Focusing on purposes helps strip away nonessential aspects of a problem.
3. The Solution-After-Next Principle: Having a target solution in the future gives direction to near-term solutions and infuses them with larger purposes.
4. The Systems Principle: Every problem is part of a larger system of problems, and solving one problem inevitably leads to another. Having a clear framework of what elements and dimensions comprise a solution assures its workability and implementation.
5. The Limited Information Collection Principle: Excessive data-gathering may create an expert in the problem area, but knowing too

much about it will probably prevent the discovery of some excellent alternatives.

6. The People Design Principle: Those who will carry out and use the solution should be intimately and continuously involved in its development. Also, in designing for other people, the solution should include only the critical details in order to allow some flexibility to those who must apply the solution.

7. The Betterment Timeline Principle: The only way to preserve the vitality of a solution is to build in and then monitor a program of continual change; the sequence of Breakthrough Thinking solutions thus becomes a bridge to a better future.

The challenge to management and Quality Improvement Teams is when the effort should be focused in part or totally on developing a completely new solution. There is no simple answer to this challenge, but some part of every team effort should be focused on unconstrained breakthrough thinking to seek possible breakthroughs. If customer needs are skillfully discussed during quality function deployment or hoshin planning efforts, the planning effort can lead to strategic breakthroughs. However, technological and other breakthroughs are typically initiated by scientists or professionals who conceive of a whole new idea. After all, what eye patient or even ophthalmologist would have asked for laser surgery in 1970? Science fiction writers had discussed the concept of power beams for years, but it was considered beyond practical use. Yet today laser surgery is a regular part of treating eye disorders.

UMMC Integrated TQM Model

To build on the models of others, UMMC has developed an integrated TQM model (see Figure 2.1 in Chapter Two) that illustrates the integration of philosophy, analytical skills, people skills, and a supportive structure and organization. We have also developed a more detailed version of this model that incorporates the specific methods, tools, and techniques involved for each of the four major dimensions.

Critical Paths of Care

Concepts of Critical Paths

"A critical path defines the optimal sequencing and timing of interventions by physicians, nurses, and other staff for a particular diagnosis or procedure, designed to minimize delays and resource utilization and to maximize quality of care" (Coffey and others, 1992, p. 45). Critical paths have been shown to reduce length of stay, and improve cost effectiveness. There are several different terms associated with the general approach and methods of the critical path method (CPM) applied to the healthcare industry. Examples are care maps (Zander, 1991), collaborative care (Etheredge, 1989), cooperative care, and coordinated care.

Critical path methods were developed and refined in the construction and engineering fields, where they have been used for decades. For those applications, several excellent computer programs are available to compute beginning times, ending times, critical path(s), slack times, and other useful data, in addition to creating the graphic displays. Although there were some earlier attempts, the research of Sandra Twyon, Karen Zander, and others at New England Medical Center, Boston, Massachusetts, is credited with initiating the recent growth of critical paths in health care.

The critical paths are based on the fact that the care of a patient with a specific condition or procedure requires many interdependent services to be provided for the patient. If these are not appropriately coordinated and scheduled, the quality of care decreases, delays occur, additional resources are required, and costs increase. The sequence of required activities, in their precedent order, can be illustrated as a flowchart or activities to provide the required care for the patient. The term critical path comes from the fact that one sequence of activities or path through the flowchart, or sometimes simultaneous paths, requires the most time. Reducing the time of any other activities will not reduce the total time to provide the care. The critical path approach uses a collaborative effort to define the required services, products, and information; determine the precedence relationships among them; determine the appropriate time and resources required; and determine the schedule to minimize the total time and resources required.

Characteristics of Critical Paths

Different applications of critical paths have different characteristics. The name used for a particular application is of less concern than the characteristics of that application. These characteristics will be briefly described so you will have a better understanding of the range of uses (Coffey and others, 1992).

Scope. By scope we are referring to the range of application or period of care over which the critical paths will be applied. Examples include:

- Inpatient care applications. This is the most common scope of critical paths. Most of these applications are initiated at the time of admission, or time of surgical procedure, and end at the time of discharge.
- Complete episode of care. This is a logical extrapolation of the inpatient care application, but would begin at the time the patient comes to the physician's office, and would end at the termination of post-hospitalization follow-up.
- Specialized applications, such as critical paths for ambulatory surgery patients or renal dialysis patients. An example currently being developed at UMMC is a coordinated care model for managing the care of outpatients in a new cough and dyspnea clinic.
- Life/health management. This type of application of critical paths has the potential to provide the most cost-effective, high-quality approach to managing chronic conditions. Such critical paths may provide models for involving patients in the management of their long-term health and medical care.

Format. The format of a protocol of care is another characteristic that distinguishes different applications. Many industrial applications of critical path methods use a flowchart type of format, with a number of pieces of information shown on the chart, such as the beginning time, duration, ending time, and slack time shown on the figure. These charts provide a graphical picture of the many activities to be accomplished and their precedence relationships. However, the charts are very large and are often used when fastened to walls. The format currently used for most inpatient and other clinical applications is a matrix of activities by day or hour. A sample is illustrated in Exhibit 14.2 (Coffey and others, 1992). The advantage of this format is that it is small enough to be able to store in a patient's chart or at the bedside. The disadvantage is that this format does not communicate which actions require the completion of other actions before they can begin, known as precedence relationships.

Multidisciplinary Staff Actions. Several different types of staff actions are shown in typical inpatient critical paths. Sample categories of staff actions include: consults/assessments; treatments; nutrition; medications; activity/safety; teaching of the patient, family, or significant other; discharge planning; and other activities (Zander, 1991).

Problem/Outcome. Another characteristic not included in some critical paths is a listing of expected problems and outcomes (Zander, 1991).

Documentation. The approach to documentation is another characteristic. The critical paths may or may not be used as part of the permanent patient documentation.

Process for Critical Paths

The process for development and use of critical paths will vary among organizations, but the following actions are commonly involved (Coffey and others, 1992).

Gain support and approval to implement critical paths of care. This should be done carefully so all the major groups participate in the decision and understand the costs and benefits. The

Exhibit 14.2. Sample Critical Path Protocol of Care.

CRITICAL PATHWAY: Cervical Spinal Cord Injury with neurological deficit without respiratory complications
PHYSICIAN:
DATE INITIATED:
PATHWAY CODE: 9.1.1 MCLA 333.21515.20175
August 8, 1991

UNIVERSITY OF MICHIGAN NEUROSURGERY

ADMIT DIAGNOSIS: Cervical Spinal Cord Injury
DRG: 9
PROCEDURE: Spinal fusion
EXPECTED LOS: 4.5 days

	DAY 1 (Admission)	DAY 2/3 (Surgery)	DAY 4/5 (Transfer)	DAY 6/7 (Discharge)
Date				
Consults	PMR, SCI social worker, SCI nurse. Orthotics, Rehabilitation engineering	Physical, occupational therapy	Dietitian	Transfer to PMR-SCI service
Tests	Lateral C-spine, CXR, MRI, ABG, Admission Profile.	PARU: CBC, CHEM A & B, ABG, Lateral C-spine	PARU: CBC, CHEM A & B, ABG, CXR, Lateral C-spine with position change.	
Activity	Bedrest (if Stryker do not turn until lateral C-spines and resident's orders) Turn q2h. ROM q4h. Consider roto test for pulmonary management.	Hospital bed turn q2h (logroll). HOB no greater than 30 degrees. ROM q4h. Splints per OT.	ROM q4h with progression to sitting. Splits per OT.	
Treatments	Vitals, spinal motor scale checks q1h. Pin level checks q1h. Temperature q2–4h Respiratory assessment q2–4h with Respiratory parameters q2–4h Quad cough technique q3–4h	Vitals, spinal motor scale checks to q1–3h Pin level checks q1–3h	Vitals, spinal motor scale checks q4h. Pin level checks q4h	→ → → →

	Foley to DD	Discontinue Foley ISC q3–4h to maintain <300cc of urine volume.	
	Assess need for P & PD		Continue Bowel Program
	Bowel Program begun: LOC/SUPP		
	O₂ per NC	Discontinue O₂ if O₂ sat >96%.	
	Antiembolitic socks with SCD		
	IS q1h C & DB		
	Nurse Call Device (rehab engineering)		
	Prism Glasses (OT)		Assess for Hyperreflexia (BP, Sweats, HA)
	Maintain traction as ordered (check topknot q2h) Pin care q day.	Maintain Halo Vest. Pin care q day Neck dressing checked q1–3h.	
Medications	Consider Heparin SQ		Consider Heparin lock
	IVF as ordered		
	Antibiotics x24h	Discontinue antibiotics	
	Histamine Antagonists IV/NG		Histamine antagonist PO
	Narcotic Analgesics IV/IM/NG		Analgesics PO
	Benadryl PRN		
	Consider Steroid	Discontinue steroid drip	
Diet	NPO x Ice chips		Diet as tolerated (at preadmission level)
	NG to LCS if nauseated — NPO		
		Advance to clear liquids if bowel sounds present.	
Patient and family education	Teach anxiety relief measures (i.e., guided imagery, relaxation techniques). Preop education per unit policy. Orient patient and family to NICU policy, procedures, and family support group. Assess discharge needs.	Assess family/patient knowledge of injury and consequences. Assess psychological stage of injury. Assess questions/ concerns of sexuality.	Prepare for transfer to acute care unit. Reassess discharge needs. Consider rehabilitation tour. Patient and family.
			Prepare for transfer to rehabilitation unit.

Source: Reprinted from Coffey, R.J., Richards, J.S., Remmert, C.S., LeRoy, S.S., Schoville, R.R., and Baldwin, P.J., "An Introduction to Critical Paths" in *Quality in Management Health Care*, Vol. 1, No. 1, p. 49, with permission of Aspen Publishers, Inc., © 1992.

major groups include physicians, nurses, pharmacists, therapists, patients themselves, administration, and the board.

Select diagnoses/procedures for critical paths. Diagnoses or
procedures can be selected and prioritized for protocol development based on criteria such as the volume of cases, financial
impact of cases, profitability of cases, quality assurance issues,
interest of physicians and other staff, and interest of payers.
After the team is formed and current practices are documented,
there may be changes such as additional critical paths to reflect
the desired practice.

Select team to develop protocol. The team should include the
key clinicians providing care to the patients. Any member may
lead the team, although most implementations to date have had
nurses lead the team.

Select characteristics for critical path. The team must decide
the scope of the protocol, format, and other characteristics, like
those described above.

Document current process. Most critical path efforts begin by
documenting the current practices and outcomes. This is necessary to understand what is being done, before making changes.
Also, the need for multiple, more-specific critical paths may be
determined while analyzing the current practices of different
physicians and other clinicians.

Research internal and external practices. Research at this
stage is helpful to reduce the amount of subsequent protocol
changes, but is not necessary. Try to identify different practices
within your organization and other organizations. Sample critical paths from other organizations are helpful at this stage to
help the team consider alternatives. Key questions include:
What is done? Why? Does it contribute value? Why? Could it be
done an easier or faster way? Why?

Develop critical path for selected diagnosis/procedure. The objective is to arrive at a standardized critical path for patients
meeting the criteria for that protocol. At UMMC we have arrived
at multiple critical paths per DRG, based on the procedure or
level of care provided. Clearly, for varying reasons, the care of
some patients will vary from the protocol because of the patient's condition or other factors. When this happens, the varia-

tion and the reason for it are documented, along with the plan of action. The team should consult with others who will be involved in implementing the protocol to determine the types of questions they have.

Develop process to implement and manage critical paths. Different approaches can be used, but the most common approach is to designate a case manager for one or more critical paths. This person will work with staff to achieve compliance and coordinate deviations and changes. Care should be taken here that there is consensus about how the process will be managed on a day-to-day basis. Without agreement, staff may avoid using the protocol.

Define key measures of conformance and outcomes. It is impossible and wasteful to try to measure everything. Therefore, it is important to identify the key processes, decision criteria, and outcome measures to be used.

Develop data documentation/collection process. Data documentation/collection is separately addressed because it is often overlooked. It is necessary to consider carefully what data will be collected, the operational definitions, how data will be collected, who will collect it, and how the data will be used. There is no point collecting data if it cannot be used. One helpful approach is to simulate and summarize the data, then ask how the information will help the team improve the process of care. One common issue is how the protocol will be used for patient education and medical record documentation.

Educate all affected staff. Every person who may provide care to patients covered by the protocol must be educated concerning the protocol, data collection, how to handle patients who vary from the protocol, and how the protocol will be used, if at all, in documentation for the patient's record.

Implement the critical path. After all affected staff are educated, the critical path is implemented. Often a case manager is designated to track adherence to the critical path, to intervene to facilitate desired outcomes, and to document variances.

Analyze results. A number of different results should be analyzed, including changes in utilization of resources; variations from critical paths; changes in outcomes such as length of stay, readmission rates, and infection rates; and perceptions of patients and staff. At UMMC we have found documentation and analyses of variations from the critical paths to be one of the more difficult issues.

Review and revise protocol as required. The original critical path should not be considered fixed but rather as a living, evolving model. The critical paths should be reviewed and updated regularly, reflecting improvements in clinical practice and other changes. The critical paths should be seen as documenting current practice, which will continually improve.

Benefits of Critical Paths

Critical paths are expanding quickly because there are many valuable uses of such protocols. Described here are some of the key benefits of critical paths (Coffey and others, 1992).

- Provide plan or "big picture." Traditionally the physician wrote orders each day, but rarely was there any written overall care plan. Each day the nurses, pharmacists, therapists, ancillary departments, and others carried out those orders with an incomplete understanding of the plan or "big picture" for care of the patient. One exception for medical centers were those patients on research care protocols, for which there are written critical paths. The critical path provides the plan for everyone to see, which is particularly valuable when the physician is not present.
- Provide planning and coordination of care that can be shared with the patient and family.
- Reduce variation in the process and outcomes of care.
- Education. This includes education of the house officers or residents, medical students, nurses, and patients and their families.
- Improved working environment, recruitment, and retention. Nursing and other staff like being involved, which helps with recruitment and retention.
- Benchmarking. The critical paths can be compared among

different services and hospitals to determine which approach provides the best outcomes and value.

Reasons for Failure or Poor Results from Critical Paths

Critical paths are a recent development, so there has not been much reported related to failures or poor results. However, based on the work at UMMC and discussions with others, the following are reasons for failure of the process:

- Lack of Collaboration. If one group assumes ownership of the process at the expense of other participants, the others will decrease their participation and support. Although nursing, for example, serves a key role, the process should be promoted as a collaborative effort of physicians, pharmacists, therapists, support staff, and others.
- Developing a Protocol for Too Large a Group. Our experience indicates that a DRG, for example, is too broad a group for a specific critical path of care. There are multiple critical paths per DRG at UMMC, with most surgical critical paths based on the procedure(s) performed.
- Lack of Prioritization. Developing an effective critical path protocol requires substantial time of all parties involved and requires refinement as experience is gained with the protocol. To avoid overcommitment of staff, it will be necessary to prioritize which critical paths will be done first.
- Adopting External Critical Paths. Some organizations are now offering critical paths for sale. These provide an excellent starting point for discussions by the team for each protocol, but are of questionable value if they do not go through the review process necessary to achieve full understanding and buy-in.

Action Step: Establish a team to investigate critical paths, if they are not in use. TQM tools, such as brainstorming and flowcharting, can help the team develop the critical path.

Selected References on Critical Paths

Some useful references on critical paths are *Collaborative Care: Nursing Case Management*, edited by Mary Lou Salome Etheredge (1989); "Professional Nursing Case Management Improves Quality, Access and Costs," *Nursing Management* (1989), by Phyllis Ethridge and Gerri S. Lamb; and "Care Maps: The Core of Cost/Quality Care," *The New Definition*, by Karen Zander (1991). Many healthcare organizations are working on critical paths. Some with more experience include Alliant Health System, Louisville, Kentucky; New England Medical Center, Boston, Massachusetts; the Toronto Hospital, Toronto, Ontario, Canada; University of Michigan Medical Center, Ann Arbor, Michigan; and Vanderbilt University Hospital and Clinics, Nashville, Tennessee.

Quality Function Deployment

Quality function deployment (QFD) is used primarily for design or redesign of products or services. It is an integrated process relating customer requirements to the planning and deployment of quality, technology, cost, and reliability characteristics. There are a number of definitions and interpretations of QFD. Bob King states that "QFD is a system for designing product or service based on customer demands and involving all members of the producer or supplier organization" (King, 1989a, p. 1-9). Yoji Akao, who was a primary developer of QFD in Japan, provides a more involved definition of QFD "as converting the consumers' demands into 'quality characteristics' and developing a design quality for the finished product by systematically deploying the relationships between the demands and the characteristics, starting with the quality of each part and process. The overall quality of the product will be formed through this network of relationships" (Akao, 1990, p. 3). In its simplest form, QFD begins with statements of desired quality in the customers' words, then translates these into quality characteristics of the product or service provided by your organization. Through a series of more detailed characteristics, weights and priorities, and comparisons, the customers' desires are translated into design characteristics for the product or service to cost effectively meet those desires.

The purpose of this section is to define and provide a basic understanding of quality function deployment as an important advanced tool for TQM. References are provided at the end of this section for a more complete and advanced understanding of QFD.

Why use quality function deployment? The primary reason is to meet and exceed your customers' expectations at a reduced cost. Akao states: "In many of the published cases, the use of quality function deployment has cut in half the problems previously encountered at the beginning stages of product development and has reduced development time by one-half to one-third, while also helping to ensure user satisfaction and increasing sales. However, if applied incorrectly, quality function deployment may increase work without producing these benefits" (Akao, 1990, p. 3). When new products or services are developed, whether in healthcare or other industries, it is common to experience numerous start-up problems leading to a series of costly redesigns. These typical start-up problems have made all of us leery of being the first person to buy a new product or use a new service. Figure 14.3 illustrates the relative amount of time and resources spent using a traditional design process versus a QFD design process (King, 1989a, p. 1-2). Using a traditional approach, little time is spent defining the customer requirements for the product, consequently design takes less time. However, there is often a long redesign period after the new product or service is initiated. Using QFD, substantially more time is spent up front understanding the customer requirements and desires and the relative priorities among them. Hence the complete design process takes less time. By carefully meeting the customer requirements, there should be much less time needed for redesign after the product or service is initiated. Overall, there is a substantial reduction in the time and cost to achieve an acceptable product or service.

Although first introduced in Japan in 1966, the concept of quality function deployment did not receive significant attention by U.S. industrial organizations until the late 1980s. QFD

Figure 14.3. Comparison of Traditional and QFD Systems.

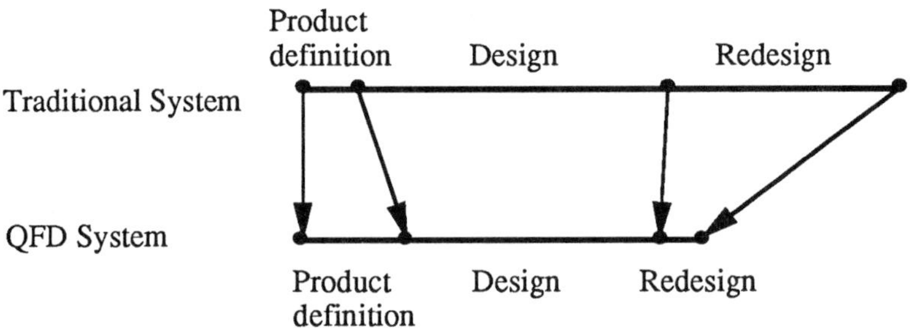

Source: King, 1989, p. 1-2.

has been used by only a few healthcare organizations, beginning about 1990.

Concepts of QFD

QFD is a formalized process to listen to the voice of the customer. Customers' requirements, stated in their words, are assigned relative weights related to the characteristics of your processes for producing services, products, or information. Relative weights are also assigned to competitors' performances relative to the customers' requirements. The relative weights are then used to prioritize those things that need improvement. The relative weights can then be extended to prioritize resources, research and development efforts, and other activities. Using QFD places the effort and resources where you will gain the greatest customer benefit at least cost.

Quality function deployment, like other TQM methods, should be used as a tool to help you better meet the needs of your customers and should be tailored to the specific situation. We will address only the basic approach in this section; references for more complete coverage of QFD are given below. In its most complete form, QFD can include as many as thirty detailed, interrelated matrices of information. However, the most important first step is to define the relationships of customer requirements, system characteristics, and competitor comparisons.

This is sometimes called the A–1 chart (King, 1989a, pp. 4-1 to 4-10) or the 1–1 chart (Akao, 1990, pp. 16–49). The basic structure and functions of the different portions of the QFD A–1 chart are illustrated in Figure 14.4. You begin by listening to *what* your customers want, in their own words. These are listed down the left column of the chart. Then you consider *how* the characteristics of your system contribute toward what the customers want. The characteristics of your process are listed at the top of the chart, then the relative measures are listed within the chart. Finally, comparisons with competitors will provide information of *how much* of each customer criterion will be required to meet or exceed their capabilities. These are listed at the right of the chart. Most experience to date of UMMC, St. Clair Hospital, Pittsburgh, Pennsylvania, and other healthcare organizations has been with this basic chart. More extensive applications of QFD are certain to follow in the future.

Process for QFD

The process to complete the initial QFD chart includes the following steps. These may be done in different sequences, and

Figure 14.4. Structure and Functions of Basic QFD Chart.

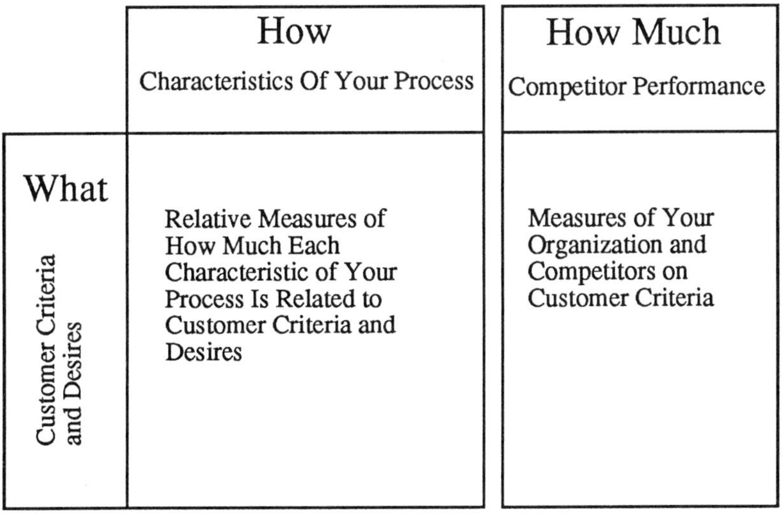

How Characteristics Of Your Process	How Much Competitor Performance
What Customer Criteria and Desires	Relative Measures of How Much Each Characteristic of Your Process Is Related to Customer Criteria and Desires	Measures of Your Organization and Competitors on Customer Criteria

each step should be revisited as other steps are completed. The requirements, process characteristics, competitor comparison, and the various weights change steadily as customers' perceptions change and the services and products of your organization and your competitors change. It is important to look outside your organization to identify your customers' requirements and the current capacities and plans of competitors.

Secure leadership commitment. Leadership commitment for a QFD project is the first step, as with any other portion of TQM or other corporate undertaking.

Identify project to use QFD. Normally quality function deployment is used for a new or substantially changed product or service, although the same approach can be used to improve a current service. At UMMC we were planning a new unit in which to perform endoscopies, endoscopic radiology, cardiac biopsies, adult bronchoscopies, and other procedures. Developing this new medical procedures unit (MPU) offered an excellent opportunity to use QFD. At St. Clair Hospital they wanted to improve the emergency services provided to patients.

Form and train team. The characteristics of a QFD team are similar to those of a quality improvement or benchmarking team: five to six members including people who are most familiar with the process, a team leader trained and as experienced as possible with QFD, a positive, "can do" attitude, attention to detail, good listeners, and ability to implement or influence change. For a team to be successful, it must have sufficient time, support, and resources to complete the QFD project. You may want to use an external consultant, as we did, to train the team members about QFD. We would suggest initially focusing on the basic charts and not spending too much time on the intricate extensions to technology deployment, cost deployment, and reliability deployment, unless they are of particular concern to your team. The many charts are confusing until the team becomes familiar with the basics. Based on our experience also, we suggest you begin by training a large QFD team, since some people will drop out for various reasons.

Determine customer requirements and desires. The purpose is to determine what potential customers of the service or product would like, in their own words. These may be demands, requirements, or desires. Note that there are frequently multiple customers. For example, the UMMC Medical Procedures Unit has multiple customers, including patients, patient families, physicians, and employees. These customer requirements are entered along the left side of the sample basic QFD matrix illustrated in Figure 14.5, in the column labeled "a." Example customer desires may be full recovery, no pain, a short wait time, and courteous staff.

Different methods can be used to gain this input, but direct face-to-face discussions will provide the most information. Some information can be gathered by questionnaires or telephone surveys. At UMMC we used focus groups of physicians, nurses, and patients to identify and discuss different customer requirements in their terms. Each group had different requirements.

Care should be taken to probe topics involving the three types of quality described by Noriaki Kano: expected quality, one-dimensional quality, and exciting quality (refer to Figure 2.3 in Chapter Two). Customers often do not raise requirements related to expected quality, such as safety, which are absolute requirements. Expected quality characteristics must be identified, either with the customers or by your staff, because failure on these requirements will result in serious problems and lost customers. Also, customers normally do not raise requirements related to exciting quality because they have not thought about it. In this case, you may want to test different potential ideas to see what the customers think. Look for things that are unexpected and excite the customers.

Determine relative importance of customer requirements. The next step is to determine the customers' perceptions of the relative importance of each of their requirements. These customer weights are used to determine priorities for changes, investments, and other improvements. The relative importance of the different customer requirements can be obtained from questionnaires, telephone surveys, and personal interviews. It is often good to discuss the priorities with focus groups of people who identified the requirements, then follow up with a broader

Figure 14.5. Sample Basic QFD Chart.

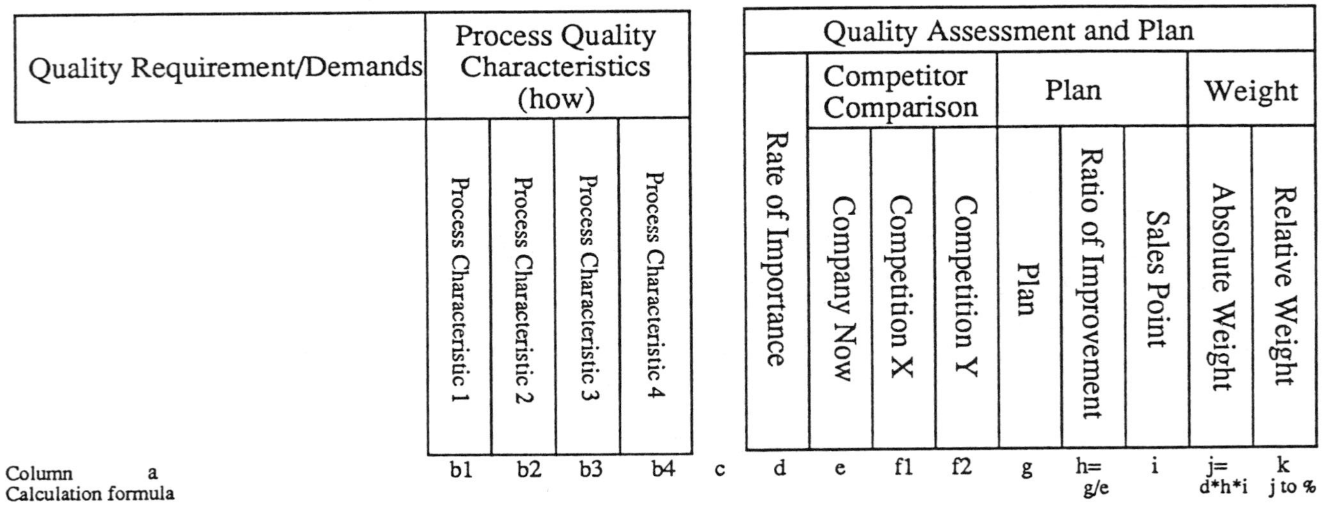

		Column / Calculation formula
Quality Requirement/Demands		a
Process Quality Characteristics (how)	Process Characteristic 1	b1
	Process Characteristic 2	b2
	Process Characteristic 3	b3
	Process Characteristic 4	b4
		c
Quality Assessment and Plan	Rate of Importance	d
	Competitor Comparison — Company Now	e
	Competitor Comparison — Competition X	f1
	Competitor Comparison — Competition Y	f2
	Plan — Plan	g
	Plan — Ratio of Improvement	$h = g/e$
	Plan — Sales Point	i
	Weight — Absolute Weight	$j = d*h*i$
	Weight — Relative Weight	$k = $ j to %

Scale	Customer Requirements								"1-5"	"1-5"	"1-5"	"1-5"	"1-5"		"1-1.5"		
1	Customer requirement 1	O / 42			O / 42				3	4	3	3	4	1	1	1	3	14
2	Customer requirement 2		O / 69	◎ / 207					4	5	4	5	5	1	1.2	4.8	23
3	Customer requirement 3	△ / 44, 396	◎ / 396	O / 132					5	4	5	3	5	1.25	1.5	9.4	44
4	Customer requirement 4	△ / 19			◎ / 171				3	3	3	3	4	1.33	1	4	19
	Total	105	465	339	213	1122								Total		21.2	100
	Percentage (%)	9	41	30	19	99											
	Company now	9															
	Competitor x																
	Competitor y																
	Plan																

Scales:

Column b: Main Correlations:
◎ 9 = strong correlation
O 3 = some correlation
△ 1 = possible correlation

Columns d–g: 1–5, with 5 = most important

Column i: Sales Point: 1, 1.2, 1.5, with 1.5 = most important

Source: King, 1989a, p. 4-3.

survey of customers to determine customer priorities. These ratings of importance are entered to the right of the process characteristics, as illustrated in column "d" of Figure 14.5. A scale of 1–5 is commonly used, with 5 being the most important.

Evaluate process quality characteristics. The design characteristics of a system are commonly stated in terms different from those that customers use. The first step is to identify the key quality characteristics of the process required to produce a service or product desired by the customers. These are entered as headers above columns "b1," "b2," etc. Columns are added to address all the key process characteristics. For example, key characteristics might be the qualifications of staff, medications used, type of seating, and guest relations training.

For each of your key process quality characteristics, the team assesses the correlation between that characteristic and each of the customer requirements. For simplicity, only three levels of correlation are used: strong correlation (weight = 9), some correlation (weight = 3), and possible correlation (weight = 1). If there is no correlation, that cell of the matrix is left blank. For visual impact, symbols are entered in the upper left portion of each cell, as illustrated in the "b" columns of Figure 14.5.

Compare your organization to competitors. Most often quality is viewed relative to comparable services and products available elsewhere. Therefore, QFD includes a comparison of your organization's current performance to that of competitors for each of the customer-stated requirements. Your customers' perceptions are most important when comparing your services and products relative to those of your competitors'. Therefore, this comparison should include customer input through focus groups or surveys. This information may be gathered at the same time as the customers' ratings of relative importance of different customer requirements. Based on input from your customers, physicians, managers, and staff, the team enters relative weights for your organization and each competitor. For simplicity, a scale of 1–5 is used, with 5 being the best performance. Sample numbers are illustrated in column "e" for your organization, and in columns "f1" and "f2" for two competitors (see Figure 14.5).

Develop plan of where to focus attention. The whole purpose of these QFD activities is to focus attention and resources on the requirements most valued by customers and where your organization compares least favorably to competitors. Based on the rating of importance by the customers and the relative comparison of your current services and products to your competitors' for each of the customer requirements, the QFD team develops a plan for the future relative performance, on the same scale of 1–5. These values are illustrated in column "g" of Figure 14.5. Note that the plan is a judgment of the team, based on comparison with competitors for each customer requirement. The next step is to develop a ratio of improvement, which is simply the planned performance level divided by the current performance level, as illustrated in column "h" of Figure 14.5. This ratio is used later to develop a weight that translates to the relative emphasis that should be placed on each of your process characteristics. The sales point is a ratio representing the judgment of the QFD team as to the relative importance for sales emphasis of the different customer requirements. The convention is to use weights of 1.5 for a strong sales point, 1.2 for a lesser sales point, and 1.0 for all others. These are illustrated in column "i" of Figure 14.5.

The customers' ratings of importance (col. "d") are then multiplied by the ratio of importance (col. "h") and the sales point (col. "i") to generate an absolute weight for each of the customer requirements. These absolute weights are then standardized to a total weight of 100, by dividing each of the absolute weights in column "j" by the total weight at the bottom of column "j" and entering the relative weights in the respective rows of column "k."

The relative weight of each customer requirement is then multiplied by the correlation value of each process quality characteristic, and entered in the respective cells of the "b" columns. Using the first customer requirement, row 1, and the first process characteristic, column "b1," for example, the relative weight of 14 from column "k" is multiplied by the sum correlation weight of 3 for the first process characteristic to yield a weight of 42. The weights for all customer requirements are then summed for each process quality characteristic to yield a total. The percentage weight to each of the process quality characteristics is calculated by dividing the weights in each of the "b" columns by the total in column "c."

The purpose of the basic QFD matrix is to translate direct qualitative inputs from customers about their requirements and the relative importance of those requirements to the relative emphasis your organization should place on the different process quality characteristics. The specific process quality characteristics of your current services and products are compared with your competitors' quality characteristics by your QFD team, in order to develop specific changes that will most cost effectively meet and exceed your customers' requirements for a new or revised service or product.

Initially QFD appears to be very complex, and it can be, if carried to great levels of detail. However, the basic chart described above is fairly quickly understood. Our experience indicates that the process takes several months to learn the approach and to gather input from the various customer groups. However, once used, the participants begin to think critically about the processes, facilities, and personnel providing services. The power comes from the detailed discussions with customers about their requirements and desires, comparisons with competitors, and consideration of how the organization can meet the customer requirements most effectively. The initial comparisons may be based on customer perceptions, but more detailed benchmarking may be appropriate later.

Action Step: Assign a cross-functional team to use the QFD approach when your organization is planning a new or revised service. The customer input and results will be worth the investment.

Reasons for Failure or Poor Results from QFD

Quality function deployment is sufficiently new in healthcare that there is little experience with success or failure. However, based on comments from industry representatives and the nature of QFD, the following are seen as potential reasons for failure or poor results.

- Lack of leadership support. As with any other aspect of TQM, leadership support is necessary for success.
- View as a one-time activity. QFD, like other TQM methods, is most useful when integrated into continuous improvement.
- Do not get direct customer input. There is a temptation to talk to a few patients who are friends and conclude that the team understands the real requirements of the customers.
- Omit some customer groups. For many of the processes in healthcare organizations, there are multiple customer groups, each with their own requirements.
- Omit expected quality and/or exciting quality indicators. These can be easily omitted because the customers do not normally think about them. Your team must raise and probe these types of quality indicators.
- Rush through the process. QFD is a complex, time-consuming process, but it has proven results. If you rush through the steps, you may increase the work without increasing the benefits.

Selected References on QFD

The following are excellent references on QFD: *Quality Function Deployment: Integrating Customer Requirements into Product Design*, edited by Yoji Akao (1990); and *Better Designs in Half the Time: Implementing Quality Function Deployment in America*, by Bob King (1989a).

Training programs on QFD are also offered by GOAL/ QPC, Methuen, Massachusetts; Japanese Business Consultants, Inc., Ann Arbor, Michigan; American Supplier Institute, Dearborn, Michigan; and other organizations.

Sample hospitals that have used quality function deployment include Bethesda Hospital, Cincinnati, Ohio; New England Memorial Hospital, Stoneham, Massachusetts; St. Clair Hospital, Pittsburgh, Pennsylvania; and UMMC.

Hoshin Planning

Hoshin planning is a combination of strategic planning and policy deployment throughout your organization. The general term *hoshin planning*, or *hoshin kanri*, is used because this approach was first developed and applied as an integrated system in Japan. "The word hoshin can be translated as 'policy' or 'target and means.' The word kanri is translated as 'planning' but also means 'management' and 'control.' So sometimes you'll see 'policy management,' sometimes you'll see 'policy control.' A literal translation that would make sense to people is 'target and means management.' (The significant aspect of hoshin planning is its strong focus on the means, the process by which targets are reached.) Another name is 'Management by Policy (MBP)' which is used in Japan to distinguish it from 'Management by Objectives (MBO)' " (King, 1989b, p. 1-3). Some organizations call this type of effort policy deployment. "What hoshin provides is a planning structure that will bring selected critical business processes up to the desired level of performance. Hoshin kanri operates at two levels: First, at what Juran called 'breakthrough' management or the strategic planning level; and, second, at the daily management level on the more routine or fundamental aspects of the business operation. Hoshin kanri has been called the application of Deming's plan-do-check-act to the management process" (Akao, 1991, p. xxii).

> Hoshin Planning is a system. It is a component of the TQM system that allows an organization to plan and execute strategic organizational breakthrough. Its key elements are:
>
> - A planning and implementation process that is continuously improved throughout the year (P-D-C-A).
> - Focus on key systems that need to be improved to achieve strategic objectives.
> - Participation and coordination by all levels and departments as appropriate in the plan-

ning, deployment of yearly objectives and means.

- Planning and execution based upon facts.
- Goals and action plans which cascade through the organization based upon the true capability of the organization [GOAL/QPC, 1989, p. 1].

"Hoshin Planning is the one element of TQM that is most consistently applied in Japanese companies of all sizes and in all industries" (GOAL/QPC, 1989, p. 5).

Hoshin planning includes many of the elements of traditional strategic planning, such as determining the needs of the community, strengths and weaknesses of your organization and competitors, and major strategies and objectives. In hoshin planning the strategies are often called breakthrough strategies. Each organization has used a somewhat different approach to strategic planning in the past, but some of the differences between hoshin planning and traditional strategic planning include the following:

- Gaining input from all levels of the organization to develop the strategic plans.
- Prioritizing among strategies and alternatives, so everyone understands the priorities and the reasons for them. A form of prioritization matrix can be used for this (see Exhibit 12.2 in Chapter Twelve).
- Communication of the strategic plans to every employee. Although an organization's executives determine its strategy, this is seldom communicated to department heads or employees for them to use in prioritizing their own activities.
- Development of departmental and even personal goals that help accomplish the organization's strategic goals.
- Focus on key systems and critical success factors to achieve the departmental and organizational goals.
- Developing and using measurements to determine how well each department and the organization is doing according to its goals.

A hoshin planning model is illustrated in Figure 14.6. The capability, planning information, and commitment flow up the organization, and the strategic direction and focus flow down the organization. A key advantage of hoshin planning is to develop a process to align and communicate the most important strategies, goals, capacities, and measurements throughout the organization. The process promotes a common focus for the whole organization.

Process for Hoshin Planning

There are a number of different approaches to implement hoshin planning. As with other components of TQM, hoshin planning can be initiated at the corporate, divisional, or departmental levels. However, it is most effective if implemented throughout the organization. The process suggested here is one useful approach (cf. GOAL/QPC, 1989).

Determine reason to use hoshin planning. As with TQM and all its other components, your organization must answer the question "why." The primary reasons to undertake hoshin planning are to focus effort and resources on those few strategies and processes that will best achieve the organization's survival and vision, and to develop an effective process to align the goals and efforts of the organization.

Secure leadership commitment. Leadership commitment to undertake hoshin planning is the first step, as with any other portion of TQM or other corporate undertaking.

Gather internal input. Ideas and data from managers, physicians, and staff within your organization are key to understanding the current capabilities and ideas for improvements. Example information from managers and staff could include data on capabilities, comparisons with competitors, key processes, and ideas for breakthroughs. Approaches like *Breakthrough Thinking* (Nadler and Hibino, 1990) can be used to gather breakthrough ideas from all employees. Quality function deployment projects can provide very useful inputs to the planning process.

Gather external input. Data and ideas from external sources

Figure 14.6. Hoshin Planning Model.

Strategic Planning Process

Leadership Solicits Internal/External Inputs on:
- Capabilities
- Comparisons to competitors
- Breakthrough strategies and success factors
- Key processes

Department Managers Solicit Internal/External Inputs on:
- Capabilities
- Comparisons to competitors
- Breakthrough strategies and success factors
- Key processes

Individuals Provide Inputs on:
- Capabilities
- Comparisons to competitors
- Breakthrough strategies and success factors
- Key processes

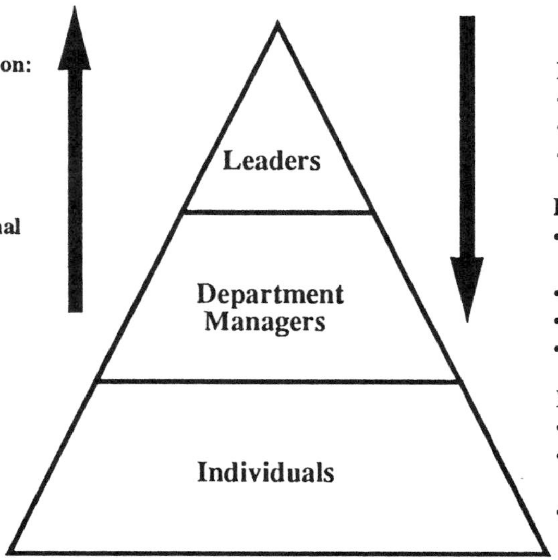

Policy/Plan Deployment Process

Leadership Determines and Communicates:
- Breakthrough strategies
- Critical success factors
- Measures of goals
- Key processes
- Strategic goals

Department Managers Establish:
- Department goals based on organizational goals
- Key processes for department
- Critical success factors for department
- Measures of department goals

Individuals:
- Personal goals based on department goals
- Relate personal processes to department and organizational key processes
- Measures performance related to department measures

Leaders

Department Managers

Individuals

are equally important. Information about the requirements of current and potential customers, capabilities and plans of competitors, and capabilities and plans of suppliers are all useful. In particular, you should be focusing on major changes and paradigm shifts in the environment, since hoshin planning addresses a planning horizon of three to five years. Customer input is also solicited for quality improvement projects, but that input tends to relate to current and near-term customer requirements. Hoshin planning focuses on the longer term.

Establish organizational vision. This may have already been done as part of other TQM efforts. The vision should be based on the internal and external inputs, and should reflect as closely as possible a vision for the organization that will provide a positive motivation for the future. The vision should be positive, since people are not motivated by negative visions. Reducing costs, for example, may be necessary, but it is negative and cannot serve as a motivating vision.

Establish 3–5-year plan. As part of the planning effort, the long-term vision is translated into a 3–5-year plan with specific goals and a plan or means to achieve them. Particular attention is paid to breakthrough strategies and key processes for success. In some cases it is equally important to identify those portions of the business or activities that will be diminished or discontinued. There is a tendency to tell managers and staff that they should continue everything they are doing, no matter whether it is required by customers or not, and to put extra effort toward the organization's key strategies.

Often external factors play a key role in the plan. The expectations of employers, government, and third-party payers are currently having a major impact on the plans of healthcare organizations. Although UMMC has achieved substantial improvements in quality, customer satisfaction, cost effectiveness, working environment, and competitive position, for example, we are being expected to do much more. Our projections are that we must hold our costs constant over a four-year period of continuing inflation to remain cost competitive. This external expectation is a key part of our strategy for the next few years, along with continuous quality improvement.

No matter what other strategies are pursued, continuous quality improvement must be included. Without continuous quality improvement, any organization's future is at risk.

Develop annual objectives. Measurable annual objectives toward the long-term goals are important to communicate the expectations. However, it is very important to develop a plan for how the annual objectives can be achieved, with input from departments and staff. Goals without plans for achievement are unlikely to produce lasting change and contradict Deming's fourteen points (1986).

Deploy to departments. For departments to contribute meaningfully to the organization's vision and objectives, they must develop plans and objectives that support the organizational direction. First, the organization's vision, mission, goals, and objectives must be communicated to every division, manager, department, and staff person. Next, each department's mission and objectives should be developed to support the organization's breakthrough strategies.

Deploy to individuals. Every individual should be given a copy of the vision, mission, goals, and objectives for both the organization and his or her department. The performance plan for each person should then relate his or her plans and activities to achieving the larger departmental and organizational strategies and objectives. In this way at least a portion of every person's effort contributes to the organization's major goals. A portion of that person's time may be spent in supporting other ongoing activities. Of particular importance to individuals is what efforts can be eliminated or reduced, if they do not add value for customers. It is hard to align individuals to the organizational strategies and objectives if they perceive everything as additional work. It gives the impression that management is demanding everything rather than prioritizing the really important activities.

Implement. Simply having plans is inadequate. There must be a coordinated implementation effort to achieve the objectives, with the key processes regularly measured. Implementation will also involve changes for unexpected events.

Monitor progress. The principle of deployment is that every department and individual can measure progress each month related to the departmental and organizational goals. This keeps the focus on the priorities and provides regular feedback on progress.

Align reward and recognition with strategic objectives. One of the key difficulties of implementing any portion of TQM is that existing reward and recognition mechanisms are inconsistent with the proposed actions. If, for example, the strategic objective is to become the recognized high-quality provider, then groups and individuals must be rewarded for improving quality. On the other hand, if managers are recognized and rewarded for increasing revenues or indirectly "building empires," they will be focusing their efforts on empires rather than quality. A key component of alignment related to hoshin planning is to align the group and individual reward and recognition system with the strategic goals.

Conduct annual review. The annual review serves multiple purposes. First, it documents the progress toward the key departmental and organizational goals. Second, it provides a mechanism to recognize and reward efforts toward the goals. Third, it provides input to revise plans and to develop the next 3–5-year plan.

Reasons for Failure or Poor Results from Hoshin Planning

To date very few healthcare organizations have begun implementing hoshin planning. Consequently, there is little information about reasons for failure or poor results. However, based on the hoshin planning process, some cautions can be offered.

- Lack of leadership commitment.
- Do not obtain or use input from internal managers and staff. Participation is the key to commitment for any change involving people. If people help to develop the change, they will be committed to that change and will work hard to implement it.
- Failure to communicate the strategic plans and goals to managers and staff. If they do not know the priority issues

and objectives for the organization, they cannot direct their objectives to support them.

- Failure to align reward and recognition systems with the stated organizational priorities.

Action Step: Use hoshin planning methods to deploy your goals and strategic plans throughout your organization.

Selected References on Hoshin Planning

The following references can be used for a much more complete presentation on hoshin planning: *Hoshin Kanri: Policy Deployment for Successful TQM*, edited by Yoji Akao (1991); *Hoshin Planning: The Developmental Approach*, by Bob King (1989b); and *Hoshin Planning: A Planning System for Implementing Total Quality Management (TQM)*, by the GOAL/QPC Research Committee (1989).

Sample healthcare organizations that have implemented hoshin planning to varying degrees include Bethesda Hospital, Cincinnati, Ohio; Bryn Mawr Hospital, Bryn Mawr, Pennsylvania; Meadville Medical Center, Meadville, Pennsylvania; and Our Lady of Lourdes Medical Center, Camden, New Jersey.

PART FOUR

Reflections

Chapter Fifteen

Beyond the Glitter

There are many emotional peaks and valleys experienced when implementing a Total Quality Management Process. This chapter describes the highs, lows, and many frustrations that we and our friends encountered along our quality journeys. While the peaks are exhilarating, the reality shocks you will face when well-laid plans fail or resistance flares up are depressing. If you are the TQM champion and/or executive officer, your role is to nurture and breathe energy into the process when institutional energy and commitment are declining. We will present ideas and experiences from UMMC and other healthcare organizations so that you can learn from our missteps, anticipate possible friction points, and prepare strategies to address them.

First Steps Create Exhilaration

Following five one-day training sessions during 1989, called TQ 101–105, many of our managers grasped the potential of TQM and expressed hope that the process would help us begin our organizational transformation. The ability of quality to positively motivate was working. We heard people say, "This makes sense!" or "I've always managed this way." It seemed obvious to the TQM champions and our training and development staff that the managers would take this learning back to their units and begin to use the tools and techniques in their daily work.

Our curriculum planners worked hard to develop hands-on sessions to give the workshop attendees the opportunity to practice these new skills. We also developed a series of management actions to make sure managers could assimilate quality knowledge and begin to utilize it. We were swept away on a wave of enthusiasm. One could almost feel the excitement. What we found next, however, was a shock. We had confused knowledge with skill building. Learning the theory of quality was not enough; managers needed action plans and additional training to begin. There were many barriers to implementation, some of which came in rapid-fire succession, and others that took longer to develop. As we analyzed our problems, we drew the analogy to buying your first house. It looked great, it belonged to you, and it was all very exciting, until you had the first heavy rain. Then the basement began to leak, the paint peeled, the plumbing broke down, and the septic tank overflowed. You had scraped together all your resources for the purchase and had no money left to fix the problems. The enthusiasm and excitement expressed by our managers following TQ 101–105 clouded the long-term perspective of our leadership. Although we had created awareness of the new philosophy and new techniques, a long-term plan for supporting the new culture was not in place. The excitement motivated us but also caused us to neglect the details, which soon became apparent.

As we surveyed our problems and compared them to our high hopes, we were anxious. Would we be able to overcome the barriers? Could TQM work in healthcare? Today we know the answer is yes! Yes, TQM does work; and yes, the barriers are surmountable. We hope that by sharing the lessons we learned we can help you avoid the same errors, and help you save some of your resources for the elimination of barriers.

Post-Training Depression

While our audiences were interested and involved at the training sessions, the evaluations were far from outstanding. Many did not grasp how the principles of quality could help them in their daily work. Some did not understand the focus on statistical thinking. Many felt we were already a quality institution and could not see how this process would help. Even among those who gave us high marks, unless they were active quality team members, the course work did not stimulate them to adopt the quality process tools and techniques in their daily work. Today it is easy for us to see that while the theory was exciting and uplifting, the process for change was threatening and not clear. Even though we felt we had educated all managers about how to use tools and techniques outside the team experience, there was reticence to change, and our customers (the managers) did not feel comfortable. A common question from our managers was, "Now what do I do?" We found we had set our expectations too high. We assumed our managers to be able to utilize immediately the tools and techniques of TQM in their departments. We should have expected that people would have difficulty applying the knowledge. If knowledge by itself led to action we would all be thin, nonsmoking, healthier people. Just as human nature can keep us from changing personal habits to lead healthier lives, familiar work habits can keep us from adapting the new quality philosophy. "People can see the potential but they don't have the courage, conviction, or knowledge to commit themselves to translating the potential into results" (Shafer, 1991, p. 18). What seemed so simple at first glance is extremely complex. Our managers needed assistance in translating the lessons into actions. They needed to know when and how to utilize the process in daily work. They needed more time to explore the concepts and see how they could be applied.

We have discussed among friends and associates what happens to each person exposed to quality concepts to allow them to have a personal "Aha!" experience—that point when they can see exactly how the process can help them achieve personal or institutional goals. No commonality can be found in the responses. Sometimes it is a conference when a speaker says something that clears away the fog, sometimes it is a book, sometimes an experience with a team, and sometimes it just feels right; it is seen as the way to manage. If we knew the magic formula to cause this to happen, we would gladly share it with all of you. We believe the key is to create enough flexible opportunities for many to have the "Aha!" experience, especially among the managers of your organization who will be leading the process.

Drucker pointed out that "the greatest challenge to U.S. business in this decade, especially for large companies, will be the development of its management people. And we are totally unprepared for it" (Drucker, 1988, p. 25). As managers of managers and staff, we need to lead the way and model the new behaviors. We need to counsel, coach, and develop those who work for us. Many times our managers are crying out for assistance. One study of 261 managers in eighteen organizations found that "the managers needed more guidance, clearer feedback, more carefully established goals, more discussion of their management styles and more useful performance appraisals" (Longenecker and Giola, 1991, p. 81). Review your management education courses. If your program is old and needs to be updated, speak with a local community college, business school, or leading area businesses. Develop a program based on helping managers adjust to the ambiguity of the current healthcare environment. Include change theory and exercises on decision making. These elements may be necessary before you begin TQM education.

Action Step: Make sure your early expectations are realistic. Practical knowledge of "how" to begin must accompany the education and training in theory. Make practical tools and aids available to managers to support the quality process. Create opportunities for the "Aha!" experience.

Management Resistance

When our educational program began, we found we could divide management reaction into three categories, as illustrated in Figure 15.1.

One-third felt the process held tremendous potential. They gave us high marks on the evaluations of the seminars, showed their enthusiasm, and actually began to implement techniques in their departments. Another third were fence sitters

Figure 15.1. Rule of Thirds.

1/3	1/3	1/3

Total Quality is the right approach.	Fence sitters: I'll do if my boss does.	This will never work.

and had a wait-and-see attitude about the process. They gave us mediocre evaluations and tended to keep their feelings to themselves, but they were not enthusiastic about TQM. The final third displayed all the outward signs of resistance. Their evaluations were negative, and while they may have understood the concepts, they were not about to buy in.

As the Total Quality Council reviewed the evaluations and impressions, we brainstormed reasons why this resistance was expressed and developed some strategies to overcome resistance. These issues and the strategies we developed may help you deal with resistance in your organization.

Insecurity

With the turmoil in our industry today, many managers are concerned about the future. When managers are insecure, they exhibit certain symptoms. The first is a lack of flexibility. Managers give the impression: "There is only one way to do things — my way!" The second symptom is overanalysis of the data. There is so much fear present that managers are afraid to make a mistake. When TQM is suggested as a strategy, the red flags go up for this group. Why isn't my input needed anymore? Why do we need to ask employees for input? What is my role? These are the unspoken questions. When employee teams begin to bring forward their ideas for improvement, insecurity in this group will tend to increase. People wonder, "Will senior management think I haven't been doing my job? If this process is successful, will the organization still need me?" Peter Grazier points out: "Historically, insecurity has remained in check because managers have been in charge of the flow of information. Participative management concepts by their very nature, bring latent insecurity to the surface" (1989, p. 94). What concerns are your managers dealing with? A good way to determine this is to ask them. Arrange small focus groups where concerns can be raised and strategies can be explored. When the pyramid is turned upside down to put the employees in touch with the customers, managers are still caught in the middle, as Figure 15.2 illustrates. After TQM implementation, the managers still have the role of coordinator, coach, educator, and facilitator.

Managers must be reassured that the goal of the process is to keep talented people, not eliminate them. The most effective way to eliminate management positions is through attrition. When a manager leaves the organization, the questions should be: Do we need to replace this person? Could a self-directed work team be formed? Could the duties of this manager be combined with others? While the managers' role may change, their value to the organization will not. Quality improvement comes from attacking process problems, not people. Through quality improvement techniques, we can unleash creativity and innovation and improve our effectiveness. It will be possible to free the manager from the restrictive bureaucracy and allow change to take place.

Figure 15.2. Managers Caught in the Middle.

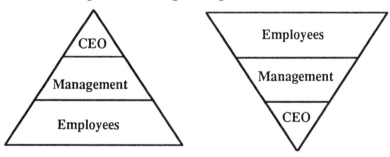

Before Transformation   **After Transformation**

Action Steps:
1. Demonstrate the need for change.
2. Make sure all levels of managers are included in the planning process.
3. Give managers the tools and techniques to be successful.
4. Make the commitment to place managers in nonmanagement positions, if management reductions are necessary.

Personal Values in Conflict with Quality Approach

Most of our managers learned the command and control style of management based on the historical military model. This is the only style they know. When managers give all the directions, employees conclude they are not being paid to think about improvement. Employees learn not to offer ideas or suggestions. Donald Petersen and John Hillkirk described the effects of this management style: "In most work places, the problem is not this glaring. The managers don't routinely berate or belittle people. They might even say they're interested in hearing their workers' ideas. But it is quite clear that most of the time, the leaders' opinions are the only ones that really count" (1991, p. 4). The change from a top-down type of management to an employee-centered type of management does not happen overnight. There must be time, education, and appropriate organizational support for managers to assess their current management style, see how this style may be negatively impacting business goals, build new skills, and develop a personal action plan for change.

Action Step: Develop values clarification exercises to demonstrate why the new management philosophy and empowerment are necessary. Provide guidance and support for managers so they can evaluate and adjust their style.

One interesting exercise we used, to illustrate the importance of empowerment, was to have managers brainstorm a list of the positive reasons they should be empowered by their superiors. The title at the top of the flipchart should read

Reasons Why My Boss Should Empower Me. The list usually includes
such items as:

- I'm closer to the work and I know what the problems are.
- I have good ideas.
- I have money-saving ideas to contribute.
- I could contribute more than I do.
- My boss doesn't understand what could be done.
- My technical skills are better.
- I am the one doing the work.
- I want to learn and develop.

The group facilitator then takes a second color marker
and changes the title on the flipchart slightly. First the facilitator
crosses out the words "my boss" and "me," and then substitutes
the words "I" and "others." The title now reads, *Reasons Why I
Should Empower Others.* This exercise is a very powerful tool to
show the paradox of empowerment. We all want to be empowered by our bosses but have trouble empowering others.
Peter Block writes: "While empowerment is a state of mind it is
also the result of position, policies, and practices. As managers
we become more powerful as we nurture the power of those
below us" (1987, p. 64). Allowing managers to talk about empowerment and the organizational requirements for employee
involvement may help you avoid the paradox.

Ego Protection

Becoming a manager is an exciting and challenging career
move. There are usually several perquisites that accompany a
new job as well. Among other things a promotion can mean an
office, a secretary, a salary increase, and a special status in the
organization. It is not hard to understand why people become
used to this new status and attention. Most managers would
define their main strength as being an effective problem solver.
Deming would remind us that many times problem solving is
merely "tampering." When we as managers respond inappropriately to an apparent special event and we take action,

operating on faulty data, we may actually make the problems worse. In healthcare we seem proud of the fact we are fire fighters, until people begin to realize that they have solved the same problems year after year without achieving resolution. Many managers defend fire fighting. They feel important when they can calm a crisis. These same individuals claim they have no time for learning the new ways because they have to get their normal work done. A major barrier is convincing managers that TQM is not additional work, but the way they should do all work. Getting to root causes means problems will be much more effectively solved. Also, we have observed that too few managers have learned how to listen to others and integrate suggestions in their planning process. Managers have taken their responsibilities seriously, and they become the center of attention and control for their department. Grazier hit the nail on the head: "Managers consequently see themselves as the provider of answers to any and all questions" (Grazier, 1989, p. 100).

Our jobs support the attainment of career goals and, more important, our financial well-being. Our status and ego are all wrapped up in what we do. For many of us, our jobs are critically important. Many think of themselves as synonymous with their current positions. Think about the questions a stranger asks on meeting you: Who are you? What do you do? It should not come as a surprise that any plan to change our job may be seen as a threat. If we see a challenge or threat to our ego and security, the response may be turf-guarding and ego protection. Each person's knowledge, skill, and ability to contribute to the organization should be viewed as separate from his or her current position, both by the person and the organization. Make sure people see their value to the organization beyond their current jobs. Let managers explore the new philosophy and experience autonomy and freedom. Begin to break down barriers to empowerment through focus sessions. Bring in customers to discuss the strengths and weaknesses of your services. Ask them to identify the characteristics of a healthcare provider of choice.

Action Step: View employees' value separately from their current jobs, and encourage everyone else to do the same. This is necessary if you wish to become a flexible, learning organization.

Action Step: Begin your process with managers serving both as team leaders and team members. Let them experience empowerment before they empower others. Recognize that fears and anxieties exist. Allow time for issues to surface and talk about strategies to overcome these issues.

Managers Feel Excluded

In many organizations there clearly is a "Father Knows Best" style of management that exists from the top of the hierarchy to the front-line supervisor. Historically, those at the top have left other managers out of the planning process. The strategic initiatives of the organization were discussed by a few trusted executives and then communicated downward with a trust-me attitude. The exclusionary behavior is modeled at every level. Many times, as important messages travel downward in the organization, the messages become garbled and inconsistent. Few managers or employees could repeat a consistent, let alone the original, message. To be a TQM organization many people in the organization must contribute to the planning process. In the early stages of planning, solicit input from mid- and front-line managers. Discuss the rudimentary process and ask them to help shape the plan. Once the plan is clear, think about how to communicate it. We recognized our communication problems and began to script messages and develop slides and other presentation materials for important communications in 1991. These presentations were then given by the associate hospital directors (vice presidents), or their direct reports, to both hospital and Medical School groups, using a common set of presentation materials. The messages now are more consistent. Each line administrator can use examples from his or her division, and front-line employees have a chance to question, contribute, and play a role in planning. The central message was tailored to each division and allowed many more people to hear the message and play a role. Hoshin planning, discussed in Chapter Fourteen, is a complex yet proven strategy for organizational planning that uses this philosophy.

Action Step: Involve your managers in the planning process. Help them share important information with appropriately consistent tools and formats.

TQM Requires That Leaders Change First

How management behaves and models the desired behaviors during the change process and beyond will be the key to your organization's success with TQM. Roland Dumas (1990, p. 79) wrote about his experiences as a consultant for Zenger-Miller. He analyzed how training dollars were spent on quality efforts: "80 percent of the outside expenditures went for technical training and installing new systems, such as cost of quality. Less than 20 percent of the money was related to management leadership and involvement in the programs. When respondents were asked where the major problems were the ratios reversed. Eighty percent of the problems were associated with management leadership, support, and involvement, and twenty percent related to technical skills. In other words the Pareto Principle was stood on its head; 80 percent of the effort was going to fix 20 percent of the problem." Make sure you are preparing your managers to lead the transformation.

In summary, the keys to reducing management resistance are:

- Preparing managers for the renewal strategy with educational offerings
- Clearly articulating the rationale for change
- Involving managers actively in the planning process
- Developing further education based on individual needs
- Highlighting the importance of meeting all customers' needs, internal as well as external
- Allowing time for skill building and practice of new skills through role playing
- Developing or purchasing tools to assess personal management style and developing an institutional methodology to change management style to meet new cultural demands

- Providing assistance with the management style change process
- Facilitating the experience of empowerment from executives to managers below them *before* expecting them to empower employees
- Asking senior managers to teach and model skills for lower-level managers
- Creating an atmosphere of openness through sharing important data on organizational performance with all workers
- Creating opportunities for executives and senior managers to model key quality skills
- Developing the means for increased management visibility—management by walking around
- Scripting important messages for broad communication; following up in print media
- Developing reward and recognition strategies to reinforce new behaviors
- Providing the opportunity for everyone to develop creative and innovative problem-solving skills
- Integrating empowerment into management performance planning objectives

Tools to Smooth the Way

TQM is not a robust process; it is very fragile. While most organizations look to their managers to implement TQM, managers are poorly equipped to carry out this role. To educate and support our managers for this critical role we found we needed many new management tools and techniques. The tools and techniques described below helped us keep our process on track.

Expectations of Management

One of our first discoveries was that we had never spelled out our organizational expectations for managers. It was as if we expected new managers to learn what was required by osmosis. A task team, led by the associate director for inpatient services, developed the initial draft of our Management Expectations, which were then submitted for broad management review and input.

An interesting lesson occurred during the development of this document. When an external consultant visited the Medical Center, we shared with pride our newly developed Management Expectations. He pointed out that he understood our zeal to include the humanistic side of management, but informed us that we had omitted such mainstays of management performance as meeting budget, plans for the future, and other established basic management expectations. The team quickly reconvened and reworked our expectations, which appear in Exhibit 11.1. (We completed our book *Transforming Healthcare Organizations* [1990] during the early stages of developing these expectations, so that the last one, "Coordinate resources and activities to meet society's expectations as well as our own objectives of quality and efficiency," was not included there.)

Management Action Tool

The second tool developed in 1989 is called the Management Action Tool (MAT). The MAT was based on the Management Expectations. The purpose was to give the managers a series of actions to begin to use TQM concepts, tools, and techniques in their daily work. The MAT has been revised several times as our knowledge of TQM evolved. This tool, listing Manager Actions, is explained in Chapter Eleven.

The Manager's Guide to TQM

As we watched managers struggle to begin the process in their departments, we identified the need for a guidebook for managers (University of Michigan Medical Center, 1991b). The purpose of the guidebook was to give suggestions on how to begin using quality tools and techniques in daily work. A task team of employees, led by the lead team facilitator for professional services, began their work in 1990. We first conducted a management needs assessment to determine what the managers, the customers for this process, desired. This process identified the quality issues managers were having difficulty implementing. The team brainstormed ideas, gathered resources, and developed the first draft of the guide. The first draft was then pilot tested with a small group of managers. The pilot managers were interviewed to see which techniques were helpful and which were not. The guide was then reorganized and edited based on customer feedback. The highlights include:

- Steps to build an environment of continuous improvement
- Exercises to begin to solicit employee input
- Practical steps for managers to introduce basic management and TQM concepts

Our facilitators report that the guide has been very helpful to managers who want to begin to utilize the process in their departments. Using a tool like this helps to integrate TQM skills into daily work. The table of contents of the guide is listed in Exhibit 15.1.

Action Step: Make sure appropriate tools and techniques are available to help managers with the implementation process. Frequently ask managers and team leaders what is working well and what can be improved.

Exhibit 15.1. Contents of Manager's Guide to Begin Total Quality Process.

1. Introduction
2. Explaining the Need to Change
3. Understanding and Learning to Live by Expectations of Management
4. Describing and Communicating Departmental Mission — Values
5. Identifying Processes, Customers, and Requirements
6. Understanding Process Capability
7. Evaluating and Prioritizing Potential Improvements
8. Assessing the QI-Readiness of Your Work Unit
9. References

Leadership for Total Quality and MAAP

In 1991 we found our managers required additional educational support to create a new culture. Working with an internal consultant from human resources and with an external consultant, we designed a course to help managers understand how their style and management behavior affected the culture. We used the Life Styles Inventory, a tool developed as a companion piece to the Cultural Audit by Human Synergistics, Plymouth, Michigan.

A prerequisite for the course required that each manager fill out a questionnaire that described his or her personal management style. A second step was to ask five people, a combination of peers and subordinates, to fill out the same form describing how they viewed the manager's style. The people completing the questionnaires mailed them to the consultant for scoring, and the information was completely confidential. After the questionnaires were scored, a small group of managers attended a one-and-a-half-day seminar to learn about the management styles. They learned how the style they described compared to the style described by others, and how their style affected the overall culture. The information was presented in a constructive manner, with the goal of helping the managers to understand better who they are and why they act the way they do. Managers were given special assistance to evaluate their strengths and weaknesses and to develop specific action plans for personal change. As managers, our performance in the past was normally judged on our contribution to the bottom line. For many this was the first time they had received honest feedback about their behaviors. The final half day was spent in preparing a Management Assessment and Action Plan (MAAP). The management characteristics from this tool are given in Exhibit 15.2. This tool helps the manager assess key management behaviors and monitor progress on these behaviors over time.

It is helpful to see your personal scores and feedback, as well as where you stand as a peer. We began this process with the top executives and clinical chairmen of the organization. We then extended the opportunity to attend the course to all man-

Exhibit 15.2. Management Assessment and Action Plan (MAAP).©

1. Accomplishes challenging, but achievable, self-set goals.
2. Thinks and plans ahead.
3. Considers options before taking actions.
4. Takes moderate risks.
5. Work is well thought out and complete.
6. Demonstrates energy and enthusiasm toward work.
7. Knows technical side of the business.
8. Makes decisions and follows through.
9. Uses a daily "To Do" list.
10. Demonstrates that quality is a high priority.
11. Invests in own growth.
12. Creates enjoyment in his or her work.
13. States ideas in a clear way.
14. Thinks in independent and innovative ways.
15. Will take a stand for values and beliefs.
16. Identifies the needs of others and strives to meet them.
17. Involves subordinates in decisions when appropriate.
18. Constructively resolves conflicts.
19. Promotes others' professional development.
20. Gives undivided attention when listening.
21. Provides positive rewards to others in a variety of ways.
22. Makes taking time with people a high priority.
23. Helps others think through alternatives.
24. Provides a lot of feedback.
25. Looks for and praises positive aspects of performance.
26. Provides constructive input for improving performance.
27. Treats people in a friendly, pleasant way.
28. Does things to make everyone feel a part of the group.
29. Freely expresses himself or herself.
30. Considers impact on others before acting.

Source: Management Vector Analysis, Jackson, Michigan, 1991.

agers and supervisors. The evaluations of the course have been outstanding, although the information gained often indicates substantial change is required. It was surprising to see how many of our managers had never been given feedback on their strengths and weaknesses.

The CEO Annual Report on Quality

Beginning in January 1992 and each January thereafter, an annual report that chronicles the progress of the TQM process at the medical center will be produced. The report format includes an executive summary, the milestones in the process, updates on structure, team efforts, education, rewards and recognition, quality indicators, and any other quality information. This report is presented to the hospital executive board and then distributed to all employees with a cover letter from the CEO. This is an important communication tool for the organization. The major milestones from our process are illustrated in Table 15.1.

These types of tools, combined with appropriate management education, skill building, and practice time, give managers the assistance required to make major changes.

Problems in Developing a Customer Focus

We experienced many problems as we tried to develop a customer-focused organization. Most of our problems related to the fact that healthcare has not been customer focused. Our systems and processes were established with the providers as the main customers.

Negative Reaction to the Term Customer

When we began in 1987, there was an extremely negative reaction to the word *customer*. It was difficult for many people to see the term as indicating a complex new relationship with both internal and external customers. Most viewed the term as a synonym for patient. We spent time and important organizational energy debating whether or not *customer* was a good word. One UMMC team leader actually assigned a team member, who was against the use of the term, to research the meaning of the word in the current literature. The team member was given several articles to read and an assignment of reporting back to the team. After investigating the literature, he reported that his understanding had been less than comprehensive; he could see that the term described a relationship and was not just a term from industry that did not fit the healthcare milieu. He now understood its significance. Sometimes the reaction to the word

Table 15.1. Milestones in the UMMC Total Quality Process.

Milestones in the Total Quality Process	Start Date	How the Milestone Contributed to Total Quality Process
National Demonstration Project	Sep. 87	Joined a research study which demonstrated that industrial quality control principles were applicable to healthcare.
Admission/Discharge Pilot Project	Sep. 87	Provided evidence that UMMC could benefit from implementation of Total Quality principles.
Total Quality Task Force	Sep. 87	Served as driving force behind initiation of the Total Quality Process at UMMC.
Innovation & Creativity Task Force	Sep. 87	Identified environmental barriers to creativity and innovation, reviewed literature and other educational materials and reached a set of recommendations.
Vision & Values Task Force	Sep. 87	Developed formal "Statement of Quality" via employee focus groups, served as initial statement about the values encouraged through the Total Quality Process.
Work Reorganization Task Force	Sep. 87	Developed plan to evaluate levels of training and competency required to perform tasks. Led to department/nursing unit specific efforts, which produced several redesigned processes.
Total Quality Council	Dec. 88	Reconfigured Total Quality Task Force as a Council, continued to serve as driving force behind initiation of the Total Quality Process.
Physician Orientation	Jan. 89	Created initial physician awareness of UMMC's involvement in the Total Quality Process.
Statement of Quality	Mar. 89	Developed by Vision & Values Task Force, prominently displayed in organization as reminder of UMMC's Quality Values.
Total Quality 101–103	Mar. 89	Marked the move from organizational awareness to organizational knowledge.
Departmental Quality Indicators	Mar. 89	Asked departments to begin identifying both internal and external customers' requirements and create valid indicators to monitor progress.
Communication & Materiel Task Force	May 89	Developed plan to improve communication with staff at all levels of the organization.
Reward & Recognition Task Force	May 89	Developed plan to reward and recognize both individual and team contributions to organizational effectiveness.
Training & Education Task Force	May 89	Developed comprehensive plan to train personnel at all levels of the organization.
Work Force Diversity Task Force	May 89	Developed plan to make managers and workers sensitive to issues related to a diverse work force.

Table 15.1. Milestones in the UMMC Total Quality Process, Cont'd.

Milestones in the Total Quality Process	Start Date	How the Milestone Contributed to Total Quality Process
Clinical Departmental Grand Rounds	Oct. 89	Increased physician awareness of benefits of the Total Quality Process at the UMMC.
Employee Orientation	Oct. 89	Assured that every existing and new UMMC employee had a rudimentary understanding of the Total Quality Process.
Expectations of Management	Nov. 89	Informed individual managers of the management style and practices expected of them to support the Total Quality Process.
Manager's Guide	Feb. 90	Provided step-by-step instructions to begin the Total Quality Process in an individual department.
Healthcare Forum/Witt Award	Apr. 90	Recognized UMMC's efforts to achieve organizational excellence through the Total Quality Process.
Team Leader, Facilitator, and Member Training purchased from Qualtec	May 90	Provided formal process for education in TQ principles for team members, leaders, and facilitators. Also supplied formal team storyboard process.
Institutional Quality Indicators	Jul. 90	Development of Quality Indicators encouraged UMMC to evaluate customer requirements.
UMMC Vision Statement	Jul. 90	Aligned efforts of the organization with the future desired characteristics of the Medical Center.
Corporate Lead Team	Sep. 90	Established to coordinate the Total Quality Process throughout the Medical Center. Replaced TQ Council.
Divisional Lead Teams	Sep. 90	Serve to sanction, support, and recognize team efforts. Help to prioritize opportunities for improvement within.
Cultural Assessment	Oct. 90	Identified optimal desired "Constructive" Culture. Identified our position relative to the ideal.
Quality Improvement Video	Oct. 90	Enhanced orientation of employees to the Total Quality Process.
UMMC Goals	Oct. 90	Provided basis for employees to evaluate their own work and decide if they were helping UMMC move toward shared goals.
Total Quality Process Plan	Dec. 90	Developed by Corporate Lead Team as tool to educate UMMC about Strategic Plan for integration of the Total Quality Process at UMMC.
Quality Function Deployment Training	Dec. 90	Initiated training relative to Quality Function Deployment techniques for the development of new products and services taking customer requirements into consideration "up front."

Table 15.1. Milestones in the UMMC Total Quality Process, Cont'd.

Milestones in the Total Quality Process	Start Date	How the Milestone Contributed to Total Quality Process
Awareness Sessions	Jan. 91	Designed to integrate the various pieces of the Total Quality Process for employees.
Centralized Facilitators	Jan. 91	Assisted in implementation of the Total Quality Process through facilitation of Divisional Lead Teams and individual Quality Improvement Teams. Facilitators also enhance educational process.
Leadership for Total Quality	Jan. 91	Produced individualized action plan for each participating manager relative to behavioral changes required to produce an optimal culture supportive of the Total Quality Process.
Quality Function Deployment Project in Medical Procedures Unit	Feb. 91	Began utilization of QFD techniques to design processes for the new Medical Procedures Unit.
Applied Management Practices Group	Mar. 91	Developed Applied Management Practices Group to consult on Total Quality to other healthcare organizations.
Chairs' Retreat	Apr. 91	Developed a plan for the Clinical Quality Improvement Initiative.
Total Quality Exposition	May 91	Served as first celebration of Total Quality achievements especially those made by Quality Improvement Teams.
Clinical Quality Improvement Initiative	Jun. 91	Marked beginning of comprehensive program to provide high-quality, cost-effective clinical care.
Cost/Benefit Analysis	Oct. 91	Indicated that the Total Quality Process made sense not only as a Transformation Strategy, but financially as well.
Departmental Quality Indicators	Oct. 91	Departmental indicators were largely developed. The process required was as useful as the indicators themselves.
Gainsharing Program	Oct. 91	Aligned employee incentives with organizational goal of cost effectiveness.
Nursing Mutual Gains Contract Ratification	Jan. 92	Marked success of collaborative problem-solving approach to negotiations with unions.

Source: University of Michigan Hospitals, 1992, pp. 6–8.

customer may not be vocalized. Spend time explaining the significance, and resistance will be diminished.

We began to use the supplier-customer arrow graphic,

previously presented in Figure 2.2, to illustrate the new relationship we were trying to create and the importance of customer satisfaction to our organizational success. Today the word *customer* is a common and accepted term in our organizational vocabulary. We have also noted, during presentations throughout the United States, that the term is now gaining wide use and acceptance in healthcare.

Listening to the Voice of the Customer?

Our second series of reality shocks, related to the development of a customer focus, also occurred early in the process. One of the final assignments for managers at the completion of our training sessions was to identify major processes within their department, list the customers, and define their requirements. Many units and departments did begin to identify customers and determine requirements. What surprised us, however, was that many were not talking to the customers to determine if their assumptions were valid. You cannot understand customer requirements if you depend on assumptions or customer surveys alone. You must validate the accuracy of your assessment by directly asking the customer in telephone interviews, focus groups, and one-on-one conversations. The kinds of questions we should be asking customers include:

- What are we doing well?
- What do we need to improve?
- What are your requirements?
- Have we met your requirements?
- How could we better meet your requirements?
- What do we provide that you do not require? This is an important and often overlooked question, because we frequently provide things the customers do not care about.
- Did you realize the outcome you expected?
- What factors would cause you to choose us for healthcare?
- What factors would cause you to choose someone else?

If we wish to improve, we must learn how to listen more effectively. Managers and employees should be involved in customer conversations. There is no better way to assess if your quality process is having the desired results on customer satisfaction.

New Customer-Oriented Training

When patients come to your organization, they rarely see the CEO or senior executives. While physicians play a key role in patient care, many other employees interact closely with the patient. Patients spend the most time with the front-line employees. From the door attendants, to the clericals, to the technicians, each employee encounter has a significant bearing on how your customers will evaluate you. Guest relations training is a good beginning in determining customer needs, but more sophisticated training is required. In healthcare we are so accustomed to making decisions for the customer that a complete change in approach is required. An article by Erie Chapman helped provide insights for our employees. Chapman's premise, summarized in Exhibit 15.3, is that we tend to treat patients like prisoners and that a major change is needed to involve patients in their care and allow them to be controllers of their own destiny (1990, p. 18).

The Chapman article can become the subject for focus groups of employees to talk about the customer friendliness of the organization. Obviously in an industry with such a poor service history, we need more than the guest relations programs

Exhibit 15.3. Patients and Prisoners: The Parallels.

- Have clothes taken away
- Are assigned a number
- Turn over their valuables
- Are assigned a stranger as a roommate
- Are allowed to see family on limited basis
- Lead lives according to institution's schedule
- Give up control over lives
- Enter bleak, cold environments

Source: Chapman, 1990.

of the past. Common courtesy is essential, but there is much more that must be done.

Questions About Customer Orientation

Many healthcare organizations claim they are customer focused. How do you determine how you measure up? The following list of questions can be used with employees to demonstrate customer awareness.

- Do you understand the word *customer*?
- Who are your personal customers?
- What strategies does your organization have in place to challenge the basic principles that govern a patient's hospital stay?
- Are your processes customer focused or provider focused?
- Is the customer respected, and are customer needs met above all else?
- How do you test for customer-oriented policies and practices?
- Are your employees placed in wheelchairs or on crutches as a part of their orientation process to understand how difficult it is to traverse your environment?
- What other type of sensitivity training occurs for health professionals?
- Are customers asked to evaluate the demeanor and sensitivity of the providers?
- What else could be done to make the customer interface more acceptable to patients and families?

We become so used to the life and death situations in our business, that we tend to forget the impact that our words and actions have on our customers. One of the most helpful things for our employees to keep in mind is that most of our customers would rather be elsewhere. Healthcare, particularly hospitalizations or surgical procedures, would be avoided by most if possible. We have to try much harder than most industries to delight our customers.

Learning to Listen

The listening process must begin with developing an awareness of customers. First the customers must be identified, and then strategies developed to open lines of communication. Two successful strategies we utilized to create customer awareness were open forums for unhappy customers and a special showing of the movie "The Doctor." The first strategy was arranged through our patient relations office. We identified families whose experience with our organization had been negative. Clearly their requirements had not been met. The chief of nursing affairs met with the families and then invited them to come to a special session to tell the story of their experiences to our staff. For most of the staff, hearing these stories was very painful. However, they all expressed their gratitude for understanding the perspective of the patient and family members. All attendees felt the direct learning method is critical in developing customer sensitivity and better customer-focused processes.

There is no doubt that listening to the voice of the customer creates a competitive advantage, but it requires a major shift in thinking. You must continually evaluate how well you listen to the customers of your organization.

Action Step: Encourage employees to talk to external customers. Encourage them to ask patients: How was your visit? What went well? What went poorly? What could be improved?

Action Step: Encourage managers and executives to make rounds and ask internal and external customers what their requirements are and how they are being satisfied. Then communicate the information and initiate changes to make improvements.

Customer Complaints

Some organizations believe that a reduction in the number of complaints is a key sign of success. While this is important, we would add a note of caution. Patients do not like to voice complaints to healthcare organizations. There is a fear that if they voice their complaints, they may be treated differently or even receive worse care. They feel trapped. Also, a significant number of patients will not complain but will simply go to a new provider. Keep in mind that hearing complaints allows you to find problems and fix them. If you focus on reducing the number of complaints, you may also reduce your early warning system. Solicitation of problems is a key strategy in customer satisfaction. Ask your patients for complaints and, more important, actively solicit ideas, potential for improvement, and compliments. Be prepared to take action on these suggestions immediately.

Track and trend patient concerns. Assign a group of staff to manage concerns as quickly as possible. Use the data on a routine basis to identify areas of improvement.

Issues with Teams

A number of issues and lessons have been learned about team efforts to improve quality.

Early Team Success Is Encouraging

By 1989 there were three pilot teams making excellent progress. As these teams reported back, our educational process was in full swing. We developed the educational curriculum for the first phase and began to educate our executives, medical staff leadership, managers, and supervisors. We essentially jumped right into the process. Many managers were inspired by the success, anxious to use their new skills, and so they rushed to set up teams. However, the quality council recognized that things were out of control. We had no idea of how many teams we had, what they were working on, how much they were costing, or what results they were achieving. We found that many teams did not share their results. They had saved dollars but were afraid the organization would seize the dollars and punish them by reducing departmental budgets rather than rewarding them for their efforts.

Inadequate Training

Early in our process, we realized our team leaders and facilitators needed more specialized training. Although we had extensive training and development resources to speed our process along, we decided to utilize the team training process of Qualtec Quality Services. This training is based on the successful process that Florida Power and Light (FP&L) used to compete for and win the Deming Prize, Japan's highest quality award. FP&L is the only American company to receive this honor. Purchasing FP&L training materials allowed us to avoid developing our own, which our director of training and development estimated would take a year or more.

Qualtec training required a definition of roles and responsibilities of team members and specific training. Upon purchase, the question arose whether teams could continue without training. The risk was that unprepared team leaders might be unsuccessful, claim they had tried TQM, and that it did not work in their departments. The quality council tried to strike a balance between supporting innovation and creativity of untrained teams and encouraging appropriate team training. Our response was to allow the teams already formed to continue. Practicing team leaders were the first persons eligible for the training sessions. We developed formal definitions for the teams. A Quality Improvement Team must meet the following criteria: have a trained team leader, and a trained team facilitator, meet regularly once a week for an hour or every other week for two hours, and follow the seven-step quality improvement process. Teams that did not meet all four criteria were called Improvement Teams. As our process developed, there were other types of teams that evolved, one was called a Quality Project Team. This type of team also used quality tools and techniques to solve institutional problems. All three of these teams are problem-solving or opportunity-improvement teams. Finally, natural work teams are evolving. These teams are work teams that have regularly scheduled meetings, the size is five to ten members, and they manage normal business utilizing team concepts. Chapter Eight contains additional information on teams.

Time for Training as a Barrier

Our goal was to educate all managers and clinical leaders as team leaders and facilitators. This process called for five days of training each for team leader and facilitator programs. When we analyzed how long it would take us to accomplish our goal, there was a three-year time frame. We quickly realized another timing barrier in the institution. Given the time required to train managers as leaders and facilitators, we chose to support full-time facilitator/trainers to support our aggressive training initiative. These facilitators teach the courses and serve as experts until such time as all managers have completed training as leaders and facilitators.

Success in Spite of Problems

Our first teams deserve high accolades for perseverance. There was no structure for support, no system of reward or recognition, and little effective leadership for the process. In many ways it proved to us how effective teamwork can be, because the teams thrived in spite of the lack of support.

Some Early Mistakes

Despite significant success, the first years of our Total Quality Process were fraught with mistakes. Although we were learning by doing, the process was very painful. As we look back, the power of the process enabled us to thrive in spite of our flawed approaches. The following list contains some of our early mistakes.

- The process for rolling out TQM across the organization was unclear and ill-defined. There was no strategic plan, and people were not sure where we were going.

- Goals for the teams and the TQM process were fuzzy.
- There was not an effective training program for team leaders or facilitators.
- The facilitators (our management engineering staff) became the team leaders by default because they had the most sophisticated skills in the area of statistical process control.
- Accountabilities for the teams were unclear, particularly for cross-functional teams.
- The teams were isolated from each other; no support groups existed to share strategies and experiences.
- Few teams were working on issues that were critical to organizational success.

Once the mistakes were identified, we took steps to create the education and support systems necessary.

Action Step: Develop a strategic plan early in your process.

More Team Problems

We reached a point, in our fourth year, where many teams were stalled. We were puzzled. We pleaded and pushed, and yet many teams seemed unable to find time to meet, and forward momentum was slow. Our consultant from Qualtec suggested that we needed to develop a more effective monitoring system. This reinforced what many of us believed—that what you measure, you improve. The lead teams began to ask why teams were not meeting, did they need any help, and what was restricting progress. The answers indicated that many teams were not meeting regularly. Lack of regular meeting times leads to loss of momentum. If weekly meetings are problematic, every other week for two hours seems to work just as well. We developed some measuring techniques so the lead teams have something to focus on and problems can be diagnosed and solved. Measurements include: time spent in each step, team trained, meetings that are canceled, meetings the facilitator misses, meetings with poor attendance. Data are collected on team progress using the form illustrated in Exhibit 15.4. Then summary graphs of the following are developed:

- Active versus proposed quality teams, as illustrated in Figure 15.3.
- Types of active teams, as illustrated in Figure 15.4.
- Types of active and proposed teams, as illustrated in Figure 15.5.
- QI story steps of active teams, as illustrated in Figure 15.6.
- Completed QI stories, as illustrated in Figure 15.7.

Develop Questions to Ask About Team Progress

While these steps may appear bureaucratic in the beginning, changing the way you do business is a major undertaking, and these practices can be discarded as the organization learns the new ways. The new rules also make clear to managers the level of senior management commitment. It is not enough to start teams; the teams must complete the process or they become like the committees of old. Getting to root causes and applying appropriate countermeasures will yield ultimate success.

Action Step: Monitor and communicate team progress. Develop specific measures and report results to the organization. Determine indicators of team achievement. Recognize and reward teams upon completion or achievement of significant steps and goals.

Lack of a Strategic Plan

As stated several times, we did not have a strategic plan when we began. We started with a pilot team. Our COO developed a rudimentary plan that we used to explain what we felt lay ahead, as illustrated in Figure 15.8.

Many other healthcare organizations also spent inadequate time in planning their approach. For example, the COO from the University of California San Diego Medical Center told us they also had jumped right into the team process without effective planning and ultimately had to refocus to get the

Exhibit 15.4. Status Report of Active Teams/Completed Storyboards.

Team Location	IT	F	X	T	P	T	1	2	3	4	5	6	7	NA	C	Facilitator	Comments
Active Teams/Completed Storyboards																	
		Type					Step in Process										
Clinical Quality Improvement (7 Teams)			x		x											D. Guglielmo	Formed 8/91
			x		x											L. Price	Formed 8/91
			x		x	x										W. Behnke	Formed 8/91
			x		x											R. Coffey	Formed 8/91
	x				x											A. Perry	Formed 9/91
	x				x											A. Perry	Formed 9/91
	x				x											M. D. Staples	Formed 9/91
Financial Services (19 Teams)			x		x											L. Clevenger	Formed 6/89
	x													x		NA	Formed 9/91
	x													x		NA	Formed 9/91
				x											x	N. Gilbert	Formed 10/89
				x											x	N. Gilbert	Formed 10/89
				x											x	N. Gilbert	Formed 10/89
				x											x	N. Gilbert	Formed 10/89
				x											x	N. Gilbert	Formed 10/89
				x											x	N. Gilbert	Formed 10/89
	x													x		NA	Formed 9/91
	x													x		NA	Formed 9/91
				x											x	T. Bates	Formed 10/89
	x													x		T. Bates	Formed 6/91
	x													x		NA	Formed 9/91
	x													x		NA	Formed 9/91
	x													x		NA	Formed 9/91
	x													x		W. Behnke	Formed 9/91
				x											x	W. Behnke	Formed 10/89
	x													x		NA	Formed 9/91

Figure 15.3. Active Versus Proposed Quality Teams.

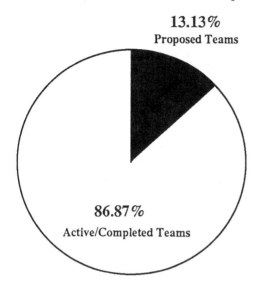

13.13%
Proposed Teams

86.87%
Active/Completed Teams

N = 99 Teams

14 of 99 Completed
13 of 99 Proposed
72 of 99 Active

Figure 15.4. Types of Active Teams.

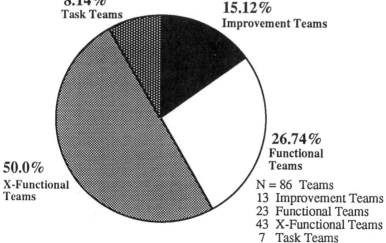

8.14%
Task Teams

15.12%
Improvement Teams

26.74%
Functional
Teams

50.0%
X-Functional
Teams

N = 86 Teams
13 Improvement Teams
23 Functional Teams
43 X-Functional Teams
7 Task Teams

Figure 15.5. Types of Active and Proposed Teams.

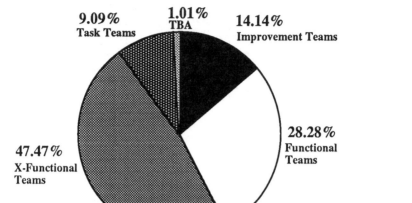

N = 99 Teams
    14 Improvement Teams
    28 Functional Teams
    47 X-Functional Teams
     9 Task Teams
     1 TBA

Figure 15.5. QI Story Steps of Active Teams.

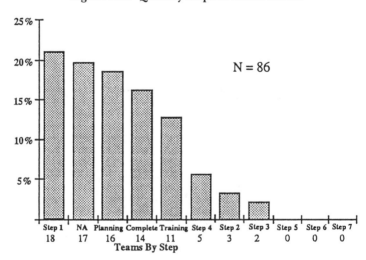

Figure 15.7. Completed QI Stories.

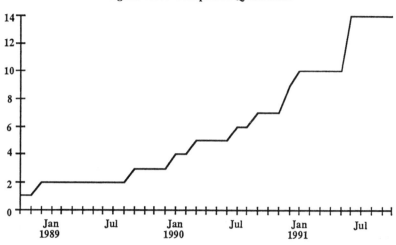

process back on track. Several other organizations told us their process went off track because of a lack of leadership commitment. One organization had a poor understanding of the resources required, and the board called a halt to the process. Another admitted they pushed the threshold for change too

Figure 15.8. Phases for UMMC TQ Process.

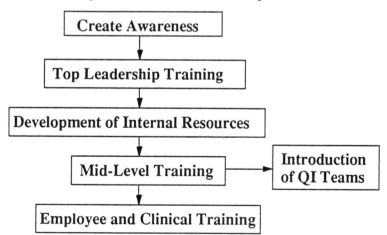

fast—the organization just wasn't ready. While each story of failure gives a slightly different focal point, they all showed lack of strategic planning. Henry Ford Health System, Detroit, Michigan, on the other hand, is a good example of an organization that developed a strategic plan first. They spent eighteen months planning before any teams were implemented. They made sure the elements were in place before they rolled the process out in the environment. While any strategic plan may need to be altered based on findings, having the plan in place can help you avoid a multitude of problems. On the other hand, do not fall into the trap of paralysis by analysis. You learn from doing and improving.

When our process at UMMC experienced institutional confusion, the Total Quality Council reviewed what had been accomplished to date and developed a more comprehensive roadmap. It is far more difficult to plan retrospectively. However, our second planning process led to the development of a TQM rollout plan and a five-year strategic plan. More careful planning of TQM is indicative of lessons learned during the rollout.

Today, on an annual basis, the Corporate Lead Team holds a planning retreat with all ten Divisional Lead Team Leaders and members to brainstorm and multivote goals for the next year. This process is educational for lead team members; they know their goals must flow from the organizational goals.

The Divisional Lead Teams also hold planning sessions to determine how the team will focus attention for the year and for the longer term. These plans are then shared across the organization.

Leadership Issues. There were several early teams that failed because we assigned employees to lead the teams, and their managers did not have TQM knowledge and experience. As a consequence, managers have served as team leaders in all areas until they gain experience with the quality improvement process. Then employees will be trained and serve as team leaders, while managers facilitate teams.

Team Demand Exceeds Capability. In 1989 we learned that our process was out of control. We had no idea of how many teams were functioning, what they were working on, or if they had completed appropriate training. We called this our "nuclear explosion" phase. The problem became apparent as we began planning for a team leaders' meeting. Each quarter our COO meets with team leaders to learn progress and issues, sustain the forward momentum, create a support network, and keep the process on track. We thought we had about thirty teams at the time. The meeting was scheduled for a small conference room. The staff became concerned when over 200 people called to say they were coming. The COO was calm, however, and said: "Get a larger room and send around a sign up sheet. Ask for the name of the team leader, their phone number, and the team they are leading. Maybe then administration will have some concept of what is going on with the team effort." We learned a valuable lesson: once you teach people the skills, they will begin to use them. You must have some basic definitions and a process to track what is happening with the team efforts.

While the team efforts were hampered by a variety of organizational barriers, they continued to tackle institutional problems with amazing success and meet the goals we had set for our Total Quality Process. The steps we took to remove the barriers to team progress were successful, and in late 1991 it was clear to all that the team approach was becoming engrained in our culture.

Other Quality Process Pitfalls

Hitting the Wall

There are times during the implementation process when, just like a runner, you hit the proverbial "wall." Your process seems to run out of steam or energy. Multiple barriers arise and can seem overwhelming. Skepticism, resistance to change, control orientation, fiscal crisis, and people who see TQM as just more work are some of the barriers that make up the wall. If you recognize these barriers and try to remove or address them one by one, you can keep the process on track, as illustrated in Figure 15.9. Anticipating the barriers and recognizing them early is key. With careful planning you can keep the process on track.

Figure 15.9. Elements of the "Wall."

	Control Oriented Managers	Budget Crisis	
Resistance	Results Slow	Apathy	Ineffective Training
CEO Change	Fear	Champion Leaves	Lack of Trust

Total Quality. The very term *Total Quality* can seem overwhelming. "The Total Quality challenge can seem too big, too amorphous, too limitless and therefore limiting" (Gaspari, 1991, p. 6). This is why planning and communication are so essential. Defining the steps, laying out a plan, and continually reinforcing progress with reports to the organization can focus attention and help allay anxiety. Progressing with small, easily understood steps makes communication easier. Articulation of milestones on a large Gantt chart posted in a public place can make the process more understandable to employees. A Gantt chart typically plots the duration of each of a set of activities along a horizontal line. Thus, the Gantt chart resembles a horizontal bar chart, with the bar for each activity illustrating its beginning time, duration, and ending time.

Action Step: Make sure the process is understandable. Communicate the plan and progress in manageable elements for the employees.

A Common Language. While it is necessary to develop a common language for the process and define the terms for use in your organization, keep in mind that quality jargon can pose a significant barrier to TQ progress. There are Japanese terms, statistical terms, and many other unfamiliar words. Many quality enthusiasts become zealots and seem like missionaries to the people who are not quite on board. Early in our process, one of our physicians made the remark that TQM sounded like a quasi-religious experience to him! Did we really think people were going to live by the quality values? We did, but the fact that he was so put off by the terminology caused us to think about ways to reduce some of the intensity. To enhance organizational learning, try to keep jargon and missionary zeal to a minimum. Define the terms for use in your organization, and establish a glossary of terms for distribution to all employees.

Action Step: Define the terms you will use in your organization in a clear and cogent way. Keep jargon to a minimum. Use examples applicable to your organization where possible.

Reduce Bureaucracy to Find Time. As noted earlier, most American managers learned how to manage "by the rules." Many times we find ourselves using these rules even when they no longer fit. Doing it right for many means doing it by the book! When Jack Welch took over as CEO of General Electric in April 1981, the focus on bureaucracy changed. Welch considers bureaucracy "evil" because it threatens productivity and encourages people to look at the company and its procedures rather than at customers and the competition (Bardwick, 1991, p. 22). In a speech at the third annual National Forum for Quality Improvement in Health Care in Atlanta (Oct. 23, 1991), Donald Berwick pointed out that "in TQM, knowledge replaces control." To be successful the educational process must refocus management attention on meeting the customer requirements rather than on feeding the institutional bureaucracy.

Many managers believe they are simply too busy to learn the necessary skills for TQM implementation. We would suggest that finding the time will make a big difference in their management lives. There is a big investment of time on the front end as TQM tools and techniques and behaviors are learned. However, once the tools are learned, managers find that teams are getting to root causes and are permanently solving problems. Managers are not dealing with solving the same problem time after time. Fire-fighting behavior is replaced with quality-by-planning and quality-by-design. To be successful, however, the pursuit of quality must become routine. Once fully implemented, the quality process will yield service or product quality, cost effectiveness, enhanced productivity, and problems that stay fixed.

Action Step: Find time for quality by getting rid of bureaucratic practices such as unnecessary reports, paperwork with multiple-level signatures, meetings that do not add value, and doing things that can be eliminated.

The Budget Crisis. The precarious economic conditions in healthcare can be a distraction in some organizations and a complete deterrent in others. If you are on the verge of financial crisis, it is not the time to begin a Total Quality Management process. You will need to solve the financial crisis, and then begin the planning for TQM. Most healthcare managers today are consumed with budget issues. They wonder how they can provide the same level of service with fewer resources. Teaching the concepts of the cost of poor quality, and how to reduce rework, complexity, and error, can help managers grasp the cost-reducing potential of a TQM approach. Utilizing these techniques is far more effective than the across-the-board cut mentality that may be required in an emergency.

Action Step: Stress the potential cost savings generated by addressing the cost of poor quality. Teach all employees the concepts of waste prevention and how they can help the organization save scarce resources.

Resistance. There will be resistance to the quality efforts. To think employees or managers will quickly abandon old values and behaviors in favor of new ones is naive. You should expect resistance. The resistance will be evident in the management ranks and among the employees. The key to turning resistance into support is to recognize that people do not resist something they think can help them personally and help the organization. The educational process can help provide the rationale for adopting the new philosophy. Getting people involved in planning the change process can also help reduce resistance. When people understand how the change process can help them in their daily work, they want to participate instead of resist. Through your educational programs stress the WIIFM (what's in it for me) approach.

Action Step: Set up corporate task teams that can work on keeping progress visible for employees. Demonstrate management commitment to TQM, and apathy will be replaced with enthusiasm.

Quality Indicators. When we tried to introduce the concept of departmental quality indicators, our managers balked. When we began to investigate the resistance, what we heard was fear. Managers were afraid that their supervisors would use these indicators to point out that they were not doing their jobs. We also heard that this work was duplicative of the JCAHO requirements. It was clear that we had not done a good job in explaining the purpose of developing customer-oriented indicators. Another problem was asking our managers to talk directly to customers when they were not prepared. Our design was to have most departmental indicators be customer based, not provider based. We found our managers needed mini-sessions on how to develop customer-focused quality indicators and why indicators were necessary. True progress began when the managers could see how departmental customer indicators related to the overall health of the organization. As the voice of the customer identified service and quality gaps, team and individual efforts resulted in solutions that helped the organization meet its goals. Figure 15.10 illustrates this concept.

Decentralization of the Quality Process. The line management must own the quality process. The TQ process cannot be delegated to a staff department. Each and every person must commit to the new philosophy and begin to live by the new rules of conduct. Without leadership there will be no decentralization and ownership, and the process will stall in the second, knowledge phase.

Slow Results. There may be few visible, tangible results in the first two years of the process. The only things that can be counted are the numbers of people trained and the number of teams started. To inform our staff of quality progress, we set up two team boards, one outside the cafeteria and one in the executive hallway. One format describes the team name, the team members, the team leader and facilitator, the opportunity they are working on, and the current step they are working on. If

Figure 15.10. Listen to Our Customers.

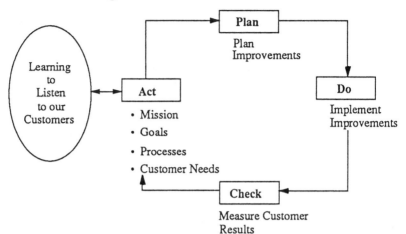

you plan to manage expectations, you must keep communication flowing. Use Gantt charts to list milestones and explain progress, as previously illustrated in Table 15.1.

The Henry Ford Health System also experienced the problem of expectations that exceeded progress. The typical employee expected immediate results when results were often slow in coming. Our friend Vin Sahney, vice president, Henry Ford Health System, described this issue in this way. "When you begin a TQM process the organizational expectations for change rise dramatically. Everyone expects to see instantaneous results. The gains from TQM tend to come slowly over time. This creates an expectations gap in the organization" (personal communication, Oct. 23, 1991). Figure 15.11 graphically depicts this concept of an expectations gap. If large gaps between expectations and results continue, physicians, employees, and customers will develop a negative reaction. The gap is best managed by presenting a realistic plan that identifies levels of employee involvement, numbers of teams, and time frames for results. You should communicate whatever evidence of progress you have. In the early stages, communicating the number of people trained, the number of teams formed, and the number of employee suggestions submitted can all create forward momentum.

Figure 15.11. TQM Expectations Gap.

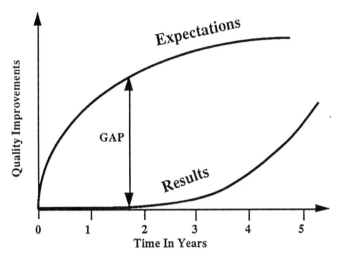

Source: Sahney, 1992, p. 78.

Action Step: Expectations must be managed. Keep communication flowing. Gantt charts that list milestones are helpful in explaining progress and keeping everyone updated.

Lack of Trust. A feeling of trust in the organization must be present before a quality initiative can take place. Some suggest that trust is the "glue" of the quality process. We suggest that large corporate issues that may have interfered with trust in the past be dealt with first. Establish some quality task teams to work on issues that people believe are barriers to the TQ process. Provide corporate support to remove these barriers, and communicate the commitment to change the organization.

Ineffective Training. Developing effective training sessions is not quite as easy as it sounds. A continuing comprehensive educational process is required, and the nature of the process will change depending on the stage of the quality process. Even organizations that have ten years of quality experience report that there are many new skills and techniques to teach. Talking with people in organizations with a quality focus will give you an understanding of the types of training required. Chapter Nine relates the training currently in place at UMMC.

Action Step: Consult with organizations that have quality experience as you plan your educational process.

 Organizational Inertia. There are many times during the process when energy can begin to wane. One of our lead teams, Professional Services, was concerned about what they perceived as a slowdown in progress with their teams and the process in general in their division. They began to brainstorm what the symptoms of the slowdown were. They then prepared a cause-and-effect diagram to determine what was causing the problems. The next step was to list some aids that could reduce the barriers. Their determination led to many things that they, as the senior managers in the division, could do to eliminate the inertia. The lesson here is that there will be slowdowns, and you should expect them. When they occur, you should take the necessary steps to diagnose what the causes are and provide leadership to overcome the barriers.

 Ineffective Internal Communications. Poor communication is thought to be responsible for many problems: poor marriages, strained family relationships, business and other problems. While a TQM approach helps reduce barriers and begins to improve communication across departmental barriers, there is much more required to learn to communicate more effectively.

 If you are a department manager, you can begin to improve your communications by holding regular staff meetings where time is allowed for free-flowing questions. Also take the time at the end of the meeting to critique it. This will demonstrate your commitment to improving communication to your staff. Circulate to all department employees memos, budget documents, and reports. If people are not interested, they will not take the time to read them, but at least they will have had the chance. Also make sure you pass down the line important management decisions and the reasons for them. The people in your department should have access to any information about the organization that will help them contribute more effectively. Employees should not have to find out information by reading about it in the newspaper first.

If you are a senior manager, you can audit how effective communications are with your people. Ask them: Do you consider yourself well informed on administrative issues? How often are announcements made that come as a complete surprise to you? How often are you asked to provide feedback on issues before decisions are made? Are you satisfied with the communication patterns in our department? What could be done to make you feel more informed? When you have the answers to these questions, ask the group to develop a new communication plan that will detail communication flow.

No matter how hard an organization tries, communication can be improved. One of the first task teams should be a communications team. The goal should be to develop a communications plan for the TQM effort.

Action Step: Assess communication patterns in your organization and develop an action plan for improvement. Set up a communications task team and develop a TQM communication program.

Visibility of Executive Leadership. During the early phases of the process, the visibility of executive leadership is key. If the senior leaders are not leading the TQM effort, people in the organization recognize that this is not an important issue. Leadership is more than the *rhetoric* of quality. Delivering a speech or introducing a videotape are not forms of active leadership. The leaders of the organization must teach quality courses, use quality tools in their meetings, ask to see graphs of relevant data, or ask quality questions on rounds. There must be a demonstration that the tools and techniques will be used by everybody but especially by the leaders.

Rate of Change. The rate of change during a TQM process is overwhelming for some and not fast enough for others. Frequent assessment of the organization can give you an idea of which phase each department is in and who needs additional help. Surveys on a departmental basis can illustrate the level of quality knowledge and practice. Also, if critical processes are flowcharted in advance of setting up teams, data can be collected that will get the teams started on the right foot.

Why Quality Programs May Fail

There are as many reasons for the failure of TQM programs as there are programs. While some reach a stumbling point, revitalization can rejuvenate the process. These are the most fixable problems. Some programs grind to an absolute halt. The organization either returns to the previous method of management or never changed in the first place. However, even these processes can be revitalized. An analysis to see what went wrong and how the mistakes can be avoided the second time around is essential. What are some of the major program derailers?

Just Another Program. The main reason for failure is that TQM is treated like just another program. Leaders do not understand the level of commitment and energy required to sustain the effort. As we have indicated several times, TQM requires very comprehensive change: organizational, cultural, attitudinal, and operational. TQM is not a new program—it is a new way of doing business. The literature on TQM advises that you think of quality as a continuous process, one that will not end, rather than a program.

Too Heavy a Focus on Teams. Teams are seen as the be all and end all. While teams are critically important in providing training and focus for employee involvement, they are just a building block. Cultural change to support the new team spirit is also essential. The goal is to have the tools and techniques of quality become a part of daily worklife. As you begin, a strong support network is required to ensure team success. Once the culture begins to change, the quality tools and techniques become the way of managing, and teamwork and data-driven decision making become comfortable.

Delegation to Staff or Quality Department. Sometimes quality efforts fail because the process is delegated to staff or a department to implement. This strategy clearly shows the organization that quality does not really matter. If executives place other initiatives higher on their agenda or delegate the process to others, it emphasizes other corporate issues are more important than quality.

Lack of Alignment. Lack of alignment with major organizational issues can also cause a process to go off-track. If the process seems like something extra, to be learned on top of everything else rather than a new way of managing, people will resist the process. The types of problems solved, as the process becomes well known, must be seen as organizationally significant to sustain momentum.

Behavioral Change Does Not Occur. Change may be superficial rather than systemic. If only a few managers change their style, the right words may be used and teamwork improves, but there is no organizational revitalization, and business continues as usual.

Lack of an Effective Strategy. An effective strategy for driving the quality process through the organization is key. If we could begin again, we would drive the process by "slice" in the organization. This means we would train everyone in the chain of command over the team. We believe the key is to empower the team to make decisions on an as-needed basis. If supervisors and managers above the teams are not trained, the team does not receive required support and progress is slowed. Figures 9.2 and 9.3 illustrated education strategies that emphasize that managers and supervisors must be trained before the staff that report to them are included on teams.

TQM Champion Leaves. Many organizations have been in the early stages of development when a key turnover occurs and the quality champion leaves the organization. The first four years are probably the most critical; after this phase the quality process tends to take on a life of its own and is not as dependent on a single champion. Before you begin the process, the champion should be asked to agree to a five-year commitment. If despite the best efforts it appears you will lose your champion, assess where you are in the process, where you are heading, and who can take on the leadership on an interim basis. If the quality champion is also the chief executive, make sure you recruit someone who has quality experience who can take over the process.

Creating a New Bureaucracy. Many organizations focus on TQM as an end, not as a means. They establish programs built on teams, charts, graphs, and information gathering. They do not link TQM to their business strategies. Their TQM process simply becomes an extra parallel process to line management. They so blindly follow processes that they forget about the internal and external customer requirements. The new "quality" rules replace old rules and stifle creativity.

Creativity and innovation must be a part of an effective quality process. Too much process can retard breakthrough thinking. Some processes should be abandoned in favor of new practices, rather than improved. Patrick Townsend and Joan Gebhardt suggest that focusing exclusively on doing things right could lead to making obsolete products perfectly (1991, p. 24). Challenge your employees to think about quality in incremental phases.

Too much process can also keep line managers from taking charge of it. If the process is too complicated, line executives will defer to the experts. Keep the process simple and usable.

Action Step: Review carefully for duplicative efforts or overgrown bureaucratic practices as your TQM process develops. Integrate creativity and innovation into your quality process.

Already a Quality Organization. Many organizations believe they are already "doing" quality. A closer examination shows they are using teams and tools and techniques, but they lack the full discipline of the process. There is a distinction between true teamwork and using quality tools. Many so-called quality teams are merely reconfigurations of committees. Table 15.2 illustrates typical differences between committees and quality teams.

Lack of Visible Action. In some organizations there is too much talk and not enough action. "Lech Walesa told congress that there is a declining world market for words. He's right. The

Table 15.2. Comparison of Committee and Quality Team.

	Typical Committee	Quality Team
Leadership	Chairperson	Team leader
Membership	Hierarchical	Equitable
	Voting/majority	Consensus
	Representatives OK	Representatives not OK
Orientation	Task oriented	Process oriented
	Formal rules (e.g., Robert's Rules)	Developed by team
	Subcommittees	Subteams
	Can be audited	Requires team approval

only thing the world believes anymore is behavior, because we all see it instantaneously. None of us may preach anymore. We must behave," said MaxDePree, chairman, Herman Miller (1990, p. 26).

Techniques to Sustain Momentum

Do Not Rush to Implement Programs Without Planning. First, make sure there is true executive commitment to the process. This is often difficult to assess because coming out and saying you're against quality is like saying you're against motherhood and apple pie. Most managers will support the rhetoric of quality, but their actions will not support the process. Second, set up a team of individuals to plan how the process will be implemented in your organization. If pilot teams are part of your plan, begin with one to three teams. More than three will be difficult to monitor and support when the organization is in a learning phase. Use these pilot teams to demonstrate how the tools and techniques can be applied.

Assure an Integrated Clinical/Administrative Plan. In the early days of TQM in healthcare, there were two developmental models that evolved. One model focused on improving administrative issues, those processes that supported patient care. Examples of organizations that followed this approach are UMMC; Alliant Health System, Louisville, Kentucky; and Rush-Presbyterian-St. Luke's, Chicago, Illinois. These efforts were led by healthcare executives.

The second approach focused on the actual process of patient care itself. Examples of organizations that pursued this approach are Intermountain Health Care, Salt Lake City, Utah; Brigham and Women's Hospital, Boston; and Harvard Community Health Plan, Brookline, Massachusetts. At each of these organizations the process was led by a physician. A recent GOAL/QPC publication illustrated several of the early health-care models and how they evolved (1992).

Today we are much more aware that an integrated model is required, one that blends improvements in administrative and clinical efforts. The reason the two models developed seemed to be determined by the background of the quality champion. Where an administrator had the lead, the process took on an administrative focus. Where the lead was played by a physician, the process took on a clinical focus. We would propose that without an integrated clinical and administrative focus you do not have Total Quality—you have partial quality.

Action Step: Develop an integrated program with a clinical and administrative focus. Identify and support administrative and clinical champions.

Chapter Sixteen

Conclusion

Total Quality Management represents a major change in organizational culture and processes. It means creating an organization focused on customer satisfaction, which leads to customer retention and eventually growth in market share. It is a pragmatic methodology for managing healthcare organizations, and is both specific and systematic. The impact of TQM is being demonstrated in a variety of industries worldwide, including healthcare. It is no longer possible to discredit TQM as a means for improvement because no successful examples exist in healthcare. *Striving Toward Improvement* presents compelling stories of six hospitals that have made the commitment to quality (Joint Commission on Accreditation of Healthcare Organizations, 1992b). Mara Melum and Marie Sinioris, in their book *Total Quality Management: The Health Care Pioneers*, feature several other healthcare organizations that are well along in their quality journeys (1992). Across the country, healthcare organizations of all sizes are improving their organizations through TQM.

To implement TQM there must be a firm commitment from the leadership of the organization to change their former way of doing business. The role of the leaders is key. They must answer the questions: Why change? Why TQM? They must create the environment where the methodologies can take root and flourish. In successful quality organizations, the leaders not only model the quality behaviors and values, they teach quality classes. They design programs to support quality and use their energies and skills to help improve the communities their hospitals serve. Leaders must continually ask: Do our quality systems support continuous improvement and innovation? If not, what changes must be made? How can we better align our organization to meet the needs of our community?

The concept of employee empowerment and involvement is also critical. Customer-focused organizations understand the requirements of both internal and external customers. Empowered employees gain satisfaction through their work because the organization recognizes and utilizes their skills. The reward and recognition systems parallel or mirror the employees' efforts to reinforce behavior. Empowered employees, therefore, create satisfied customers. TQM is not superficial change; it requires looking at referring physicians, staff physicians, managers, employees, and the communities we serve in a new way — as a chain of suppliers serving customers.

As healthcare grows from a cottage industry to a near trillion-dollar-a-year industry, there have not been the necessary adjustments in our systems to create smooth-flowing processes. In many instances systems grew and expanded without comprehensive planning. As Deming would say, a large part of the problem is the process, or how the work is done. The employees are not to blame for inefficiencies; it is the entire system that is responsible for the problem! In this era of reimbursement chaos, TQM offers a systematic means of evaluating processes, revamping the system, and renewing your organization. As two authors wrote in *Quality or Else*: "A quality program, at a minimum, lets you think about a great many seemingly disparate problems in a systematic way to see how they relate and how they could be improved without doing too much for one and making the others worse" (Dobyns and Crawford-Mason, 1991, p. 276).

While there is great evidence of a quality revolution beginning in healthcare, we are aware of no organizations that would describe their quality processes as fully developed or mature. The quality process takes time to evolve and also requires the investment of substantial resources and institutional energy. The barriers to implementation are significant. One way to anticipate barriers to successful implementation is to review the quality approaches in industry that preceded healthcare efforts by about five to seven years. Jim Clemmer, writing about barriers in a recent issue of the *Total Quality Newsletter*, said: "Many companies start with real enthusiasm for TQM, they pick an approach and do some things well, but too often what they call Total Quality Management is only partial quality management. It is not broad enough. That is why 70 percent of the programs fail" (1992, p. 7). We hope this book gives you a sense of what has to be done, how complex the process is, how to avoid potential pitfalls, and how to get the train back on track if it should derail.

TQM is not just teams, statistics, and a few new tools for problem solving; it is the creation of a new organizational culture focused on meeting and exceeding the requirements of customers. There is a tremendous temptation when implementing TQM to focus only on the parts you like or those that are easiest to accomplish. There are many examples of failed programs that illustrate that a less than "total" approach will not allow you to achieve your goals or sustain the momentum necessary for a full implementation. There are several key implementation factors that we feel bear repeating:

- The creation of a common direction
- Cultural change
- Communication
- Integration
- Achieving a balanced approach
- The role of innovation and creativity

Creation of a Common Direction

The leadership of the organization must develop and communicate a consistent, customer-oriented vision. The goal is to align the organization behind the mission, vision, and goals. Each division and department should also establish a mission and vision statement to guide them and draft departmental indicators based on the organizational indicators. This allows each person to understand how his or her job contributes to organizational success. Alignment creates organizational synergy. Deming felt so strongly about this concept that he made it number one of his fourteen points — constancy of purpose!

Cultural Change

The leadership and management of the organization must establish a supportive environment for the quality effort. Does the climate of your organization require change? Does the leadership understand the type of management support required? One important leadership requirement is involvement. Quality efforts cannot be delegated. The leaders of the organization must personally model the new behaviors, or the transformation will lack energy and credibility. Team efforts, so necessary to create seamless organizations, cannot take root in an unsupportive climate. If management is just tolerating teams rather than participating fully, the message to the organization will be clear: quality is not important! On the other hand, great progress can be made when the managers begin to model the behaviors of quality. We use phrases like "walk the talk" to illustrate the concept that your actions speak much louder than words. Personal modeling of the TQM principles will convince the organization that this change process, unlike others in the past, is real. These behavioral changes are the most difficult part of an organizational transformation. It is a difficult task to replace habits that have developed over a successful career. Some subtle actions that may be telegraphing a message different from what the executives wish include:

- No time set aside on managers' calendars for TQM meetings and celebrations.
- Quality is the last item on, or missing from, the executive meeting agendas.
- There is no priority for TQM meetings or resources.
- There is a continued focus on short-term financial goals.
- The reward and recognition program is not consistent with quality principles.

- Cost-reduction strategies seem far more important than quality efforts.

Communication

An effective communication plan is essential to the success of the quality initiative. Just as location, location, location is the key ingredient in real estate value, communication, communication, communication is the key ingredient in TQM success. Sharing progress with employees is essential. Employees must see the link between the quality efforts and changes in the organization. Effective communication is also necessary for the success of teams. Time after time, when teams reported to our lead teams, it was obvious that communication breakdowns in our organization were responsible for many system failures. People had good intentions but were only capable of seeing the world from the narrow perspective of their department. They did not understand the role of other personnel or departments. Flowcharting processes allowed us to understand where the major glitches and rework loops were and how to begin to adjust the systems. When people understand their role and the roles of others, and most importantly the communication mechanisms, all processes work more smoothly. Given the large number of services required by patients and the many functions in a healthcare organization, it is impossible to develop a smooth-flowing system without an institutional focus. The first step to improvement is flowcharting of all critical processes. We have found that flowcharting enhances communication among departments. In creating an accurate, useful flowchart, customers and suppliers enhance their understanding of their role in critical processes.

Integration

There are many facets of the TQM process that must be integrated. A short list of these includes:

- TQM requires the integration of a customer-focused continuous improvement philosophy, analytical knowledge and skills, and interpersonal or "people" knowledge and skills.
- The efforts of everyone involved—physicians, employees, administration, suppliers, and customers—must be integrated. The internal customers must be part of a chain with the goal of external customer satisfaction.
- Effective TQM also requires the integration of quality assurance and quality improvement methods. To begin, utilize TQM tools and techniques to address QA issues.
- Successful TQM also requires a fully integrated reward and recognition program. The organizational leaders should identify key behaviors and set reward and recognition strategies to reinforce these new behaviors.
- Quality and performance planning must be integrated.
- TQM methods must be integrated in personnel practices such as recruitment, promotion, and diversity management.
- TQM must be fully integrated in the strategic planning process of the organization.
- TQM must be integrated into all processes, clinical and nonclinical. Separating administrative and clinical approaches can lead to confusion and a lack of focus across departments.

Achieving a Balanced Approach

There are many issues that you will face during implementation that require a balanced approach. Some of these are:

- Skills of your employees. There must be a balance of analytical, humanistic, and customer-oriented skills. An approach too heavily focused on any one of the three will not achieve the desired effects. Organizations that focus only on analytical methods such as flowcharting, control charts, and statistical process control fail to capture the commitment of the people who must make the change. Focusing only on organizational dynamics and the things that make people feel good will restrict the analytical rigor to make quantitatively correct decisions.

- Quality planning, quality teams, and quality in operations. If you do not plan effectively for quality, your process will reach a point where you will not be able to sustain progress. A balanced approach of planning, teams, and quality in daily work will give you the best chance for success.

- A top-down and bottom-up planning effort. The energy of the organization can be captured best when the process is both top-down and bottom-up. Each department in the organization must have a quality plan for the way the quality process will roll out in their area, and each employee must have a quality mind-set. The quality process cannot be something that is thought of only by a few once in a while. Everyone in the organization must constantly ask: How can I improve on this idea, work process, or service? How can I meet and exceed the needs of my customers?

- And you must be concerned about the people in the middle, the managers who may be getting buffeted on both sides.

The Role of Innovation and Creativity

If the future success of your organization depends on your ability to continually improve, how are you helping all employees to be innovative and creative? It is quite clear that as you begin to apply the problem-solving methodologies, there are some processes that should not be improved. They should be thrown out and a new process developed. We have found some teams quickly identify that the processes they have been asked to improve are obsolete and should be redesigned. Other teams, however, stumble along wasting organizational resources. Creativity training may help your employees and managers develop a dual focus on improvement and innovation. Many employees have ideas about how to improve things; the sad thing is most managers never listen.

There is a great risk when a quality process begins that the old bureaucracy will be replaced by a new bureaucracy, one with charts, statistics, and new rules and regulations. We know from research that there is a tendency for people to resist doing things in new ways. How can you create the energy for change? In concert with TQ training, establish creativity training. Help employees break old thought patterns, challenge existing assumptions, and develop new ways of doing things. Give them new tools and techniques, and train managers to explore the potential for new methodologies in their daily work. Effective managers must know how to be active listeners, questioners, and participants in the change process.

World-Class Healthcare

As quality initiatives prove successful, healthcare executives must not be satisfied with minor adjustments to the system. We should follow the lead of manufacturing leaders and aim for world-class status. The manufacturing literature began to reflect this notion of "world class" about 1986, to indicate a superior performance exhibited by top manufacturers the world round. "There will be no safe harbor for those companies unwilling to work toward or resistant to becoming world class in the 1990's. All manufacturing must face new thresholds of performance. Directly or indirectly the standard for competition will be redefined by world class companies in each industry. In order to remain viable competitors, aspiring organizations must meet or exceed the newly established thresholds (Roth, Giffi, and Seal, 1990, p. 9).

We believe the same pressure to compete will occur within healthcare. We have already seen some hospitals competing for an international healthcare market. This tendency will increase over time, especially for the large medical centers.

Survival

In the end TQM is a matter of survival for healthcare organizations. As Tom Peters emphasized in an audiotape message: "The only three sustaining strategic directions are: superior service, superior quality of product, and constant innovation. However there is a fourth point, and it should be obvious, those three

directions are built on a base of participation by all hands"
(1984). With the public outcry about healthcare cost, we must
take action to meet the needs of our customers. This means
providing outstanding service and quality care that is continually improved for a reasonable price. This cannot be accomplished without involving every employee in the effort. We believe the concept of reducing the cost of poor quality holds great
promise for organizations. Reducing rework, waste, and steps
that do not add value can free up assets that can be reallocated
to areas of need.

There is a story told by quality experts about W. Edwards
Deming being questioned by a reporter while he was trying to
eat his breakfast. We heard the story from Paul Batalden, the
vice president for medical care at Hospital Corporation of
America, Nashville, Tennessee. The reporter wanted to know the
real secrets of quality management. He asked Deming, "What do
we have to do in the West to compete and promote Total Quality?" Deming looked up from his breakfast with a cold stare and
told the reporter to tell his readers, "Just do it, that's all, just do it."

There is no secret, no quick fix, and it is a long and at
times difficult journey. However, like any journey, it begins with
one small step. Take that step. Learn to live in the future.
Implement the management methods that will allow your organization to become the provider of choice and the employer of
choice in your area. If you have achieved this goal, focus on being
the best in the state, the best in the nation, or the best in the
world. Use the process of quality improvement to achieve not
only your organizational goals but your organizational and
personal dreams. We hope that this book will help you begin. If
you are well on your way, we hope we have encouraged you with
additional considerations and some pitfalls to avoid.

Appendix A

Self-Assessment Tool

This appendix provides a simplified self-assessment tool adapting the Malcolm Baldrige National Quality Award criteria for use by healthcare organizations. This tool can be used by your senior management team or by a department or division in your organization to determine where you stand relative to the Malcolm Baldrige National Quality Award criteria. The relationship of the Baldrige award assessment categories is illustrated in Figure A.1.

The Malcolm Baldrige National Quality Award framework has four basic elements (National Institute of Standards and Technology, 1992, p. 5):

> *Driver.* Senior executive leadership creates the values, goals, and systems, and guides the sustained pursuit of customer value and company performance improvement.
>
> *System.* The system component comprises the set of well-defined and well-designed processes for meeting the customer's quality and performance requirements.
>
> *Measures of Progress.* The measures of progress component provides a results-oriented basis for channeling actions to delivering ever-improving customer value and organizational performance.
>
> *Goal.* The basic aim of the quality process is the delivery of ever-improving value to customers.

Figure A.1. Relationship of Baldrige Award Assessment Categories.

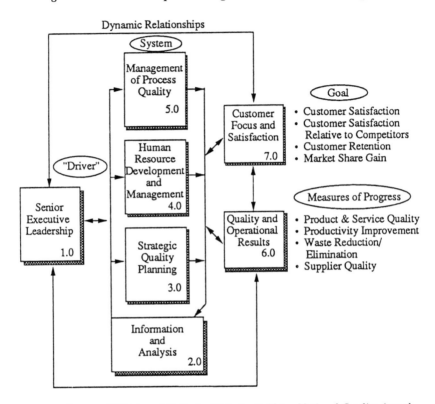

Source: *1993 Award Criteria, Malcolm Baldrige National Quality Award,*
National Institute of Standards and Technology, 1992.

Assessment Tool

The assessment tool contains separate evaluation sheets for
each of the seven major categories of the Baldrige Award, as
illustrated in Exhibit A.1.

1. Leadership
2. Information and analysis
3. Strategic quality planning
4. Human resource development and management
5. Management of process quality

6. Quality and operational results
7. Customer satisfaction

Scoring Tool

The scoring scale for each of the seven categories indicates level 1 as beginning, level 6 as growing, and level 10 as reaching maturity. Short descriptions are provided for each of the major categories in Exhibit A.1 to assist with the scoring. *To obtain a higher score, however, all descriptions for lower scores should be true.*

Maturity	10
	9
	8
	7
Growing	6
	5
	4
	3
	2
Beginning	1

A sample scoring form is provided in Exhibit A.2 to record the ratings. Using this form, the ratings are then multiplied by the relative weights of the different scoring categories to get the score for each of the seven categories. Note that customer focus and satisfaction has the largest weight of any category. A sample completed scoring form is included in Exhibit A.3 to illustrate a completed form.

Exhibit A.1. Self-Assessment Tool for Healthcare Organizations Based on Baldrige Criteria.

---

1. Leadership — 95 points
9.5 percent

This category represents the executives' personal leadership, involvement, and communication of quality goals and values throughout the organization. How the executives create and sustain a customer focus and meet community healthcare goals is key.

Rank

10	Quality is the number one priority of the leadership team of the organization and department. The leadership team establishes the strategic direction for the organization and the targets that will lead to achievement.

9	Your organization and department have assessed community healthcare needs, developed an action plan to meet those needs, and communicated your goals.

8	Leaders and department heads establish personal improvement plans to evaluate and enhance quality leadership and involvement in the quality process. The organizational leaders model quality behaviors and lead the quality effort.

7	Quality values are integrated into the daily management behaviors of leaders, as indicated by employee surveys.

6	Quality issues are part of every agenda. The quality process drives all meetings.

5	Rewards and recognition reinforce the quality improvement process. The executives and department heads participate in reward and recognition efforts formally and informally.

4	Leaders and department heads meet with customers and suppliers to determine requirements and assess satisfaction.

3	Leadership is concerned about breaking down interdepartmental barriers to the quality process. Leadership is accessible and keeps employees informed on quality progress.

2	Executives/department heads are visible advocates for quality. They lead or serve on teams and teach quality courses. They exhibit quality behaviors, such as reinforcing a customer focus, and planning and reviewing progress toward quality.

1	Organizational and departmental mission, values, vision are developed and shared broadly with all employees.

Exhibit A.1. Self-Assessment Tool for Healthcare Organizations Based on Baldrige Criteria, Cont'd.

2. Information and analysis — 75 points
7.5 percent

This category measures the effectiveness of the organization's data collection and analysis. How does the organization use data to prevent quality problems?

Rank

10	Expert systems actively support quality by planning and design and achieve on-line prevention of problems.

9	Information systems drive the organization planning process and integrate data on clinical care outcomes, community health status, availability of access to care, and issues of continuity.

8	Financial, patient care, and strategic management information systems are integrated to facilitate clinical, managerial, and improvement team efforts and decision making.

7	Current functional systems exceed the expectations of the areas served. Each employee has the information necessary to help the organization achieve quality goals.

6	The organization or department uses competitive comparisons and benchmarks to improve quality.

5	Processes are in place to ensure reliability, consistency, standardization, timely update and rapid access throughout the organization.

4	Indicators of user satisfaction are developed and monitored, and satisfaction continuously improves.

3	Information systems projects are developed and prioritized in response to customer requirements.

2	Data are reviewed, analyzed, and distributed to all who need it in a timely fashion. Data gathering cycle times are continuously shortened.

1	Data are available on operations, processes, employee factors such as safety, health, morale, and customer satisfaction.

Exhibit A.1. Self-Assessment Tool for Healthcare Organizations Based on Baldrige Criteria, Cont'd.

3. Strategic quality planning — 60 points
6 percent

This category looks at the way the organization sets and achieves goals both short and long term and how these goals are integrated into business planning.

Rank

10	Quality improvement plans are totally integrated into long-term and short-term planning processes. Plans are evaluated so the planning process can be improved and alignment occurs between organizational, departmental, and personal goals.

9	Five-year improvements are projected using indicators of quality and customer satisfaction scores.

8	Requests for key resources (capital, training, staff) are prioritized and granted based on data on customer requirements.

7	Organizational and departmental quality plans are reviewed and improved annually. The method for deployment of goals to all departments is clear.

6	Quality plans indicate the deployment process, including the method, overall plan requirements for all work units, the suppliers' roles, and the necessary resource commitment.

5	Every department has a written quality plan including a mission statement and a goal attainment plan.

4	Plans for overall operational improvement include: quality improvement, re-engineering, productivity improvement, and waste reduction.

3	Critical indicators are trended and action plans are developed for areas where improvement is needed.

2	Customers have been identified and their valid requirements have been determined. Critical indicators have been developed for these customer groups.

1	Critical processes have been identified and flowcharted.

Exhibit A.1. Self-Assessment Tool for Healthcare Organizations Based on Baldrige Criteria, Cont'd.

4. Human resource development and management — 150 points
15 percent

This category measures the level of employee involvement in the quality process. Training, performance evaluation, morale, and well-being are important indicators. Also, how the organization builds and maintains an environment for employee participation in quality excellence is key.

Rank

10	You are viewed as the employer of choice. Employee morale, satisfaction, well-being and involvement are rated high when compared to healthcare peers and others.

9	Measures of employee empowerment and involvement show favorable trends. There is evidence of mobility and flexibility in work schedules.

8	Employee surveys are conducted annually and required corrective actions are taken.

7	Trends in the effectiveness and extent of quality-related training programs are positive.

6	Improvement goals for human resource plan are developed. Indicators exist and are monitored for health, safety, and ergonomics.

5	Training programs are based on needs assessment of employees and managers. They are linked to long-term and short-term goals of problem solving, waste reduction, and process simplification.

4	Trends indicate effectiveness and extent of involvement of all employee groups. Personal growth and development plans exist for all employees.

3	A variety of recognition/reward strategies exist and occur in a timely fashion. Organizational leaders personally participate in these events.

2	The methods for effective employee contribution to organizational quality and effectiveness are identified and used in training and employee involvement.

1	Employee indicators reflect the success of empowerment and employee involvement methods.

Exhibit A.1. Self-Assessment Tool for Healthcare Organizations Based on Baldrige Criteria, Cont'd.

---

5. Management of process quality — 140 points
14 percent

This category focuses on process quality, continuous improvement, and superior quality. The systematic approaches utilized to assure quality are key.

Rank

10 Superior clinical outcomes are achieved and utilized to define quality for payer groups. Your organization is a benchmark for others.

9 QA and TQM efforts are fully integrated. Quality is built into all products and services. There is a focus on health promotion as well as treatment of disease.

8 TQ tools and techniques are utilized to conduct randomized clinical trials. Current process capabilities to achieve quality goals are assessed. When capabilities are inadequate, improvement or reengineering takes place.

7 Measures of diagnosis-specific clinical outcomes are developed and tracked.

6 Supplier quality is measured and tracked.

5 Processes are in place to assure quality of all products and services. Audits occur to check the quality system.

4 Fire-fighting management approach has been replaced with search for root causes.

3 Process improvements are sought to prevent adverse outcomes and improve clinical results.

2 Needs for changes in care processes are data driven and clinicians are responsive.

1 Tools and techniques of quality are utilized for quality assurance and to meet JCAHO requirements.

Exhibit A.1. Self-Assessment Tool for Healthcare Organizations Based on Baldrige Criteria, Cont'd.

6. Quality and operational results — 180 points
18 percent

This category includes the quantitative results of quality improvement as well as operational and supplier performance.

Rank

10	You are deemed the provider of choice by your customers and suppliers. Other healthcare organizations use your processes as benchmarks.

9	Across the institution, results of process management are benchmarked against other healthcare organizations and successful quality companies. Key measures include productivity, efficiency, and effectiveness.

8	Significant improvement trends noted in major quality indicators. Quality level of service indicates many processes are best in class.

7	Supplier quality is measured and monitored. Strategic partnerships are developed for mutual gain.

6	Positive quality results exist in most areas of the department or organization and some results are best in class.

5	Supplier quality indicators are developed.

4	Trends and current levels of quality and operational performance are positive. The organization compares favorably on performance indicators to competitors.

3	Trends and current levels in product and service level are positive.

2	Current process capability is measured and reported on regularly.

1	Institutional customer groups have been identified, valid requirements established, and indicators developed to measure product and service quality.

**Exhibit A.1. Self-Assessment Tool for Healthcare Organizations
Based on Baldrige Criteria, Cont'd.**

**7. Customer satisfaction—300 points
30 percent**

This category measures the extent of the organization's customer focus and the method
by which customer requirements are met and exceeded.

Rank

10 Customer surveys and the general public indicate best-in-class results compared to healthcare institutions and other quality institutions on some indicators. Service is perceived to be world class.

9 There is evidence that improvement results are linked to the Total Quality
Management process. Positive trends exist in financial performance and market share.

8 Positive trends are seen in all customer satisfaction indicators. Indicators
compare favorably with appropriate healthcare benchmarks.

7 The organization's supplier quality compares favorably with appropriate
healthcare benchmarks.

6 Suggestions for new product or process improvements are actively solicited
from customers with an intent to delight the customer.

5 Customer input is utilized to improve processes and develop new products.

4 Departments review satisfaction of internal and external customers using
identified indicators and take action for improvement.

3 Barriers to effective service and process improvement are identified and
eliminated.

2 Customer-based indicators are trended. A process exists to identify, reply to,
and resolve customer complaints.

1 Methods for determining current and near-term customer requirements are
defined and measures are developed to track performance.

Exhibit A.2. Sample Scoring Form for Self-Assessment Tool Based on Baldrige Criteria.

Category	Rank	Weight		Score
1. Leadership	_____ ×	9.5	= _____	out of 95
2. Information and analysis	_____ ×	7.5	= _____	out of 75
3. Strategic quality planning	_____ ×	6	= _____	out of 60
4. Human resources development and management	_____ ×	15	= _____	out of 150
5. Management of process quality	_____ ×	14	= _____	out of 140
6. Quality and operational results	_____ ×	18	= _____	out of 180
7. Customer satisfaction	_____ ×	30	= _____	out of 300

_____ = Total score

Potential total score = 1000

Exhibit A.3. Sample Completed Scoring Form for Self-Assessment Tool Based on Baldrige Criteria.

Category	Rank	Weight		Score	
1. Leadership	8 ×	9.5	=	76	out of 95
2. Information and analysis	3 ×	7.5	=	22.5	out of 75
3. Strategic quality planning	4 ×	6	=	24	out of 60
4. Human resources development and management	3 ×	15	=	45	out of 150
5. Management of process quality	5 ×	14	=	70	out of 140
6. Quality and operational results	4 ×	18	=	72	out of 180
7. Customer satisfaction	5 ×	30	=	150	out of 300

Total Score = 459.5

Potential Total Score = 1000

Note: Average Baldrige winner's score ranges from 700–800.

Appendix B

Action Steps

Action steps have been included throughout this book. These are actions that you and others in your organization can take to implement Total Quality Management. The action steps are listed together here to facilitate communication of the actions among leaders, managers, physicians, staff, customers, and suppliers of your organization.

Chapter Two: Understanding TQM

Action Step: Clearly state and demonstrate your commitment to change the organizational culture and processes to implement TQM as an approach to serve better your patients and other customers, including staff.

Action Step: Develop and communicate operational definitions for terms used in your TQM process, so that everyone in your organization can communicate effectively.

Chapter Three: Integrating TQM and Quality Assurance

Action Step: Meet with major businesses and insurance payers in your area to share information on TQM methods and projects, and discuss their expectations of your organization.

Action Step: Communicate the similarities and differences

of TQM and your traditional QA program. Develop and communicate plans for integration.

Chapter Four: Integrating TQM with Other Initiatives

Action Step: When introducing TQM or any other new process or program within your organization, communicate its relationships to previous processes and programs.

Action Step: Include all levels of managers, staff, and physicians in the planning of any new process or program. Ask them what questions they have about the new program and its relationship to past or existing programs.

Chapter Five: Organization and Leadership

Action Step: Establish a motivating vision and a plan for organizational alignment. Frequently update all levels of the organization on progress toward the vision.

Action Step: Assess the organizational structure for quality, educational process, tools, and aids to determine the capacity and capability for change.

Action Step: Assess the readiness for change. Is the support appropriate for the proposed rate of change? Are the goals clear? Does the plan require enough of a stretch for organizational change?

Action Step: Consider using a Policy Deployment Process to guide your quality planning and your organization.

Action Step: Analyze your personal leadership style. What changes will you have to make to move toward an empowering style?

Action Step: Find an external mentor and/or develop a network of advisers who are further along in the implementation process and who can assist you when transitional problems occur. Continually assess readiness for change at all levels of the organization.

Action Step: Decentralize your process. Build in the appropriate level of structure to allow TQ to permeate all levels of your organization.

Chapter Six: Organizational Culture

Action Step: Evaluate your culture. Ask:

- Have you completed a cultural assessment?
- Do you have a positive or negative climate?
- Do you have a values statement?
- Are the values communicated, understood, and upheld?
- Who are your heroes?
- How do you celebrate?
- Do positive or negative stories get repeated?
- What barriers hinder the development of a positive culture?

Action Step: Plan how you will communicate the desire to start a TQM process. What supports will be necessary to show you are serious about change?

Action Step: Communicate the rationale for change. Help people understand why change is necessary. Allow people to express anger, then provide appropriate support and education.

Action Step: Share the plans for change and progress broadly. Provide updates, consistently allow employees to give feedback, and follow up on their recommendations. Provide emotional support by making yourself available for counseling, coaching, and mentoring.

Action Step: Be patient. Provide managers and employees the flexibility to experiment with new techniques. Encourage and support risk taking.

Action Step: Provide resources to support the natural transition of a cultural change and sustain the new culture.

Action Step: Examine the transition model and determine which stage of the process your organization or department is in. Can you identify different phases by department? Determine what type of support is required to facilitate forward progress.

Action Step: Set the stage for creativity and innovation. Treat employees as your most important resource. Remove barriers to innovation and empower employees to generate ideas and implement them.

Action Step: Brainstorm the elements of the current management style in your organization. Define the paradigm you wish to create. Assess your progress at frequent intervals.

Action Step: Audit your personal response to suggestions and count how many times you say no, directly or indirectly, to employee ideas and suggestions. Keep a log and review it often. Assess your need to change in order to promote creativity in your staff.

Action Step: Consider these six steps to enhance diversity:

Step 1   Develop a plan with senior management and appoint a diversity task team.

Step 2   Collect data on current environment, practices, and policies. Develop a diversity audit to survey attitudes and practices.

Step 3   Analyze data and present it to senior management.

Step 4   Prioritize important issues.

Step 5   Develop action plans to change systems and culture. Set up task teams.

Step 6   Evaluate progress, communicate results to the organization, and begin the cycle over again.

Action Step: At a senior management meeting, discuss the concept of organizational fear. Brainstorm a list of possible fears, and then list aids to remove them. Communicate this list. Suggest that your managers repeat this exercise with their staff.

Action Step: Acknowledge that negativity exists in the organization. Create forums where people can safely identify and discuss problems that require action. Model the empowering behaviors you wish to establish.

Action Step: Evaluate your planning processes. Are there enough opportunities for employees to participate? How can you increase opportunities?

Action Step: Review your personnel policies and procedures. Do they indicate the concern necessary for a people-oriented culture? Is your personnel office viewed as supporting management or the employees?

Action Step: Survey the organization to determine how top

managers are viewed. When data are in hand, communicate the results and develop an action plan to address problems.

Action Step: Model creative problem-solving skills, such as peripheral vision, to enhance personal and organizational performance. Reward creative and innovative approaches in your managers and employees.

Chapter Seven: Physician Involvement

Action Step: Research successful clinical information systems that focus on physician resource utilization rather than costs across relatively homogeneous patient populations. Support a physician advocate who will investigate the steps your organization must take to implement such a system and encourage the participation of the medical staff.

Action Step: Support the development of methodologies to stabilize the processes of care within your institution. Engage the physicians in the development and approval of the selected techniques.

Action Step: Discuss and distribute the benefits of the stabilization of care with physicians and other clinical providers.

Action Step: Expose clinical staff to successful working clinical models in healthcare. Link examples of improvements in other processes with enhancements in patient care quality.

Action Step: Explore methods for identifying issues of concern among the physicians in your organization. Investigate the potential of investigating these issues through pilot *Clinical* Quality Improvement Team efforts.

Action Step: Establish a team of interested clinicians to encourage the appropriate application of TQM in clinical areas. Select visible and realistic pilot efforts supported by the clinical leadership for pilot clinical teams to explore. Provide appropriate administrative support to ensure the success of these efforts.

Action Step: Develop a curriculum sensitive to physicians' unique time constraints. Shorten the training sessions to education in key concepts.

Action Step: Establish a hospital-funded small grants program at your institution to fund innovative approaches to clinical practices. The program should have the full support of your clinical leadership. Provide necessary analytical, staff, and financial support to ensure the program's success.

Action Step: Start a few clinical teams to gain visibility, then wait for physician ideas to come forward spontaneously. Avoid "world hunger" issues. Pick issues for which accessible and reliable data already exist.

Chapter Eight: Teamwork

Action Step: Support and recognize a continuum of quality improvement efforts, not just formal Quality Improvement Teams.

Chapter Nine: Education and Training

Action Step: Communicate the need for change broadly and frequently, in a language and context that all can understand.

Action Step: Use successful healthcare examples to demonstrate that TQM methods work in healthcare organizations.

Action Step: Use TQ methods in your own work, ask others to see how they are using the methods, and especially use the methods to make decisions.

Action Step: List the requirements for TQ education within your organization, and compare them with characteristics of past and current management programs and practices, to define similarities and differences.

Action Step: Use several inputs to determine the requirements for your TQ educational programs, and repeat the assessment at least annually.

Action Step: To demonstrate commitment, one or more corporate leaders should introduce every TQ educational program, participate as faculty in at least part of the programs, and answer questions.

Action Step: Provide educational and pilot-project experiences that use vividly relevant examples, and actively involve participants in exercises, personal plans for change, and pilot projects. Then leaders should follow up to support personal changes and projects.

Action Step: Identify internal staff who have or can develop the ability to teach analytical and people knowledge and skills, and develop a plan for your organization to become self-sufficient in providing educational programs and support for teams.

Action Step: Carefully review the credentials, experience with TQM, and experience with healthcare organizations when reviewing potential external consultants to assist with TQM education and training.

Chapter Ten: Reward and Recognition

Action Step: Set up an employee-based team to review current reward and recognition strategies and develop future plans, to overcome any existing negative perceptions. Survey employees to determine the rewards and recognition they appreciate.

Action Step: Consider an organizationwide policy to guarantee jobs that may be affected by Total Quality. If teams redesign work and cause job elimination, guarantee positions elsewhere in the organization. This allows people to get beyond the fear of survival and see that reducing the cost of poor quality is a better way to streamline an organization.

Action Step: Institute communication policies and practices that help employees understand the vision, mission, and goals of the organization and how their role helps achieve these goals.

Action Step: Give frequent verbal recognition. Establish expectations of managers and rules of conduct so management can be hard on problems, not on people. Brainstorm ideas with senior management on ways to reduce job stress and avoid burnout. Spend time thinking of ways to bring "joy" back to work.

Action Step: Develop new forums for large cross sections of employees, where they can listen, ask questions, and give input on organizational strategies and plans.

Action Step: Build mastery milestones into your recognition program. Remove barriers that preclude workers from performing their functions expertly. Give positive feedback and recognition for new skills and jobs well done. This will help to keep people energized and goal-oriented.

Action Step: Analyze your organization. What is the mood? Is play encouraged? Is the climate appropriate for creativity and innovation? Is humor used to enhance play and reduce stress?

Action Step: Develop a creative environment where confidence and self-esteem can be built by participative decision making, risk taking, and support. Managers should think of ways to encourage employee involvement. For example, brainstorming exercises with the staff can generate many cost-saving and improvement ideas. Implement ideas quickly and recognize and reward progress to sustain momentum.

Action Step: Involve as many employees as possible in team efforts where they have a chance to learn how to determine root causes and permanently change the processes in their department. Communicate how these efforts are affecting the organization as a whole. This allows employees to see how their efforts relate to the larger corporate goals.

Action Step: Managers must address those systems that block effective performance. The best approach to smooth out those systems is to form employee improvement teams, flowchart the processes, and make the required changes. Every system and process should be evaluated.

Action Step: Regularly encourage and reward team behaviors. Discuss team efforts with team members. Visit storyboards to review and comment on progress.

Action Step: Set up a series of employee discussions where potential rewards are generated by brainstorming sessions, and then multivote to determine what the most important motivators are in your organization.

Action Step: Have the Total Quality Council establish a Reward and Recognition Task Team, early in the process, to develop a reward and recognition program. Audit the organization to see if the rewards listed by employees are the rewards present in your organization.

Action Step: Develop a budget for the reward and recognition program. Consider milestones you wish to achieve, and recognize these milestones with events and rewards.

Action Step: Determine what level in the organization will be responsible for rewards and recognition. Do you need a central and a decentralized budget? How will you communicate about rewards and recognition given?

Action Step: Determine how to share your reward and recognition policies with all employees. Consider a special employee forum when the Reward and Recognition Task Team has completed its work in order to share the results of the policy. Also use newsletters, journals, and bulletin boards.

Action Step: Develop mechanisms for large groups of employees to give feedback on the program. Are the reward and recognition strategies meeting multiple needs? Are there other strategies that need to be added?

Action Step: Make use of focus groups and surveys to understand customer requirements and modify your program.

Action Step: Make rounds to identify and recognize quality improvement storyboards and other quality improvement efforts.

Chapter Eleven: TQM Actions in Daily Operations

Action Step 1: Understand and live by values, vision, mission, goals, and management expectations.

Action Step 2: Demonstrate commitment, sponsorship, participation, and common understanding for improvement of quality and cost effectiveness.

Action Step 3: Develop mission and goals for your department(s).

Action Step 4: Identify and understand functions and processes within your department(s), and involving other departments.

Action Step 5: Identify internal and external customers and suppliers for processes.

Action Step 6: Determine customer requirements.

Action Step 7: Choose key measures/indicators.

Action Step 8: Measure and understand process capabilities.

Action Step 9: Encourage ideas and "theories" of how to improve.

Action Step 10: Investigate methods to manage workload/demand.

Action Step 11: Evaluate and prioritize opportunities.

Action Step 12: Develop standard, approved method to perform each function.

Action Step 13: Check ideas for improvement.

Action Step 14: Take action, if within your control.

Action Step 15: Ask for help to start a Quality Improvement Team.

Chapter Fourteen: Advanced Applications of TQM

Action Step: Discuss in detail the degree of external cooperation your leadership will support, including the types of processes, information, strengths, and weaknesses you are willing to share with whom.

Action Step: Join a network of organizations implementing TQM. Joining a regional network provides substantial benefits at low cost.

Action Step: Contact your suppliers and ask whether they have experience with TQM and are willing to work together to help improve your quality and cost effectiveness.

Action Step: Identify a key process needing improvement and a potential benchmarking partner. If you join a network, one or more of those organizations may be willing to participate.

Action Step: Establish regular communication opportunities and forums with each of your key customer groups. Use focus groups, surveys, personal interviews, and other feedback methods to listen and dialogue.

Action Step: Meet with representatives of key business, industrial, and service organizations within your area to obtain and understand all applicable quality guidelines used for their suppliers.

Action Step: Evaluate your progress on quality improvement annually using a combination of internally and externally developed criteria.

Action Step: Establish a team to investigate critical paths, if they are not in use. TQM tools, such as brainstorming and flowcharting, can help the team develop the critical path.

Action Step: Assign a cross-functional team to use the QFD approach when your organization is planning a new or revised service. The customer input and results will be worth the investment.

Action Step: Use hoshin planning methods to deploy your goals and strategic plans throughout your organization.

Chapter Fifteen: Beyond the Glitter

Action Step: Make sure your early expectations are realistic. Practical knowledge of "how" to begin must accompany the education and training in theory. Make practical tools and aids available to managers to support the quality process. Create opportunities for the "Aha!" experience.

Action Steps:

1. Demonstrate the need for change.
2. Make sure all levels of managers are included in the planning process.
3. Give managers the tools and techniques to be successful.
4. Make the commitment to place managers in nonmanagement positions, if management reductions are necessary.

Action Step: Develop values clarification exercises to demonstrate why the new management philosophy and empowerment are necessary. Provide guidance and support for managers so they can evaluate and adjust their style.

Action Step: View employees' value separately from their current jobs, and encourage everyone else to do the same. This is necessary if you wish to become a flexible, learning organization.

Action Step: Begin your process with managers serving

both as team leaders and team members. Let them experience empowerment before they empower others. Recognize that fears and anxieties exist. Allow time for issues to surface and talk about strategies to overcome these issues.

Action Step: Involve your managers in the planning process. Help them share important information with appropriately consistent tools and formats.

Action Step: Make sure appropriate tools and techniques are available to help managers with the implementation process. Frequently ask managers and team leaders what is working well and what can be improved.

Action Step: Encourage employees to talk to external customers. Encourage them to ask patients: How was your visit? What went well? What went poorly? What could be improved?

Action Step: Encourage managers and executives to make rounds and ask internal and external customers what their requirements are and how they are being satisfied. Then communicate the information and initiate changes to make improvements.

Action Step: Develop a strategic plan early in your process.

Action Step: Monitor and communicate team progress. Develop specific measures and report results to the organization. Determine indicators of team achievement. Recognize and reward teams upon completion or achievement of significant steps and goals.

Action Step: Make sure the process is understandable. Communicate the plan and progress in manageable elements for the employees.

Action Step: Define the terms you will use in your organization in a clear and cogent way. Keep jargon to a minimum. Use examples applicable to your organization where possible.

Action Step: Find time for quality by getting rid of bureaucratic practices such as unnecessary reports, paperwork with multiple-level signatures, meetings that do not add value, and doing things that can be eliminated.

Action Step: Stress the potential cost savings generated by addressing the cost of poor quality. Teach all employees the concepts of waste prevention and how they can help the organization save scarce resources.

Action Step: Set up corporate task teams that can work on keeping progress visible for employees. Demonstrate management commitment to TQM, and apathy will be replaced with enthusiasm.

Action Step: Expectations must be managed. Keep communication flowing. Gantt charts that list milestones are helpful in explaining progress and keeping everyone updated.

Action Step: Consult with organizations that have quality experience as you plan your educational process.

Action Step: Assess communication patterns in your organization and develop an action plan for improvement. Set up a communications task team and develop a TQM communication program.

Action Step: Review carefully for duplicative efforts or overgrown bureaucratic practices as your TQM process develops. Integrate creativity and innovation into your quality process.

Action Step: Develop an integrated program with a clinical and administrative focus. Identify and support administrative and clinical champions.

REFERENCES

The Advisory Board Company, Governance Committee. *Aligning Hospital-Physician Interests: Strategies for Physician Enfranchisement*. Washington, D.C.: The Advisory Board Company, 1991a.

The Advisory Board Company, Governance Committee. "Clinical Utilization." Presentation. Washington, D.C.: The Advisory Board Company, Spring 1991b.

Akao, Y. (ed.). *Quality Function Deployment: Integrating Customer Requirements into Product Design*. (G. H. Mazur, trans.) Cambridge, Mass.: Productivity Press, 1990.

Akao, Y. (ed.). *Hoshin Kanri: Policy Deployment for Successful TQM*. (G. H. Mazur, trans.) Cambridge, Mass.: Productivity Press, 1991.

Albrecht, K., with Albrecht, S. *The Creative Corporation*. Homewood, Ill.: Dow Jones-Irwin, 1987.

Allen, R. F., and Kraft, C. "Transformations That Last: A Cultural Approach in Transforming Work." In J. Adams (ed.), *Transforming Work*. Alexandria, Va.: Miles River Press, 1984.

American Dental Association. *National Practitioner Data: Questions & Answers*. Chicago: American Dental Association, 1990.

American Hospital Association. *Practice Pattern Analysis: A Tool for Continuous Improvement of Patient Care Quality*. Chicago: American Hospital Association, 1991.

Anderson, K. "Health Care Costs More, Serves Fewer!" *USA Today,* Mar. 11, 1991, p. B1.

AT&T. *Statistical Quality Control Handbook.* Indianapolis, Ind.: AT&T Technologies, 1984.

Aubrey, C. A., and Felkins, P. K. *Teamwork: Involving People in Quality and Productivity.* White Plains, N.Y.: 1988.

Auld, D. "Baxter Quality." Speech. Deerfield, Ill.: Baxter International, June 1991.

Bardwick, J. *Danger in the Comfort Zone.* New York: AMACOM, 1991.

Barker, J. A. *Discovering the Future: The Business of Paradigms.* St. Paul, Minn.: ILI Press, 1989.

Barker, J. A. *Future Edge: Discovering the New Paradigms of Success.* New York: William Morrow, 1992.

Bennis, W., and Nanus, B. *Leaders: The Strategies for Taking Charge.* New York: HarperCollins, 1985.

Berg, D. "Uncommon Sense: In Defense of Disorder and Discontent." *Journal of Quality and Participation.* Sept. 1991, p. 51.

Berry, T. H. *Managing the Total Quality Transformation.* New York: McGraw-Hill, 1991.

Bertrand, K. "In Service Perception Counts." *Business Marketing,* Apr. 1989, p. 46.

Berwick, D. M. "Continuous Improvement as an Ideal in Health Care." Sounding Board. *New England Journal of Medicine,* 1989, *320,* 53–56.

Berwick, D. M. Presentation at third annual National Forum for Quality Improvement in Health Care, Atlanta, Ga., Oct. 23, 1991.

Berwick, D. M., Godfrey, A. B., and Roessner, J. *Curing Health Care: New Strategies for Quality Improvement.* San Francisco: Jossey-Bass, 1990.

"Better Safe Than Sorry Strategy Wastes Billions a Year in Unneeded Medical Care." *Ann Arbor News,* Jan. 8, 1992, p. B3.

Bhote, K. R. *Next Operation as Customer (NOAC): How to Improve Quality, Cost and Cycle Time in Service Operations.* AMA Management Briefing. New York: American Management Association, 1991.

Biesada, A. "Benchmarking: As Competition Is Heating Up, So

Is the Search for World-Class Performers." *Financial World,* Sept. 17, 1991, pp. 28–47.

Block, P. *The Empowered Manager: Positive Political Skills at Work.* San Francisco: Jossey-Bass, 1987.

Bohl, D. L. (group ed.). *Blueprints for Service Quality: The Federal Express Approach.* AMA Management Briefing. New York: American Management Association, Membership Publications Division, 1991.

Boyle, R. "Wrestling with Jellyfish." *Harvard Business Review,* 1984, *62*(1), 74–83.

Brassard, M. *The Memory Jogger Plus + : Featuring the Seven Management and Planning Tools.* Methuen, Mass.: GOAL/QPC, 1989.

Buzzell, R. D., and Bradley, T. G. *Principles Linking Strategy to Performance.* New York: Free Press, 1987.

Camp, R. C. *Benchmarking: The Search for Industry Best Practices That Lead to Superior Performance.* Milwaukee, Wis.: American Society for Quality Control, Quality Press, 1989.

Cannie, J. K., and Caplin, D. *Keeping Customers for Life.* New York: AMACOM, 1991.

Center for Quality Management. *The Seven Step Method: A Problem-Solving Process for Continuous Improvement,* developed by Analog Devices. Cambridge, Mass.: Center for Quality Management, 1991.

Chapman, E. "Hospitals and Prisons." *Healthcare Forum Journal,* Nov./Dec. 1990, pp. 18–20.

Clark, A. "Intermountain Health Care: In Heavy Pursuit of a Clinical Approach to Total Quality Management." *Strategic Health Care Marketing,* Nov. 1991, pp. 1–3.

Classen, D. C., Evans, S. R., and Pestotnik, S. L. "The Timing of Prophylactic Administration of Antibiotics and the Risk of Surgical Wound Infection." *New England Journal of Medicine,* 1992, *326*(5), pp. 281–286.

Clemmer, J. "5 Common Errors Companies Make Starting Quality Initiatives." *Total Quality Newsletter,* Lakewood Publications, 1992, *3*(4), 7.

Coffey, R. J. "Comparing TQM and Traditional QA: Considerations for Health Care Organizations." *Competitive Times,* no. 2. Methuen, Mass.: GOAL/QPC, 1991, pp. 9–10.

Coffey, R. J., Eisenberg, M., Gaucher, E. M., and Kratochwill, E. W. "Total Quality Progress at the University of Michigan Medical Center." *Journal for Quality and Participation*. Jan./Feb. 1991, pp. 22–31.

Coffey, R. J., and others. "An Introduction to Critical Paths." *Quality Management in Health Care*, 1992, *1*(1), 45–54.

Coile, R. C., Jr. *The New Hospital: Future Strategies for a Changing Industry.* Rockville, Md.: Aspen Systems, 1986.

Cousins, N. *Anatomy of an Illness as Perceived by the Patient: Reflections on Healing and Regeneration.* New York: W.W. Norton, 1979.

Covey, S. R. *The 7 Habits of Highly Effective People: Powerful Lessons in Personal Change.* New York: Simon & Schuster, 1990.

Creps, L. B., Coffey, R. J., Warner, P. A., and McClatchey, K. P. "Improvement of Quality Through the Integration of Total Quality and Quality Assessment." *Quality Review Bulletin (QRB): Journal of Quality Improvement*, Joint Commission on Accreditation of Healthcare Organizations, Aug. 1992.

Crosby, P. B. *Quality Is Free: The Art of Making Quality Certain.* New York: McGraw-Hill, 1979.

Deal, T. E., and Kennedy, A. A. *Corporate Cultures: The Rites and Rituals of Corporate Life.* Reading, Mass.: Addison-Wesley, 1982.

Deal, T. E., Kenn, A. A., and Spiegel, A. H., III. "How to Create an Outstanding Hospital Culture." *Hospital Forum*, Jan./Feb. 1983, *26*, 21–28, 33–34.

deBono, E. "Quality Is No Longer Enough." *Journal of Quality and Participation*, 1991, *14*(5), 13.

Deming, W. E. *Out of the Crisis.* Cambridge: Center for Advanced Engineering Study, Massachusetts Institute of Technology, 1986.

Deming, W. E. *Notes on Management in a Hospital.* Washington, D.C.: W. Edwards Deming, Sept. 20, 1987.

Denison, D. R. *Corporate Culture and Organizational Effectiveness.* New York: Wiley, 1990.

DePree, M. "Today's Leaders Look to Tomorrow." *Fortune*, Mar. 26, 1990, p. 26.

Dixon, G., and Swiler, J. *The Total Quality Handbook.* Minneapolis, Minn.: Lakewood Books, 1990.

Dobyns, L., and Crawford-Mason, C. *Quality or Else: The Revolution in World Business.* Boston: Houghton Mifflin, 1991.

Donabedian, A. "The End Results of Health Care: Ernest Codman's Contribution to Quality Assessment and Beyond." *The Milbank Quarterly,* 1989, *67*(2).

Drucker, P. F. *Managing in Turbulent Times.* New York: HarperCollins, 1980.

Drucker, P. F. "Tomorrow's Restless Managers." *Industry Week,* 1988, *18,* 25.

Dumaine, B. "What the Leaders of Tomorrow See." *Fortune,* July 3, 1989, pp. 48–62.

Dumas, R. A. "Organization-Wide Quality Programs." In G. Dixon and J. Swiler, *The Total Quality Handbook.* Minneapolis, Minn.: Lakewood Books, 1990.

Eisenberg, J. M. *Doctors' Decisions and the Cost of Medical Care.* Ann Arbor, Mich.: Health Administration Press Perspectives, 1986.

Ellwood, P. M. "A Technology of Patient Experience." Special report, Shattuck lecture — Outcomes Management. *New England Journal of Medicine,* 1988, *318,* 1549–1556.

Ernst & Young Quality Improvement Consulting Group. *Total Quality: An Executive's Guide for the 1990's.* Homewood, Ill.: Dow Jones-Irwin, 1990.

Espinosa, J. "Physicians Can Be Brought into Hospital's TQM Effort, with 'Empowering' Approach." *QI/TQM,* 1992, *2*(1), 11–12.

Etheredge, M.L.S. (ed.). *Collaborative Care: Nursing Case Management.* Chicago: American Hospital Publishing, 1989.

Ethridge, P., and Lamb, G. S. "Professional Nursing Case Management Improves Quality, Access and Costs." *Nursing Management,* 1989, *20*(3).

Fisher, R., and Ury, W. *Getting to Yes: Negotiating Agreement Without Giving In.* New York: Penguin Books, 1983.

Ford Motor Company. *Continuing Process Control and Process Capability Improvement.* Dearborn, Mich.: Corporate Quality Education and Training Center, Corporate Quality Office, Ford Motor Company, Dec. 1987.

Ford Motor Company. *Worldwide Quality System Standard Q-101, for Manufacturing Operations and Outside Suppliers of Production and Service Products*. Dearborn, Mich.: Ford Motor Company, 1990.

Franklin, D., Panzer, R., Brideau, L., and Griner, P. "Innovations in Clinical Practice Through Hospital-Funded Grants." *Academic Medicine*, 1990, *65*(6), 355–360.

Freidson, E. "Professional Dominance and the Ordering of Health Services." In *Professional Dominance: The Social Structure of Medical Care*. Chicago: Athterton Press, 1970.

Galli, H. "Health Care's 'Quality Dividend.'" *Boston Globe*, July 30, 1991, p. 1.

Garnick, D. W., Hendricks, A. M., and Brennan, T. A. "Can Practice Guidelines Reduce the Number and Costs of Malpractice Claims?" *Journal of the American Medical Association*, 1991, *226*(20), 2856–2860.

Garvin, D. A. *Managing Quality: The Strategic and Competitive Edge*. New York: Free Press, 1988.

Gaspari, J. "Limits Can Be Liberating." *Journal of Quality and Participation*, 1991, *14*(5), 6.

Gaucher, E. "Trained Teams." In M. M. Melum and M. K. Sinioris (eds.), *Total Quality Management: The Healthcare Pioneers*. Chicago: American Hospital Publishing, 1992.

General Motors Corporation. *Targets for Excellence, for General Motors Manufacturing Divisions and Outside Suppliers of Production Material and Service Products*. Detroit, Mich.: Suppliers Development Administration, General Motors Purchasing Activities, Sept. 1990.

Gibson, R. M., Waldo, D. R., and Levitt, K. R. "National Health Expenditures, 1982." *Health Care Financing Review*, 1983, *5*, 1–30.

Gilbert, N. *Quality Improvement Teams: Some Lessons Learned, May 1989–May 1991*. Internal University of Michigan Hospitals report. Ann Arbor: University of Michigan Hospitals, June 1991.

Gitlow, H. S., and Gitlow, S. J. *The Deming Guide to Quality and Competitive Position*. Englewood Cliffs, N.J.: Prentice-Hall, 1987.

GOAL/QPC. *The Memory Jogger: A Pocket Guide of Tools for Continuous Improvement.* (2nd ed.) Methuen, Mass.: GOAL/QPC, 1988.

GOAL/QPC. *Putting the T in Health Care TQM: A Model for Integrated TQM: Clinical Care and Operations.* A GOAL/QPC Health Care Application Research Committee report. Methuen, Mass.: GOAL/QPC, 1992.

GOAL/QPC Research Committee. *Hoshin Planning: A Planning System for Implementing Total Quality Management (TQM).* Methuen, Mass.: GOAL/QPC, 1989.

Grazier, P. B. *Before It's Too Late: Employee Involvement . . . An Idea Whose Time Has Come.* Chadds Ford, Penn.: Teambuilding, 1989.

Grostick, C. *University of Michigan Hospitals End-Stage Renal Disease Team.* Speech. Ann Arbor, Mich., Jan. 1991.

Halder, R. "Total Quality at the San Diego Naval Hospital." Personal communication at University of California, San Diego, June 16, 1991.

Harvey, J. B. *The Abilene Paradox.* Lexington, Mass.: Lexington, 1988.

Headrick, L. A., and others. "Teaching Medical Students About Quality and Cost of Care at Case Western Reserve University." *Academic Medicine*, 1992, 2(3), 157–158.

The Healthcare Forum. *The 1992 Commitment to Quality Award: Call for Entries.* San Francisco: Healthcare Forum, 1991.

Hilts, P. J. "Say Ouch: Demands to Fix U.S. Health Care Reach a Crescendo." *Wall Street Journal*, May 19, 1991, sec. 4, p. 1.

Hospital Corporation of America. *Hospitalwide Quality Improvement Process, Strategy for Improvement, FOCUS–PDCA.* Nashville, Tenn.: Hospital Corporation of America, 1989a.

Hospital Corporation of America. *Quality—Learning the New Way.* Nashville, Tenn.: Hospital Corporation of America, 1989b. Videotape.

Hospital Corporation of America. *Quality—The New Way.* Nashville, Tenn.: Hospital Corporation of America, 1989c. Videotape.

Hudson, T. "Clinical Quality Initiatives: The Search for Meaningful and Accurate Measures." *Hospitals*, Mar. 5, 1992, pp. 26–40.

Huge, E. C. *Total Quality: An Executive's Guide for the 1990's*. Homewood, Ill.: Business One Irwin, 1990.

Imai, M. *Kaizen: The Key to Japan's Competitive Success*. New York: Random House, 1986.

Inc. Executive interview. Apr. 1989, p. 49.

InterStudy. *An Introduction to InterStudy's Outcomes Management System Development Plans*. Excelsior, Minn.: InterStudy, Mar. 1990a.

InterStudy. *Status Report—Outcomes Management System Data Protocols (TyPEs)*. Excelsior, Minn.: InterStudy, Mar. 1990b.

James, B. C. "How Do You Involve Physicians in TQM?" *The Journal for Quality and Participation*. Jan./Feb. 1991, pp. 42–47.

Joint Commission on Accreditation of Healthcare Organizations. *Transitions: From QA to CQI, Using CQI Approaches to Monitor, Evaluate, and Improve Quality*. Oakbrook Terrace, Ill.: Joint Commission on Accreditation of Healthcare Organizations, 1991a.

Joint Commission on Accreditation of Healthcare Organizations. *The Transition from QA to CQI: An Introduction to Quality Improvement Health Care*. Oakbrook Terrace, Ill.: Joint Commission on Accreditation of Healthcare Organizations, 1991b.

Joint Commission on Accreditation of Healthcare Organizations. *1992 Joint Commission Accreditation Manual for Hospitals*. Chicago: Joint Commission on Accreditation of Healthcare Organizations, 1991c.

Joint Commission on Accreditation of Healthcare Organizations. *1992 Joint Commission Accreditation Manual for Hospitals, Volume II, Scoring Guidelines*. Chicago: Joint Commission on Accreditation of Healthcare Organizations, 1991d.

Joint Commission on Accreditation of Healthcare Organizations. *Building the Foundation for Corporate Quality Improvement*. Educational retreats held multiple locations in United States. Chicago: Joint Commission on Accreditation of Healthcare Organizations, 1992a.

Joint Commission on Accreditation of Healthcare Organizations. *Striving Toward Improvement: Six Hospitals in Search of*

Quality. Chicago: Joint Commission on Accreditation of Healthcare Organizations, 1992b.

Joint Commission on Accreditation of Healthcare Organizations. *1993 Joint Commission Accreditation Manual for Hospitals,* Vol. 1. Oakbrook Terrace, Ill.: Joint Commission on Accreditation of Healthcare Organizations, 1992c.

Joint Commission on Accreditation of Hospitals. *Supplement to the Accreditation Manual for Hospitals.* Chicago: Joint Commission on Accreditation of Hospitals, 1975.

Juran, J. M. *Juran on Planning for Quality.* New York: Free Press, 1988.

Juran, J. M. *Juran on Leadership for Quality.* New York: Free Press, 1989.

Juran, J. M., and Gryna, F. M. *Quality Planning and Analysis.* New York: McGraw-Hill, 1980.

Juran, J. M., and Gryna, F. M. *Juran's Quality Control Handbook.* (4th ed.) New York: McGraw-Hill, 1988.

Juran Institute. *Total Quality Management: A Practical Guide.* Wilton, Conn.: Juran Institute, 1991.

Juran Institute. *Quality Improvement for Health Care: Team Preparation.* Wilton, Conn.: Juran Institute, 1992.

Kano, N. "Attractive Quality and Must-Be Quality." (GOAL/QPC, trans.) Paper presented at the 12th annual meeting of the Japan Society of Quality Control (JSQC), 1982. Methuen, Mass.: GOAL/QPC, 1984.

Kano, N., Seraku, N., Takahashi, F., and Tsuji, S. "Attractive Quality and Must Be Quality." *Quality,* 1984, *14*(2), 39–48.

Kanter, R. M. *Men and Women of the Corporation.* New York: Basic Books, 1977.

Kanter, R. M. "The New Managerial Work." *Harvard Business Review,* Nov./Dec. 1989a, pp. 85–92.

Kanter, R. M. *When Giants Learn to Dance.* New York: Simon & Schuster, 1989b.

Kerns, D. T. "Definition of Benchmarking." In R. C. Camp, *Benchmarking: The Search for Industry Best Practices That Lead to Superior Performance.* Milwaukee, Wis.: American Society for Quality Control, Quality Press, 1989, p. 10.

Kilmann, R. H. *Managing Beyond the Quick Fix: A Completely Inte-*

grated Program for Creating and Maintaining Organizational Suc-cess. San Francisco: Jossey-Bass, 1989.

King, B. *Better Designs in Half the Time: Implementing Quality Func-tion Deployment in America.* (3rd ed.) Methuen, Mass.: GOAL/QPC, 1989a.

King, B. *Hoshin Planning: The Developmental Approach.* Methuen, Mass.: GOAL/QPC, 1989b.

Kouzes, J. M., and Posner, B. Z. *The Leadership Challenge: How to Get Extraordinary Things Done in Organizations.* San Francisco: Jossey-Bass, 1987.

Kratochwill, E., and Gaucher, E. "National Demonstration Proj-ect on Industrial Quality Control and Health Care Quality: The Progress of the Original Twenty-One Participating Orga-nizations." *The Journal for Quality and Participation,* Jan./Feb. 1991, pp. 32–34.

Kriegel, R. J., and Patler, L. *If It Ain't Broke. . . Break It, and Other Unconventional Wisdom for a Changing Business World.* New York: Warner Books, 1991.

Kritchevsky, S. B., and Simmons, B. P. "Continuous Quality Improvement: Concepts and Applications for Physician Care." *Journal of the American Medical Association,* 1991, *266,* 1817–1823.

Kübler-Ross, E. *On Death and Dying.* New York: Macmillan, 1969.

Laffel, G. "Implementing Quality Management in Health Care: The Challenges Ahead." *Quality Progress.* Nov. 1990, pp. 29–32.

Laffel, G., and Blumenthal, D. "The Case for Using Industrial Quality Management Science in Health Care Organizations." *Journal of the American Medical Association,* 1989, *262,* 2869–2873.

Larson, C. E., and LaFasto, F.M.J. *Teamwork: What Must Go Right/What Can Go Wrong.* Newbury Park, Calif.: Sage, 1989.

Lawler, E. E., III. *Pay and Organization Development.* Reading, Mass.: Addison-Wesley, 1981.

Lawler, E. E., III. *High-Involvement Management: Participative Strat-egies for Improving Organizational Performance.* San Francisco: Jossey-Bass, 1991.

Leebov, W. *Service Excellence: The Customer Relations Strategy for Health Care.* Chicago: American Hospital Publishing, 1988.

Locke, E. A., and Latham, G. P. *Goal Setting: A Motivational Technique That Works.* Englewood Cliffs, N.J.: Prentice-Hall, 1984.

Longenecker, C., and Giola, D. "Ten Myths of Managing Managers." *Sloan Management Forum,* Fall 1991, p. 81.

Maccoby, M. *Why Work?* New York: Simon & Schuster, 1988.

McCormick, B. "AMA Not Ready for New Quality Philosophy." *American Medical News,* July 22, 1991, p. 5.

McLagan, P. "Leadership Beware: Your Quality Process May Be a Bloated Bureaucracy," *Total Quality Newsletter,* 1991, *2*(12), 2–3.

McMahon and others. "The Integrated Inpatient Management Model: A New Approach to Clinical Practice." *Annals of Internal Medicine,* 1989, *111*, 318–326.

Management Systems Department, University of Michigan Hospitals. *Structured Flowcharting: How to Develop and Document "Critical Path" Flowcharts.* Ann Arbor: Management Systems Department, University of Michigan Hospitals, May 1989.

Marszalek-Gaucher, E., and Coffey, R. J. *Transforming Healthcare Organizations: How to Achieve and Sustain Organizational Excellence.* San Francisco: Jossey-Bass, 1990.

Martin, J., Sitkin, S. M., and Boehm, M. "Founders and the Elusiveness of Cultural Legacy." In P. J. Frost and others (eds.), *Organizational Culture.* Beverly Hills, Calif.: Sage, 1985.

Melum, M. M., and Sinioris, M. K. *Total Quality Management: The Health Care Pioneers.* Chicago: American Hospital Publishing, 1992.

Merry, M. D. "Total Quality Management for Physicians: Translating the New Paradigm." *Quality Review Bulletin,* Mar. 1990, pp. 101–105.

Nadler, G., and Hibino, S. *Breakthrough Thinking: Why We Must Change the Way We Solve Problems, and the Seven Principles to Achieve This.* Rocklin, Calif.: Prima Publishing & Communications, 1990.

Naisbitt, J., and Aburdene, P. *Megatrends 2000: Ten New Directions for the 1990's.* New York: William Morrow, 1990.

National Association of Suggestion Systems. *1990 Annual Statistical Report.* National Association of Suggestion Systems, 1990.

National Institute of Standards and Technology. *1993 Award*

Criteria, Malcolm Baldrige National Quality Award. Gaithersburg, Md.: National Institute of Standards and Technology, United States Department of Commerce, 1992.

Oakley, E., and Krug, D. *Enlightened Leadership.* New York: Simon & Schuster, 1993.

O'Leary, D. "Moving Healthcare Toward CQI: The Joint Commission's Plans for the Future." *The Quality Letter,* Nov. 1991, pp. 12–16.

Organizational Dynamics, Inc. *Implementing Total Quality Management.* Burlington, Mass.: Organizational Dynamics, 1990.

Panzer, R., Black, E., and Winchell, M. (eds.). *Improving Patient Care Through Enhanced Clinical Analysis.* Rochester, N.Y.: Strong Memorial Hospital, University of Rochester Medical Center, Oct. 1991.

Parker, G. M. *Team Players and Teamwork: The New Competitive Business Strategy.* San Francisco: Jossey-Bass, 1990.

Pellegrino, E. "Altruism, Self-Interest and Medical Ethics." *Journal of the American Medical Association,* 1987, *258,* 1939–1940.

Peters, T. *The Excellence Challenge.* Chicago: Nightingale-Conant, 1984. Audiotape.

Peters, T. *Thriving on Chaos: Handbook for a Management Revolution.* New York: Knopf, 1987.

Peters, T. J. "Making It Happen." *Journal of Quality and Productivity,* 1990, *12*(1), 7.

Peters, T. J., and Waterman, R. H. *In Search of Excellence.* Cambridge, Mass.: HarperCollins, 1982.

Petersen, D. E., and Hillkirk, J. *A Better Idea: Redefining the Way Americans Work.* Boston: Houghton Mifflin, 1991.

Pinchot, G., III. *Intrapreneuring.* New York: HarperCollins, 1985.

QI/TQM Newsletter, 1991, *1*(2).

Qualtec, Inc. *Team Member Manual: Participant Workbook.* Miami, Fla.: Florida Power & Light, 1988.

Qualtec, Inc. *Facilitator Skills Training Course.* (3rd ed.) Miami, Fla.: Florida Power & Light, 1989a.

Qualtec, Inc. *Team Leader Training Course.* (2nd ed.) Miami, Fla.: Florida Power & Light, 1989b.

Reverby, S. "Stealing the Golden Eggs: Ernest Amory Codman and the Science and Management of Medicine." In *Bulletin of the History of Medicine,* Johns Hopkins University Press, 1981, 156–171.

Rhodes, P. B. "Physician Payment Reform: What RBRVS Will Mean to You." *Healthcare Forum Journal,* Sept./Oct. 1991, pp. 63–66.

Roth, A. V., Giffi, C. A., and Seal, G. M. *Operating Strategies for the 1990's: Elements Comprising World Class Manufacturing.* Ann Arbor, Mich.: National Center for Manufacturing Sciences, Jan. 1990.

Russell, W. F., and Branch, T. *Second Wind.* New York: Random House, 1979.

Ryan, K. D., and Oestreich, D. K. *Driving Fear out of the Workplace: How to Overcome the Invisible Barriers to Quality, Productivity, and Innovation.* San Francisco: Jossey-Bass, 1991.

Sahney, V. "Implementation, Observed Barriers, and Management of Continuous Quality Improvement." In *National Quality of Care Forum, Bridging the Gap Between Theory and Practice.* Chicago: Hospital Research and Educational Trust, 1992. (AHA catalog no. 169510.)

Salvendy, G. (ed.). *Handbook of Industrial Engineering.* New York: Wiley, 1982.

Sandrick, K. "New Quality Systems Have Broad Impact on Physicians, Clarify Causes of Problems." *ACP Observer.*

Schein, E. H. *Organizational Culture and Leadership.* San Francisco: Jossey-Bass, 1985.

Scherkenbach, W. W. *The Deming Route to Quality and Productivity: Road Maps and Roadblocks.* Washington, D.C.: CEEPress Books, George Washington University, 1988.

Schick, F. L. (ed.). *Statistical Handbook on Aging Americans.* Phoenix, Ariz.: Oryx Press, 1986.

Schieber, J., and Poullier, J.-P. "International Health Spending: Issues and Trends," *Health Affairs,* Spring 1991, 106–116.

Scholtes, P. R., and others. *The Team Handbook.* Madison, Wis.: Joiner Associates, 1988.

Scott, C. D., and Jaffee, D. J. "From Crisis to Culture Change." *Healthcare Forum,* 1991, *34*(3), 32–42.

Senge, P. M. *The Fifth Discipline: The Art and Practice of the Learning Organization.* New York: Doubleday, 1990.

Shafer, R. H. "Results Improvement Is the Key to Creativity and Empowerment." *Journal for Quality and Participation.* 1991, *14*(5), 18.

Shaw, G. B. *The Irrational Knot,* 1905.

Sheldon, A. *Managing Doctors.* Homewood, Ill.: Dow Jones-Irwin, 1986.

Shortell, S. "Adding Value Is a Must for Survivors and Thrivers." *Healthcare Executive,* 1990, *5*(3), 17–19.

Smith, L. "A Cure for What Ails Medical Care." *Fortune,* 1991, *124*(1), 44–49.

"Solutions to the Health-Care Crisis." *Money,* July 1991, *20*(7), 74–75.

"Some Helpful Advice from Five Health Experts." *Money,* July 1991, *20*(7), 76–77.

Thomas, R. R., Jr. *Beyond Race and Gender: Unleashing the Power of Your Total Work Force by Managing Diversity.* New York: AMACOM, 1991.

Thompson, R. E. "Changing the Medical Staff Organizational Model in United States Medical Centers: A Critical Component of Continuous Quality Improvement." *Insight,* 1992, *2*(1), 1.

Townsend, P. L., with Gebhardt, J. E. *Commit to Quality.* New York: Wiley, 1990.

Townsend, P. L., and Gebhardt, J. E. "Creating More Creativity." *Journal of Quality and Participation,* 1991, *14*(5), 24.

Troy, K. L. *Recognizing Quality Achievement: Noncash Award Programs.* Report No. 1008. New York: Conference Board, 1992.

Tuckman, B. W. "Developmental Sequence in Small Groups." *Psychological Bulletin,* 1965, *63*(6), 384–399.

U.S. Department of Labor. *Opportunity 2000: Creative Affirmative Action Strategies for a Changing Work Force.* (Prepared by Hudson Institute, Indianapolis, Ind.) Washington, D.C.: Employment Standards Administration, U.S. Department of Labor, 1988.

U.S. General Accounting Office. *Management Practices: U.S. Companies Improve Performance Through Quality Efforts.* Report to the Honorable Donald Ritter, House of Representatives, GAO/ NSLAD-91-190 Management Practices. Washington, D.C.:

National Security and International Affairs Division, U.S. General Accounting Office, May 1991.

University of Michigan Hospitals. *Overview and Introduction to TQM, TQ101*. Training program manual. Ann Arbor: University of Michigan Hospitals, 1991a.

University of Michigan Hospitals. *Learning Cycle, Measurement, and Deming's 14 Points, TQ102*. Training program manual. Ann Arbor: University of Michigan Hospitals, 1991b.

University of Michigan Hospitals. *Tools & Techniques, Tampering, and Learning Principles, TQ103*. Training program manual. Ann Arbor: University of Michigan Hospitals, 1991c.

University of Michigan Hospitals. *Total Quality Leadership Program*. Ann Arbor: University of Michigan Hospitals, 1992.

University of Michigan Medical Center. *Mission of Corporate Lead Team; Notes from Corporate Lead Team*. Ann Arbor: University of Michigan Medical Center, 1990.

University of Michigan Medical Center. *Employee Suggestion Program*. Ann Arbor: University of Michigan Medical Center, Summer 1991a.

University of Michigan Medical Center. *Manager's Guide to Begin Total Quality Process*. Ann Arbor: University of Michigan Medical Center, Oct. 1991b.

University of Michigan Medical Center. *Costs, Benefits, and Return from UMMC Total Quality Process: July 1987 Through June 1991*. Ann Arbor: University of Michigan Medical Center, Feb. 1992a.

University of Michigan Medical Center. *Total Quality Leadership Program*. Ann Arbor: University of Michigan Medical Center, 1992b.

Veatch, R. "CQI Revisited." *The Quality Letter*, May 1990, pp. 2–8.

Walton, M. *The Deming Management Method*. New York: Putnam, 1986.

Walton, M. *Deming Management at Work: Six Successful Companies That Use the Quality Principles of the World-Famous W. Edwards Deming*. New York: Putnam, 1990.

Walton, R. E. "From Control to Commitment in the Workplace." *Harvard Business Review*, 1986, *63*, 76–84.

Wennberg, J. E. "Dealing with Medical Practice Variations: A Proposal for Action." *Health Affairs*, Summer 1984, 7–32.

Wennberg, J. E., Barnes, B. A., and Zubkoff, M. "Professional Uncertainty and the Problem of Supplier-Induced Demand." *Social Science Medicine*, 1982, *16*, 811–824.

Wennberg, J. E., and Gittelsohn, A. "Small Area Variations in Health Care Delivery." *Science*, 1973, *182*, 1102–1108.

Wennberg, J. E., and Gittelsohn, A. "Health Care Delivery in Maine: I. Patterns of Use of Common Surgical Procedures." *Journal of the Maine Medical Association*, 1975, *36*(5), 123–130.

Wennberg, J. E., and Gittelsohn, A. "Variations in Medical Care Among Small Areas." *Scientific American*, 1982, *264*(4), 120–134.

Wennerker, M. B., Weissman, J. S., and Epstein, A. M. "The Association of Payer with Utilization of Cardiac Procedures in Massachusetts." *Journal of the American Medical Association*, 1990, *264*(10), 1255–1260.

Whiteley, R. C. *The Customer Driven Company: Moving from Talk to Action*. Reading, Mass.: Addison-Wesley, 1991.

Whiting, R. "Benchmarking: Lessons from the Best-in-Class." *Electronic Business*, Oct. 7, 1991, pp. 128–134.

Wiggenhorn, W. "Motorola U.: When Training Becomes an Education." *Harvard Business Review*, July/Aug. 1990, pp. 71–83.

Wigton, R. S. "Ideas for Medical Education." *Academic Medicine*, 1992, *2*(3).

Wilensky, G. R., and Rossiter, L. F. "The Relative Importance of Physician-Induced Demand for Medical Care." *Milbank Memorial Fund Quarterly*, 1983, *61*, 252–277.

Wyszewianski, L. *The Clinical Efficiency and Quality Initiative: A Proposal to the University of Michigan Medical Center*. Ann Arbor: University of Michigan Medical Center, 1991.

Yankelovich, D. *New Rules — Searching for Self-Fulfillment in a World Turned Upside Down*. New York: Random House, 1981.

Zander, K. "Critical Paths: Marking the Course." *Definition*, 1987, *2*(3), 1–4.

Zander, K. "Care Maps: The Core of Cost/Quality Care." *The New Definition*. South Natick, Mass.: Center for Case Management, 1991, *6*(3), 1–3.

INDEX

agement, 326–328; and goals, 344; and implementation, 122, 132, 133; milestones in, 518–520; mistakes in, 527–528; phases for, 533; and physician involvement, 195, 200–201, 204, 205; pitfalls of, 535–544; results of, 539–541; and rewards, 281, 290, 305; and teamwork, 224, 232
Townsend, P. L., 87, 141, 290, 298, 322, 546
Toyota, and benchmarking, 457
Training. *See* Education
Travelers, and benchmarking, 457
Troy, K. L., 281
Trust, need for, 541
Tsuji, S., 34
Tuckman, B. W., 235–239, 400
Twyon, S., 469

U

UARCO, in partnership, 488
Union leaders, education for, 263
United Kingdom, healthcare spending in, 6–7
U.S. Department of Health and Human Services, 334
U.S. Department of Labor, 169
U.S. General Accounting Office, 22–23
U.S. Quality Councils, 448
University of California San Diego Medical Center, hospital planning at, 529
University of Michigan Medical Center (UMMC): Administrative Forum at, 172–173; Admission/Discharge Team at, 19, 122, 244; Clinical Improvement Team at, 203; and clinical models, 48–50; Clinical Quality Improvement (CQI) initiative at, 201–205; Clinical Quality Improvement Lead Team (CQILT) at, 202–203, 206; Corporate Lead Team at, 132, 219, 223, 224, 232, 234, 312, 344, 534; cost effectiveness at,

90, 93; cost of poor quality at, 12, 23; critical paths at, 470, 472–473, 474, 476, 477, 478; cultural audit at, 160–161; culture change at, 155, 160–161, 165, 170–171, 172–173, 178; customer concept at, 32; daily operations at, 321–322, 323, 324–328, 330, 335–336, 344; Departmental and Local Lead Teams at, 223; diverse workforce at, 170–171; Divisional Lead Teams at, 223, 309, 344, 534; education at, 253, 256, 260, 263–279; Employee Appreciation Week at, 312; employee suggestion program at, 84, 85, 87; and errors, 14; expectations of management at, 326–328; experiences of, 501–548; guest relations at, 82–83; hoshin planning at, 494; implementation at, 121–122, 123–124, 128, 130, 132, 133; Innovation Program at, 88; Integrated Inpatient Management Model at, 221; integrated model at, 27, 468–469; leadership education program at, 41–42; management identification at, 178; Material Management Department of, 135–136; Medical Procedures Unit of, 483; milestones for, 518–520; organizational change at, 99–100, 102, 109; physician involvement at, 199–208, 213; Professional Services Lead Team at, 542; publications of, 380, 382, 383, 388, 391, 394, 396, 401, 513, 517; quality assurance at, 70, 74, 75–76; quality function deployment at, 481, 482, 483, 489; quality improvement methods at, 359, 362–363, 371, 395; QI process of, 46–47; quality results at, 23–25, 40; Quality Roadmap at, 47, 193; quality tools at, 107; reward and recognition at, 283–284, 285–286, 288, 294–296, 300–301,